The RMT Review Guide
Developed by the American Association
for Medical Transcription

Cindy Stroh, CMT, FAAMT, Managing Editor

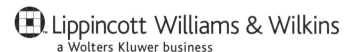
Lippincott Williams & Wilkins
a Wolters Kluwer business
Philadelphia · Baltimore · New York · London
Buenos Aires · Hong Kong · Sydney · Tokyo

Publisher: Julie K. Stegman
Senior Product Manager: Eric Branger
Managing Editor (LWW): Amy Millholen
Editor: Laura Bryan
Proofreader: Kristin Wall
Manufacturing Coordinator: Dana Jackson
Cover: Jason Delaney
Interior Design: Melissa Olson
Frontmatter Design: Hearthside Publishing Services
Compositor: Maryland Composition
Printer: Quebecor World

Copyright © 2007 American Association for Medical Transcription
100 Sycamore Avenue
Modesto, CA 95354-0550
www.aamt.org

Lippincott Williams & Wilkins
A Wolters Kluwer Health Company
351 West Camden Street
Baltimore, MD 21201-2346
www.stedmans.com
stedmans@lww.com

Printed in the United States of America

Library of Congress Cataloging-in-Publication Data

The RMT review guide/developed by the American Association for Medical Transcription; Cindy Stroh, managing editor.
     p. ; cm.
 Includes bibliographical references.
 ISBN 0-7817-6513-7
 1. Medical transcription—Examinations—Study guides. I. Stroh, Cindy. II. American Association for Medical Transcription. III. Title: Registered medical transcriptionist review guide. [DNLM: 1. Medical Records—Examination Questions. 2. Certification—Examination Questions. WX 18.2 R627 2007]
 R728.8.R57 2007
 610.76—dc22

                                                    2006010112

The publishers have made every effort to trace the copyright holders for borrowed material. If they have inadvertently overlooked any, they will be pleased to make the necessary arrangements at the first opportunity.

To purchase additional copies of this book, call our customer service department at **(800) 638-3030** or fax orders to **(301) 824-7390**. International customers should call **(301) 714-2324**.

Visit Stedman's on the Internet: http://www.stedmans.com.

Visit the American Association for Medical Transcription on the Internet: http://www.aamt.org.

06 07 08 09 10
1 2 3 4 5 6 7 8 9 10

"[Those] who succeed are the efficient few. They are the few who have the ambition and willpower to develop themselves."

Herbert N. Casson

The above quotation makes me think of transcriptionists. In a production-oriented environment, we (yes, I'm an MT) have to be efficient, using all the tools at our disposal to quickly turn around quality document after quality document, perhaps for many different clients or institutions, each with their own preferences and specifications. Attention to detail is our middle name. Many people may think MTs are not ambitious, that there is no upward career mobility in the field of medical transcription, but I disagree. Not only do we strive for that perfect report, we revel in learning new things, we confront change, we study to improve and prepare ourselves for whatever we might encounter as our industry changes. And there are any number of ways that we MTs can advance our careers—as QA specialists and editors, supervisors and managers, teachers, service owners, and association leaders, to name a few. Finally, we have the willpower to accomplish the goals we've set for ourselves, our profession, and our association.

Development of the Registered Medical Transcriptionist exam is just one such accomplishment for the AAMT. By purchasing this book, you are demonstrating that you have the ambition and the willpower to attain the RMT credential. *The RMT Review Guide* will help you do that in an efficient manner.

Although AAMT provides a candidate guide that contains a blueprint or outline of the exam objectives with a few sample questions and explains the policies and procedures related to the RMT exam, it was felt that a preparatory guide such as *The RMT Review Guide* was needed to help candidates assess any deficiencies they may have and better prepare for the exam.

The RMT Review Guide has been organized in such a way as to permit you to structure your preparation efficiently and maximize the effectiveness of your study. The guide consists of review materials in the same question-and-answer formats that appear on the exam, so that as you study you are also practicing your test-taking techniques.

Organized by units, the guide follows the exam blueprint very closely. Unit 1 covers Medical Language, Unit 2 covers Systems/Specialties, and Unit 3 covers English Language. Each chapter follows the same format and includes learning objectives, resources for study, and review questions. In addition, the medical specialty chapters include sample reports and proofreading practice questions. By checking your answers against the provided answer keys, you can determine those areas in which you need more study.

As with most test-prep guides, this text does not provide the content you need to study, thus the "resources for study" feature at the beginning of each chapter. These resources are summarized below:

1. Bickley LS. *Bates' Guide to Physical Examination and History Taking*, 9th ed. Philadelphia: Lippincott Williams & Wilkins, 2007. ISBN#: 0781767180.

2. Chabner D-E. *The Language of Medicine*, 7th ed. Philadelphia: Saunders, 2004. ISBN#: 1416001263.

3. Cohen BJ. *Memmler's Structure and Function of the Human Body*, 8th ed. Philadelphia: Lippincott Williams & Wilkins, 2005. ISBN#: 0781742331.

4. Cohen BJ. *Memmler's The Human Body in Health and Disease*, 10th ed. Philadelphia: Lippincott Williams & Wilkins, 2005. ISBN#: 0781742323.

5. Cohen BJ. *Study Guide for Memmler's The Human Body in Health and Disease*, 10th ed. Philadelphia: Lippincott Williams & Wilkins, 2005. ISBN#: 0781751721.

6. Dirckx JH. *H & P: A Nonphysician's Guide to the Medical History and Physical Examination*. Modesto, CA: Health Professions Institute, 2001. ISBN#: 0934385343.

7. Dirckx, JH. *Human Diseases*. Modesto, CA: Health Professions Institute, 2003. ISBN#: 0934385386.

8. Dirckx, JH. *Laboratory Tests & Diagnostic Procedures in Medicine*. Modesto, CA: Health Professions Institute, 2004. ISBN#: 0934385491.

9. Fischbach FT. *A Manual of Laboratory and Diagnostic Tests*, 7th ed. Philadelphia: Lippincott Williams & Wilkins, 2004. ISBN#: 0781741807.

10. Hughes P (ed). *The AAMT Book of Style for Medical Transcription*, 2nd ed. Modesto: AAMT, 2002. ISBN#: 0935229388.

11. North JL. *Using Medical Terminology: A Practical Approach*. Philadelphia: Lippincott Williams & Wilkins, 2006. ISBN#: 0781748682.

12. Roach S. *Pharmacology for Health Professionals*. Philadelphia: Lippincott Williams & Wilkins, 2005. ISBN#: 0781752841.

13. Sabin WA. *The Gregg Reference Manual*, Burr Ridge, IL: McGraw-Hill/Irwin, 2004. ISBN#: 0072936533.

14. Turley, SM. *Understanding Pharmacology for Health Professionals*. Upper Saddle River, NJ: Prentice Hall, 2002. ISBN#: 0130417424.

15. Willis MC. *Medical Terminology: The Language of Health Care*, 2nd ed. Philadelphia: Lippincott Williams & Wilkins, 2006. ISBN#: 0781745101.

The accompanying CD-ROM contains additional multiple choice questions for all the medical specialty chapters and dictation excerpts for each medical specialty to help you prepare for the practical portion of the exam. You will be able to work in study or test mode. As you work with the dictation exercises, I suggest that you practice using your mouse to control audio playback and try the techniques suggested in the *RMT Candidate Guide*. Note, too, that the audio exercises allow for only one correct answer, but the actual exam allows for multiple variations for a single audio clip. This will be explained in more detail on the CD-ROM.

It is not possible for any single text to address all the content that may be encountered on the RMT exam. However, this guide does address all the content areas and is sufficiently thorough and complete to allow you to assess your deficiencies and seek other avenues to correct them if you feel this guide is not enough. You should *not* look at this guide as a "crash course" with which you can "ace the test." You will very likely need to access one or more of the resources suggested for further study. Use this guide to organize your approach to study, to identify weaknesses, and to confirm the knowledge you already have. It is also a good idea to use a combination of approaches to prepare for the exam, such as joining a study group, taking the online RMT Prep Course, or even taking a medical terminology or anatomy course at your local college if you have been out of school for a long time or learned on the job.

As an educator, a former medical transcription service owner, and an experienced medical transcriptionist active in AAMT, I am all too familiar with the plight of students and recent graduates of quality medical transcription education programs who have difficulty "getting their foot in the door" when it comes to employment. Similarly, I have heard from many MTs transcribing for doctors' offices and clinics that they have no opportunity to show their employers that they are not only qualified medical transcriptionists but professionals. The Registered Medical Transcriptionist exam was developed to provide these two groups with a credential that assures employers and consumers that they are qualified to practice medical transcription.

I don't want to wish you luck in taking the RMT exam. I do wish you success in your studies and preparation, in your career, and in your life. I'll see *you* in the list of Registered Medical Transcriptionists soon! But remember, the RMT is just the beginning, not the end. Finally, I do want to close with one more quotation, which needs no elaboration.

"Keep away from people who try to belittle your ambitions. Small people always do that, but the really great make you feel that you, too, can become great." Mark Twain (1835 - 1910)

Be great!
Ellen Drake, CMT, FAAMT
Director of Education and Certification
ellen@aamt.org

User's Guide

This User's Guide shows you how to best use *The RMT Review Guide* by highlighting the features of the chapters.

OBJECTIVES CHECKLIST

A checklist of objectives to assist you in self-evaluation.

CHAPTER 5

Emergency Medicine

OBJECTIVES CHECKLIST

A prepared exam candidate will know the:

❑ Basics of emergency medicine including assessment, triage, diagnostic intervention, and stabilization.

❑ Role of Advanced Cardiac Life Support (ACLS) protocol in resuscitation and critical cardiac intervention.

❑ ABCs (airway, breathing & circulation) of trauma evaluation as used on scene and in the emergency room.

❑ Fundamentals of the mental status exam as well as terminology unique to psychiatric assessment in the emergency setting.

❑ Typical first-line treatment course for most common presenting complaints in the emergency setting.

❑ Diagnostic imaging and laboratory studies related to emergency medicine.

❑ Interventional medications administered in critical treatment, particularly resuscitation, drug overdose, poisoning, envenomization, and acute trauma.

❑ Medications administered routinely for common presenting complaints.

RESOURCES FOR STUDY

1. *H&P: A Nonphysician's Guide to the Medical History and Physical Examination*
   Chapter 1: General Remarks on the History, pp. 13–24.
   Chapter 2: Chief Complaint and History of Present Illness, pp. 25–34.
   Chapter 28: The Formal Mental Status Examination, pp. 273–280.

2. *Human Diseases*
   Chapter 6: Trauma and Poisoning, pp. 73–86.
   Chapter 20: Mental Disorders, pp. 315–332.

3. *Laboratory Tests and Diagnostic Procedures in Medicine*
   Chapter 4: Measurement of Temperature, Rates, Pressures and Volumes, pp. 39–60.
   Section VI (Chapters 19–24). Note: *Information in all of these chapters is pertinent to Emergency Medicine but will also be well covered in other chapters of this text.*

4. *Understanding Pharmacology for Health Professionals*
   Chapter 16: Emergency Drugs, pp. 178–191.
   Chapter 17: Anticoagulant and Thrombolytic Drugs, pp. 185–191.
   Chapter 26: Analgesic Drugs, pp. 296–310.
   Chapter 32: Intravenous Fluids and Blood Products, pp. 373–385.

RESOURCES FOR STUDY

The chapters and pages in our selected texts to refer to when studying the material for that section.

SAMPLE REPORTS

Located in all of the systems chapters, the samples are representative of common reports encountered in medical specialties.

SAMPLE REPORTS

The following four reports are examples of reports you might encounter while transcribing cardiology, cardiac surgery, or thoracic surgery.

OPERATIVE REPORT

DATE OF OPERATION
05/01/2004

ATTENDING SURGEON
John Smith, MD.

PREOPERATIVE DIAGNOSIS
End-stage cardiomyopathy.

POSTOPERATIVE DIAGNOSIS
End-stage cardiomyopathy.

PROCEDURE PERFORMED
Heart transplantation.

ANESTHESIA
General endotracheal.

JUSTIFICATION FOR PROCEDURE
The patient is a 65-year-old man with ischemic cardiomyopathy. He had been evaluated for heart transplantation at this facility and placed on the national computer waiting list.

PROCEDURE IN DETAIL
On the night of this surgery, a suitable donor was identified. The patient had previous laryngeal cancer with radiation to the neck, and he was brought to the operating room somewhat early because difficulty with his airway was anticipated. For this reason, he underwent fiberoptic awake intubation which was accomplished without difficulty. A left subclavian Swan-Ganz catheter was placed, as was a radial arterial line and a Foley catheter. With notification from the donor site that the heart was acceptable, the anterior chest, abdomen, groin, and legs were prepped with Betadine and draped as a sterile field.

With notification from the donor site that the heart had been harvested, we began the operation by making a skin incision over the sternum. The sternum was then split in the midline with a saw. A self-retaining retractor was placed, and the pericardium was opened to the right side of the midline. Heparin was administered, and cannulation pursestrings were placed in the ascending aorta, high right superior vena cava, and low lateral right atrium. Cannulation was accomplished and the connection was made to the heart/lung machine.

With notification that the heart had arrived in town, cardiopulmonary bypass was instituted, and a vent was placed through the right superior pulmonary vein through a pursestring. With the heart in the hospital, we cross-clamped the aorta, snugged down on tapes which had been placed around the inferior vena cava and superior vena cava, and divided the superior vena cava, the

(continued)

OPERATIVE REPORT

DATE OF OPERATION
05/01/2004

ATTENDING SURGEON
John Smith, MD.

PREOPERATIVE DIAGNOSIS
Ventricular tachycardia.

POSTOPERATIVE DIAGNOSIS
Ventricular tachycardia.

PROCEDURE PERFORMED
Placement of automatic implantable cardioverter-defibrillator (AICD).

ANESTHESIA
General endotracheal.

JUSTIFICATION FOR PROCEDURE
The patient is a 75-year-old man with a history of ventricular fibrillation and tachycardia.

PROCEDURE IN DETAIL
At the time of surgery, the patient was brought to the operating room and placed in the supine position where he underwent general endotracheal anesthesia without any difficulty. The patient was prepped with Betadine scrub and Betadine paint and draped in the usual sterile fashion.

An incision was then made in the left deltopectoral fold, and a pocket was made underneath the pectoralis major muscle. A percutaneous stick was then made into the left subclavian vein and attached to the guide wire. It should be noted that, during this, some air was retrieved, and the patient had a small pneumothorax for which a left chest tube was placed at the end of the procedure without difficulty.

Once the guide wire was in, the AICD lead was implanted. This was a Corpus model #1234, serial #123456, with threshold measurements of 1.1 milliampere, 600 ohms resistance, 16 millivolt R-wave, and a 0.6 volt threshold. The patient then had inducible ventricular fibrillation with a 15-joule shock and returned to normal sinus rhythm. This was done a second time, and he returned to normal sinus rhythm once again.

After this, the patient did well, and the wound was irrigated with antibiotic solution and closed with a 3-0 Vicryl subcutaneous layer and a 4-0 Vicryl subcuticular layer. The patient was transferred to the recovery room in stable condition.

ECHOCARDIOGRAM

M-MODE ECHOCARDIOGRAM

AORTIC VALVE LEVEL
The aortic valve opening is normal. The aortic root motion is normal. The left atrial intracavitary dimensions are increased.

MITRAL VALVE LEVEL
The mitral valve opening is normal. The DE and EF slopes are reduced. The E-point septal separation is increased. There is no pericardial effusion.

LEFT VENTRICULAR LEVEL
The left ventricular and septal wall thickness is increased. The left ventricular intracavitary dimensions are increased.

IMPRESSION
1. Mild concentric left ventricular hypertrophy.
2. Dilated left ventricle.
3. Reduced left ventricular function by increased E-point septal separation.
4. Dilated left atrium.

2-D ECHOCARDIOGRAM, DOPPLER AND COLOR FLOW
The 2-dimensional echocardiographic study revealed increased left ventricular and septal thickness. The left ventricular and septal wall motion and contractility revealed generalized diffuse hypokinesia. The intracavitary dimensions of the left ventricle are increased during systole and diastole. The left atrial intracavitary dimensions are increased. The aortic root motion is reduced. The aortic root and mitral anulus are thickened. There is no evidence of intracavitary mass, thrombus or pericardial effusion.

The right ventricular wall motion and contractility are normal.

DOPPLER STUDIES
The Doppler studies reveal a regurgitant jet across the mitral valve with a jet velocity of 4.25 m/s with a gradient of 72 mmHg. The E and A velocities appeared to be fairly normal with decreased deceleration time and evidence of increased left ventricular relaxation time. However, the E and the A velocities could not be sampled. Pulmonary studies were not obtained.

Transtricuspid Doppler interrogation revealed a regurgitant jet with a jet velocity of 3.2 m/s with a calculated right ventricular systolic pressure of 50 mmHg. The transaortic and pulmonic valve Doppler studies are unremarkable, with normal velocities.

IMPRESSION
1. Left ventricular and systolic and diastolic dysfunction.
2. Mild concentric left ventricular hypertrophy.
3. Dilated left ventricle and left atrium.
4. Thickening of the aortic root and mitral anulus.

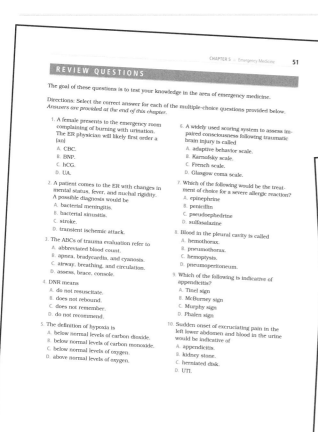

REVIEW QUESTIONS

The goal of these questions is to test your knowledge in the area of emergency medicine.

Directions: Select the correct answer for each of the multiple-choice questions provided below. *Answers are provided at the end of this chapter.*

1. A female presents to the emergency room complaining of burning with urination. The ER physician will likely first order a (an)
   A. CBC.
   B. BNP.
   C. hCG.
   D. UA.

2. A patient comes to the ER with changes in mental status, fever, and nuchal rigidity. A possible diagnosis would be
   A. bacterial meningitis.
   B. bacterial sinusitis.
   C. stroke.
   D. transient ischemic attack.

3. The ABCs of trauma evaluation refer to
   A. abbreviated blood count.
   B. apnea, bradycardia, and cyanosis.
   C. airway, breathing, and circulation.
   D. assess, brace, console.

4. DNR means
   A. do not resuscitate.
   B. does not rebound.
   C. does not remember.
   D. do not recommend.

5. The definition of hypoxia is
   A. below normal levels of carbon dioxide.
   B. below normal levels of carbon monoxide.
   C. below normal levels of oxygen.
   D. above normal levels of oxygen.

6. A widely used scoring system to assess impaired consciousness following traumatic brain injury is called
   A. adaptive behavior scale.
   B. Karnofsky scale.
   C. French scale.
   D. Glasgow coma scale.

7. Which of the following would be the treatment of choice for a severe allergic reaction?
   A. epinephrine
   B. penicillin
   C. pseudoephedrine
   D. sulfasalazine

8. Blood in the pleural cavity is called
   A. hemothorax.
   B. pneumothorax.
   C. hemoptysis.
   D. pneumoperitoneum.

9. Which of the following is indicative of appendicitis?
   A. Tinel sign
   B. McBurney sign
   C. Murphy sign
   D. Phalen sign

10. Sudden onset of excruciating pain in the left lower abdomen and blood in the urine would be indicative of
    A. appendicitis.
    B. kidney stone.
    C. herniated disk.
    D. UTI.

REVIEW QUESTIONS

Multiple-choice exam-style questions for exam practice.

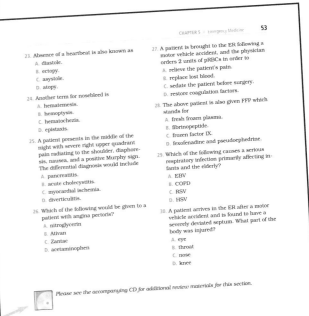

23. Absence of a heartbeat is also known as
    A. diastole.
    B. ectopy.
    C. asystole.
    D. atopy.

24. Another term for nosebleed is
    A. hematemesis.
    B. hemoptysis.
    C. hematochezia.
    D. epistaxis.

25. A patient presents in the middle of the night with severe right upper quadrant pain radiating to the shoulder, diaphoresis, nausea, and a positive Murphy sign. The differential diagnosis would include
    A. pancreatitis.
    B. acute cholecystitis.
    C. myocardial ischemia.
    D. diverticulitis.

26. Which of the following would be given to a patient with angina pectoris?
    A. nitroglycerin
    B. Ativan
    C. Zantac
    D. acetaminophen

27. A patient is brought to the ER following a motor vehicle accident, and the physician orders 2 units of pRBCs in order to
    A. relieve the patient's pain.
    B. replace lost blood.
    C. sedate the patient before surgery.
    D. restore coagulation factors.

28. The above patient is also given FFP which stands for
    A. fresh frozen plasma.
    B. fibrinopeptide.
    C. frozen factor IX.
    D. fexofenadine and pseudoephedrine.

29. Which of the following causes a serious respiratory infection primarily affecting infants and the elderly?
    A. EBV
    B. COPD
    C. RSV
    D. HSV

30. A patient arrives in the ER after a motor vehicle accident and is found to have a severely deviated septum. What part of the body was injured?
    A. eye
    B. throat
    C. nose
    D. knee

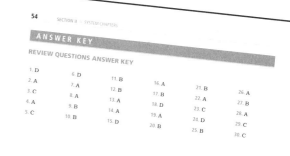 *Please see the accompanying CD for additional review materials for this section.*

CD-ROM

The CD icon indicates areas in which the reader should consult the CD included with the book for additional review materials. The CD contains hundreds of additional review questions, PLUS approximately 6 dictation exercises for each of the systems chapters.

ANSWER KEY

REVIEW QUESTIONS ANSWER KEY

1. D	6. D	11. B	16. A	21. B	
2. A	7. A	12. B	17. B	22. A	26. A
3. C	8. A	13. A	18. D	23. C	27. B
4. A	9. B	14. A	19. A	24. D	28. A
5. C	10. B	15. D	20. B	25. B	29. C
					30. C

REVIEW QUESTIONS ANSWER KEY

Answers are provided to all multiple-choice questions at the end of each chapter.

Acknowledgements

I would like to thank the following individuals who have graciously dedicated their time and expertise to help bring *The RMT Review Guide* to completion.

Contributors of review questions include Angela Kelly, CMT, FAAMT; Kim Gorman, CMT; Tammy Moore, CMT; Rebecca Sue Wester, CMT, FAAMT; and Lisa Woodley, RHIT, CMT. Without their help, this project would have been a daunting task.

I would especially like to thank my husband, Greg, for his support and encouragement to pursue and achieve higher goals.

Thanks also goes to a tremendous support team. The following people provided encouragement, guidance, and suggestions when I came upon a stumbling block: Ellen Drake, CMT, FAAMT; Laura Bryan, CMT, FAAMT; and Lea Sims, CMT, FAAMT, from AAMT; as well as Amy Millholen, Eric Branger, and Julie Stegman from Lippincott Williams & Wilkins.

I would also like to thank three very special people who have provided their friendship, as well as support and encouragement, in my taking on this project: Kim Multop, Patti Harms, and Susan Lucci, CMT, FAAMT.

Thanks goes out to each and every transcriptionist, mentor, and educator who have dedicated their time and energy to promote and enhance the medical transcription industry and help achieve the quality of excellence in documentation for patient care.

Cindy A. Stroh, CMT, FAAMT

Contributors

The publishers, author, and editors gratefully acknowledge the professionals who contributed to the content of this text.

Georgia Green, CMT, FAAMT
Westport, Washington

Kim Gorman, CMT
Eugene, Oregon

Angela Kelly, CMT, FAAMT
Clearwater, Florida

Tammy Moore, CMT
Ariton, Alabama

Rebecca Sue Wester, CMT, FAAMT
Choctaw, Oklahoma

Lisa Woodley, RHIT, CMT
Vashon, Washington

Table of Contents

Medical Language

Medical Language Fundamentals

OBJECTIVES CHECKLIST

A prepared exam candidate will know the:

☐ Common prefixes and suffixes utilized in medical language.

☐ Latin and Greek roots used in the formation of medical terms.

☐ Role and function of combining vowels in the formation of medical terms.

☐ Fundamentals of word formation with affixes, roots, and combining vowels.

☐ Methods for deconstructing words based on these fundamental parts for the purpose of identification and definition.

RESOURCE FOR STUDY

The Language of Medicine
Chapter 1: Basic Word Structure, pp. 1–30.
Chapter 3: Suffixes, pp. 75–107.
Chapter 4: Prefixes, pp. 109–138.

PREFIXES AND SUFFIXES

Prefixes with Variant Meanings

PREFIX	MEANING	EXAMPLES
ab-	from, away, off	abnormal, abdicate
ad-	to, toward	adhere, adjoin
ante-	before, in front of, earlier than	antecedent, antecubital
anti-	opposite of, hostile to	antibiotic, antisocial
be-	make, against, to a great degree	belittle, bemoan
bi-	two, twice	bicycle, bivalve
de-	away, opposite of, reduce	deactivate, devitalize
dia-	through, across	diameter, diagonal
dis-	opposite of, apart, away	dissatisfy, disjointed
en-	cause to be, put in or on	enable, engulf
syn-	with, together	synchronize, synthesis
trans-	across, beyond, through	transabdominal, transaction
ultra-	beyond in space, excessive	ultraviolet, ultramodern
un-	not, the opposite of	unable, unwind

Prefixes/Suffixes with Invariant Meanings

PREFIX	MEANING	EXAMPLES
anthropo-	man	anthropoid
auto-	self	autonomous
biblio-	book	bibliography
bio-	life	biology
centro-	center	centrofacial
centri-	center	centrifuge
cosmo-	universe	cosmonaut
heter-/hetero-	different	heterosexual
homo-	same	homosexual
hydro-	water	hydroplane
iso-	equal	isometrics
lith-/litho-	stone	lithography
micro-	small	microscope
macro-	large	macrophage
mono-	one	monocyte
neuro-	nerve	neurologist
omni-	all	omnipotent
pan-	all	panchromatic
penta-	five	pentagram
phil-/philo-	love	philanthropist
phono-	sound	phonograph

SUFFIX	MEANING	EXAMPLES
-fication/-ation	action of, process of	classification, dramatization
-gram	written or drawn	diagram
-graph	writing, recording, or drawing	telegraph, lithograph
-graphy	description of a subject or field	oceanography
-ics	the science or art of	athletics
-itis-	inflammation	tonsillitis
-latry	the worship of	idolatry
-meter	measuring device	thermometer
-metry	process of measuring	photometry
-ology/-logy	the study of	cardiology
-phore	bearer or producer	semaphore
-phobia	illogical fear	claustrophobia
-scope	observing instrument	microscope
-scopy	seeing or observing	microscopy
-ance	These noun suffixes are used	tolerance
-ation	to form abstract nouns with	adoration
-ion	the meaning of "quality, state,	incision
-ism	or condition," and action or	truism
-dom	result of an action.	kingdom
-ery		monastery
-mony		matrimony
-ment		government
-tion		sanction
-er	These noun suffixes pertain to	helper
-eer	living or non-living agents.	engineer
-grapher		photographer
-ess		princess
-ier		courier
-ster		monster
-ist		Marxist
-stress		mistress
-trix		executrix

GREEK AND LATIN ROOTS

Greek Root Words

ROOT	MEANING	EXAMPLES
aero	air	aerial, aerodynamics
aesthet	perception	anesthetic
amphi	both ways	amphibious, amphitheater
anthro	man	anthropologist
archaeo	primitive, ancient	archaeology
ast	star	asterisk, astrophysics
atmo	vapor, steam	atmosphere
auto	self	automatic, autobiography
baro	pressure	barometer
biblio	book	bibliography, bible
bio	life	biology, biography
card/cardio	heart	cardiac, cardiology
chrono	time	chronological
cosmo	world, universe	cosmopolitan
crypto	hidden, secret	cryptography

cyclo	wheel	cycle, bicycle
deca	ten	decade
demo	people	democracy
dont	teeth	orthodontist
electro	electric	electricity
ethno	race, nation	ethnicity
gam	marriage	polygamy
geo	earth	geography
graph/gram	write	telegraph, telegram
gyn	woman	gynecologist
gyro	circle	gyroscope
helio	the sun	helioscope
hema/hemo	blood	hematoma, hemophilia
hemi	half	hemisphere, hemiparesis
hetero	different	heterogeneous
holo	whole	holocaust
homo	same	homogeneous
hydro	water	hydroplane
hypno	sleep	hypnosis
hypo	under, below	hypodermic
iatry	medical treatment	psychiatry, podiatry
ideo	idea	idealogy
iso	equal, alike	isometric, isobar
kilo	one thousand	kilogram
kine/cine	move	kinetic, cinema
litho	stone	monolith, lithography
log	word	dialogue, apology
macro	large	macrocephaly
mania	madness	maniac
mech	machine	mechanical
mega	great	megaphone
meter	measure	barometer, thermometer
micro	small	microscope, microbe

Latin Root Words

ROOT	MEANING	EXAMPLES
act	do	action, reaction
agri	field, soil	agriculture
alt	high	altimeter, altitude
ambi	both ways	ambidextrous, ambiguous
amo/ami	love	amiable, amorous
ang	bend	angle, rectangle
anim	feeling	animosity, animation
ann/enn	year	annual, anniversary
apt/ept	suitable	aptitude, ineptitude
aqua	water	aquatic, aquarium
art	skill	artistic, artisan
aud/audit	hear	auditorium, audition
bene	good	benefit, benediction
brev	short	brevity, abbreviate
cap	head	cap, captain, capitol
cede/ceed	go	proceed, exceed
ceive/cept	seize	receive, receptacle
centi	100	century, centipede
cent	center	centrifuge
cert	sure	certain, certified
cide/cise	cut, kill	suicide, scissor, incise

circ	around	circle, circular
clam/claim	shout	proclaim, clamor
clar	clear	clarity, declare
cline	lean	incline, recline, decline
clud/clos/clus	shut	include, closet, seclusion
cogn	know	recognize, cognition
corp	body	corporal, corporation
counter/contra	against	counteract, contradict
cranio	skull	craniology, cranium
cred	believe	credit, incredible
curr	run	current, occurrence
dict	speak	dictate, predict
domin	master	dominate, predominate
deci	one-tenth	decibel
don/donat	give	donation, donor
duct	lead	conduct, conductor
equ	equal	equality, equilibrium
fac/fec	make, do	manufacture, affect
fic/fy	make, do	suffice, classify
fer	carry	ferry, transfer
fibor	fiber	fibrous, fibrovascular
fict	pretend	fiction, fictitious
fid	faithful	fidelity, confidence
firm	fixed	infirm, confirm
flect/flex	bend	reflection, reflex
form	shape	conform, formula
fract/frag	break	fracture, fragment
frater	brother	fraternity
fuga/fugi	flee	fugitive, refugee
grad/gress	by steps	gradually, progress
grat	pleasing, thankful	grateful, congratulate
plic/plex	interweave, fold	complicated, perplex
plur	more	plural
pop	people	population, popular
port	carry	portable, transport
pos/pon	place, put	position
post	after	postmortem, postscript
prehend	seize	comprehend
prehens	seize	comprehension
prim/princ	first	primitive, principle
pugn	fight	pugilist
put	think	reputation, disreputable
quadri/quad	four	quadrilateral, quadruplet
quer/ques/quis	seek	query, question, inquisitive
rad/ray	spoke, ray, root	radius, radiate
rect	straight	erect, rectify, direction
reg	king	regal, reign
rid	laugh	ridicule, deride
rupt	break	rupture, abrupt, bankrupt
san	healthy	sanitary, sane
scend	climb	ascend, descendant
scribe/script	write	inscribe, scripture
sect	cut	dissect, intersect
sept	seven	septuplets
sens	feelings	sensible, sensitive
serv	serve	servant, service
sess/set	sit	session, settle
sex	six	sextet
sign	mark	signature, signal
sim	like	similar, simultaneous

sist/stat	stand	insist, status
sol	alone	solo, solitary
solv/solu	loosen	dissolve, solution
spec/spic	see	spectator, suspicion
spir	breathe	spirometry, respiration
stell	star	stellate, stellar
stimu	whip	stimulation
strict	tighten	restrict, constriction
struct	build	construct, instructor
sum/sup	superior	supreme, summit
tact/tang	touch	intact, tangible
temp	time	temporary, temporal
ten/tend	hold, stretch	retentive, intend
term	end	terminal, determine
terr	land	terrain, territory
tex	weave	textile, texture
tort	twist	torture, contortion
tract	pull, drag	tractor, attraction
trans	across	transport, transdermal
trib	give	contribute, tributary
trud/trus	push	intrude, protrusion
turb	confusion	disturb, turbulence
vag	wander	vagabond, vagrant
var	different	variant, varied
ven/vent	come	convention, intervene
vert	turn	convert, reverse
vict/vince	conquer	victory, convince
vis/vid	see	vision, evidence
viv/vit	live	vivid, vitamin
voc	voice	vocal, advocate
volv	roll	revolver, revolutionary

COMBINING FORMS

When a suffix beginning with a consonant is added to a root word, a vowel (usually an o) is inserted to aid in pronunciation. Some examples are:

neur + o + logy = neurology (study of the nervous system)

cardi + o + logy = cardiology (study of the heart)

gastr + o + enterology = gastroenterology (study of the stomach and intestines)

In many textbooks, the **combining vowels** are separated from the root words with a virgule (/) such as: nephr/o, cephal/o, and hyster/o.
In this format, the root is usually referred to as the *combining form.*

A combining vowel is not necessary if the ending begins with a vowel as follows:

cyst + itis = cystitis (inflammation of the urinary bladder)

gastr + itis = gastritis (inflammation of the stomach)

card + itis = carditis (inflammation of the heart)

Some exceptions to this rule do occur in order to make medical terms easier to pronounce. These will be obvious to you as you encounter them. It is important to note in the examples above that you must often start with the suffix when attempting to define a word based on its constructed forms. Once the suffix has been defined, you should begin at the front of the word and work to the right in breaking the word down by parts.

REVIEW EXERCISES

I. For each of the combining forms, prefixes, or suffixes below, select the correct definition.

1. erythr/o
   A. blood
   B. red
   C. swelling
   D. rash

2. kary/o
   A. nucleus
   B. potassium
   C. hard, cornea
   D. humpback

3. furc/o
   A. luminous
   B. resembling
   C. fungus
   D. forking

4. ipsi-
   A. same
   B. contralateral
   C. transverse
   D. process

5. nos/o
   A. nose
   B. hospital
   C. disease
   D. none

6. –physis
   A. to grow
   B. plant
   C. role, function
   D. to bear

7. thec/o
   A. spine
   B. vertebra
   C. sheath
   D. membrane

8. hol/o
   A. heart
   B. whole
   C. hollow
   D. natural

9. myx/o
   A. mixed, combined
   B. muscle
   C. genetically altered
   D. mucus

10. eu-
   A. new
   B. good; normal
   C. out, away from
   D. inward

II. For each definition based on word parts, provide the correct formed term. *Hint: Word parts will not always be arranged in the same order as the definition provided.*

11. (pertaining to) + (the study of) + (bacteria)

12. (incomplete) + (dilation/expansion)

13. (person who) + (records) + (words/phrases)

14. (pertaining to) + (many) + (form/shape) + (nuclear)

15. (condition of) + (lung) + (dust)

16. (condition of) + (all) + (deficient) + (pituitary)

17. (stimulating the function of) + (adrenal) + (cortex)

18. (deficiency of) + (granules) + (cells)

19. (condition of) + (varied/irregular) + (cells)

20. (pertaining to) + (mind) + (body)

ANSWER KEY

REVIEW EXERCISES

1. B

2. A

3. D

4. A

5. C

6. A

7. C

8. B

9. D

10. B

11. bacteriologic

12. atelectasis

13. lexicographer

14. polymorphonuclear

15. pneumoconiosis

16. panhypopituitarism

17. adrenocorticotropin

18. granulocytopenia

19. poikilocytosis

20. psychosomatic

Foreign Influence on Medical Language

OBJECTIVES CHECKLIST

A prepared exam candidate will know the:

☐ Greek alphabet, particularly those letters that are commonly used alone or in conjunction with other terms in medical language.

☐ Rules for pluralizing Greek and Latin terms.

☐ Common French terminology encountered in medical language.

☐ Common German terminology encountered in medical language.

RESOURCE FOR STUDY

The AAMT Book of Style for Medical Transcription
Foreign terms, p. 174.
French, p. 182.
Greek letters, pp. 197–198.
Latin abbreviations, pp. 237–238.
Plurals, pp. 318–323.

OVERVIEW

The current lexicography of medical language is vast and complex. This living and constantly evolving language has been profoundly influenced over time by a diverse number of cultural and linguistic sources, many of which are still evident in the language today. While certainly the English medical terms with which we are familiar can be etymologically traced to earlier language forms, there are quite a few foreign terms that remain unaltered in circular usage today. It is important for an MT to be aware of their use and application as well as the appropriate way to document them.

GREEK LANGUAGE

Greek Alphabet

α	alpha		ω	omega
β	beta		o	omicron
χ	chi		φ	phi
δ	delta		π	pi
ε	epsilon		ψ	psi
η	eta		ρ	rho
γ	gamma		ς, σ	sigma
ι	iota		τ	tau
κ	kappa		θ	theta
λ	lamda		υ	upsilon
μ	mu		ξ	xi
ν	nu		ζ	zeta

The Greek alphabet appears frequently in laboratory data and sometimes elsewhere. Some examples are:

alpha-fetoprotein

beta blockers

gamma knife

delta wave

Omega compression hip screw

Greek plurals are fairly simple, if you know the rules, as follow:

-a changes to −ata:

   stigma to *stigmata*

   condyloma to *condylomata*

-on changes to −a:

   phenomenon to *phenomena*

   criterion to *criteria*

-s changes to −des:

   iris to *irides*

   epididymis to *epididymides*

   arthritis to *arthritides*

EXCEPT for:

−osis which changes to −oses:

   anastomosis to *anastomoses*

   diagnosis to *diagnoses*

-x changes to −ces or −ges:

   varix to *varices*

   phalanx to *phalanges*

LATIN TERMINOLOGY & USAGE

"Vox audita perit; litera scripta manet"

Latin proverb meaning: *"The spoken word perishes; the written word remains."*

Some commonly misspelled (and mispronounced) Latin terms:

et al.   *et alia—and other individuals*

etc.   *et cetera—and other things*

vice versa—with the order reversed

LATIN PLURALS

The most common plural formations include the following:

-a to −ae:

   ulna to *ulnae*

   concha to *chonchae*

-us to −i:

   radius to *radii*

   musculus to *musculi*

-um to −a:

   acetabulum to *acetabula*

   atrium to *atria*

Examples of other Latin plurals:

SINGULAR	PLURAL	SINGULAR	PLURAL
adnexa	no plural—collective noun	*labium*	*labia*
carpus	*carpi*	*matrix*	*matrices*
corpus	*corpora*	*naris*	*nares*
coxa	*coxae*	*os (mouth)*	*ora*
crus	*crura*	*os (bone)*	*ossa*
genu	*genua*	*sequela*	*sequelae*
hallux	*halluces*	*vomer*	plural not used

NOMINA ANATOMICA

Some of the most difficult Latin terminology to master is included in the Nomina Anatomica (noted as N.A. in your medical dictionary). The Nomina Anatomica is the collection of formal names given to parts of the anatomy by an official (universal) organization of scientists. Forming plurals from these names can be a challenge, and here is why:

Latin <u>nouns</u> require different endings for different uses in sentences, for differences in number (singular/plural), and even for differences in gender.

Some of the uses in sentences include the following:

Subject (nominative)
Possessive form (genitive)—basically a modifier
Indirect object (dative)
Object of verb (accusative)
Object of preposition (ablative)

Latin <u>verbs</u> are rarely seen in medical terminology, except for the participial (participle) form, which is used as an adjective. The endings for adjectives (including participles) change to agree with the noun modified, including the gender of that noun.

Examples:

curriculum vitae (course of one's career/life)—singular noun plus possessive singular form of noun

lupus erythematosus (red wolf)—masculine singular noun, masculine singular adjective

flexor digitorum longus (N.A.)—masculine singular noun, genitive plural noun, masculine singular form of adjective

(tendo) dorsalis pedis—masculine singular noun, masculine/feminine singular form of adjective, possessive singular form of noun

valvulae conniventes (N.A. plicae circulares)—feminine plural noun, masculine/feminine plural adjective, probably a participle

Some medical phrases combine Greek and Latin (or Latinize the Greek).

Examples:
Condylomata acuminata—appears to contain two similar word endings, but it is actually the plural of condyloma acuminatus. *Condyloma* needs the Greek *−a* to *−ata* rule, and *acuminatus* needs the Latin *−um* to *−a* rule.

You can see why it would be easy for the MT novice to use the wrong Latin ending inadvertently, thus creating a form which says the wrong thing.

It is recommended that MTs memorize and/or print a list of the <u>correct</u> spellings for commonly used Latin words and phrases, and use a reliable medical dictionary for the others.

The information above will, hopefully, help you to do effective research into Latin forms and endings. It will also relieve confusion due to Latin endings that are not the same (or not different) when you expect them to be.

SINGULAR AND PLURAL OF SOME LATIN NOUNS

Typical declension of noun or adjective ending in −a:

	SINGULAR	PLURAL
Nominative	vertebra	vertebrae
Genitive	vertebrae	vertebrarum
Dative	vertebrae	vertebris
Accusative	vertebram	vertebras
Ablative	vertebra	vertebris

Typical declension of noun or adjective ending in −us:

	SINGULAR	PLURAL
Nominative	humerus	humeri
Genitive	humeri	humerorum
Dative	humero	humeris
Accusative	humerum	humeros
Ablative	humero	humeris

Typical declension of noun or adjective ending in −um:

	SINGULAR	PLURAL
Nominative	ovum	ova
Genitive	ovi	ovorum
Dative	ovo	ovis
Accusative	ovum	ova

Ablative   ovo   ovis

Declension of another kind of noun:

	SINGULAR	PLURAL
Nominative	corpus	corpora
Genitive	corporis	corporum
Dative	corpori	corporibus
Accusative	corpus	corpora
Ablative	corpore	corporibus

*There are many variations in type of noun. There are also irregular nouns, which do not follow any of the rules.

FRANCO-PRUSSIAN INFLUENCES (FRENCH AND GERMAN)

FRENCH

(Definitions given here are the most common ones. Please refer to your medical dictionary for other related definitions.)

café au lait	pigmented spots seen on skin in neurofibromatosis
cerclage	encircling with a ring or loop, as in an incompetent cervix
curettage	removal of material from a wall or a cavity
déjà vu	the illusion that a new situation has been experienced before
debridement	removal of foreign matter and unhealthy tissue, as from a wound
en bloc	in a lump
en face	head on
fourchette	posterior union of labia minora
gavage	forced feeding by tube, superalimentation
grand mal	major seizure with aura, sudden loss of consciousness, and generalized convulsion
jamais vu	the illusion that a familiar situation is being experienced for the first time (opposite of déjà vu)
lavage	washing out or irrigating, especially the stomach or bowel
mal de mer	seasickness
peau d'orange	dimpling of the skin, as seen in breast cancer
petit mal	minor seizure with only momentary loss of consciousness
torsade de pointes	a ventricular tachycardia with waxing and waning QRS amplitudes. It produces an EKG pattern resembling a ballet step. Translates as "twist on the toes."

GERMAN

blitz	bombardment, as with radioactive particles or a combination of medications
dauernarkose	prolonged sleep
dauerschlaf	prolonged sleep
ersatz	synthetic or artificial
gegenhalten	involuntary resistance to passive movement, as in disorders of the cerebral cortex
grubelsucht	an obsessive/compulsive tendency to worry over trifles
leistungskern	functional part of a cell
mittelschmerz	pain between menstrual periods
schnauskrampf	a facial grimace resembling pouting
sitz (bath)	immersion of the hips and buttocks for relief of rectal, urethral, vaginal, or pelvic discomfort
steinstrasse	literally, "stone street"—residual stone fragments following extracorporeal shock wave lithotripsy

Reference: The entire section is being reprinted with permission from the author: Suzanne Gallivan, CMT.

REVIEW EXERCISES

I. For each of the singular forms below, provide the plural form.

1. criterion

2. arthritis

3. phenomenon

4. meniscus

5. urethra

6. nucleus pulposus

7. uterus

8. placenta previa

9. diagnosis

10. foramen

II. For each of the plural forms below, provide the singular form.

11. diverticula

12. epididymides

13. stamina

14. adnexa

15. biceps

16. conjunctivae

17. cerebra

18. verrucae vulgares

19. musculi trapezii

20. ganglia

ANSWER KEY

REVIEW EXERCISES

1. criteria
2. arthritides
3. phenomena
4. menisci
5. urethrae
6. nuclei polposi
7. uteri
8. placentae previae
9. diagnoses
10. foramina
11. diverticulum
12. epididymis
13. stamen
14. adnexa
15. biceps
16. conjunctiva
17. cerebrum
18. verruca vulgaris
19. musculus trapezius
20. ganglion

Abbreviations and Acronyms

A prepared exam candidate will know the:

- ☐ Definitions and terminology related to abbreviations.
- ☐ Rules and exceptions governing use of abbreviations in the medical record.
- ☐ Rules and exceptions governing the use of acronyms and brief forms in the medical record.
- ☐ Rules for capitalizing and punctuating abbreviations, acronyms, and brief forms.

OVERVIEW

The use of abbreviations in health encounter documentation is widely prevalent. There are many factors and considerations that have to be taken into account when establishing practices and policies governing their use in transcription. The primary consideration for the expansion or retention of a dictated abbreviation should be the promotion of clarity. Attention must be paid to the potential for misinterpretation when encountering abbreviations in dictation. However, it is important to note there are other potential considerations that an MT will ultimately encounter in the workplace.

Facility Policy

As with other points of style and standards, provider/client preference will often be the final word on this issue. A healthcare provider or facility that is concerned about transcription costs, particularly in a per-unit billing environment, may restrict the expansion of many abbreviations despite the standards outlined here. Other providers and facilities may be more risk-management-minded and require the expansion of all abbreviations. It is important for the MT student to be aware that variability in the application of these standards may exist in the job setting.

Productivity

It is important to note that the decision to expand an abbreviation should never be made on the basis of its impact on productivity or potential wages, even in the absence of a company policy or provider preference. Transcribing a dictated abbreviation in abbreviated or expanded form should be based on the rules and exceptions outlined in this text with consideration for facility policies. The utilization of word expansion software to increase productivity often facilitates the quick and easy expansion of any and all abbreviations encountered in dictation; however, their expansion or retention should be judiciously considered based on these principles and *not* on productivity goals.

DEFINITIONS

Abbreviation A shortened form of a word or phrase used chiefly in writing, such as *USMC* for *United States Marine Corps.* Types: *Acronyms, Initialisms, & Brief Forms*

Acronym An abbreviation formed from the initial letters of each of the successive words or major parts of a compound term or of selected letters of a word or phrase **that is pronounced as a word** (*AIDS, GERD, LASIK).*

Initialism An abbreviation formed from the initial letters of each of the successive words or major parts of a compound term or of selected letters of a word or phrase **that is not pronounced as a word but by each letter** (*ALS, CPK, HIV).*

Brief Forms An abbreviation that results in a shortened form of a single word rather than the initial letters of a series of words (*phone, exam, Pap smear, labs).*

RULES AND EXCEPTIONS

I. When and Why

Transcribe abbreviations if they are commonly used and widely recognized. Again, clarity is the goal in making these transcription decisions. Keep in mind the following rules and exceptions:

A. **Terms dictated in full.** Do not use an abbreviation when a term is dictated in full.

Exception: units of measure (*milligrams, centimeters, etc.*) (see below)

B. **Diagnosis and operative titles.** Write out an abbreviation in full if it is used in the admission, discharge, preoperative, or postoperative diagnosis; consultative conclusion; or operative title. These are critical points of information, and their meanings must be clear to ensure accurate communication for patient care, reimbursement, statistical purposes, and medicolegal documentation.

<u>**DICTATED**</u>
DIAGNOSIS: AML.

<u>**TRANSCRIBED**</u>
DIAGNOSIS: AML.

Flag report for verification.

C. **Units of measure.**

1. Abbreviate most *metric* units of measure that accompany numerals and include virgule constructions. Use the same abbreviation for singular and plural forms. Do not use periods with abbreviated units of measure. Use these abbreviations only when a numeric quantity precedes the unit of measure.

   Examples:
   She was put on 2 L of oxygen.
   An approximately 2.5 cm incision was made.

   BUT

   The wound measured several centimeters.

2. Spell out common *nonmetric* units of measure to express weight, depth, distance, height, length, and width, except in tables. Do not abbreviate most nonmetric units of measure, except in tables.

   Examples:
   The baby weighed 8 pounds 9 ounces.
   She gave the child 2 tablespoons of Motrin.

D. **Dangerous and obscure abbreviations.** Do not use abbreviations found on the "Dangerous Abbreviations" list from the Institute for Safe Medication Practices (See Appendix 4). In addition to those found on the list, avoid any abbreviation that is obscure (like *a.c.b* for *before breakfast*) or any others that are potentially dangerous. For example, *b.i.w.* is both obscure *and* dangerous. It is intended to mean *twice weekly* but it could be mistaken for *twice daily*, resulting in a dosage frequency seven times that intended.

E. **Business names.** Some businesses are readily recognized by their abbreviations or acronyms and may be referred to by same if dictated and if there is reasonable assurance the business will be accurately identified by the reader. Most abbreviated forms use all capitals and do not use periods, but be guided by the entity's designated abbreviated form.

Examples:
IBM equipment
He is an ACLU attorney.
She found the item on eBay.

F. **Geographic names.** Abbreviate state and territory names when they are preceded by a city, state, or territory name. Do not abbreviate names of states, territories, countries, or similar units within reports when they stand alone. Use abbreviations in state names in an address (such as in a letter or on an envelope).

Examples:
She was seen in an ER in Orlando, FL, a month ago.
The patient moved here 3 years ago from Canada.

G. **Units of time.** Do not abbreviate English units of time except in virgule constructions. Do not use periods with such abbreviations.

Examples:
The patient is 5 days old.
He will return in 1 week for followup.
Her IV was set to run at 10 mcg/min while in the ER.

II. Grammar & Punctuation

A. **Placement.**

1. A sentence may begin with a dictated abbreviation, or such abbreviated forms may be extended.

   DICTATED
   WBC was 9200.

   TRANSCRIBED
   WBC was 9200. *OR*
   White blood count was 9200.

2. Avoid separating a numeral from its associated unit of measure or accompanying abbreviation; that is, keep the numeral and unit of measure together at line breaks.

   ....**The specimen measured 4 cm in diameter.**
   OR
   ....**The specimen measured 4 cm in diameter.**

   NOT
   ....**The specimen measured 4 cm in diameter.**

B. **Capitalization.**

1. Capitalize all letters of most acronyms, but when they are extended, do not capitalize the words from which they are formed unless they are proper names.

   Examples:
   AIDS   (acquired immunodeficiency syndrome)
   BiPAP   (bilateral positive airway pressure)
   TURP   (transurethral resection of prostate)

2. Do not capitalize abbreviations derived from Latin terms. The use of periods within or at the end of these Latin abbreviations remains the preferred style, although it is also acceptable to drop the periods for general Latin terms.

Use lowercase abbreviations with periods for Latin abbreviations that are related to doses and dosages. Avoid using all capitals because they emphasize the abbreviation rather than the drug name. Avoid lowercase abbreviations without periods because some may be misread as words.

Examples:

e.g.	exempli gratia	*for example*
et al.	et alii	*and others*
etc.	et cetera	*and so forth*
a.c.	ante cibum	*before food*
b.i.d.	bis in die	*twice a day*

3. Do not capitalize a brief form unless the extended form is routinely capitalized.

Examples:

segmented neutrophils	*segs*
examination	*exam*
Papanicolaou smear	*Pap smear*
Kirschner wire	*K-wire*

4. Do not capitalize most units of measure or their abbreviations. Learn the obvious exceptions, and consult appropriate references for guidance.

Examples:

meter	*m*	*kilogram*	*kg*
mole	*mol*	*centimeter*	*cm*

Exceptions:

liter	*L*	*kelvin*	*K*
milliliter	*mL*	*ampere*	*A*
decibel	*dB*	*hertz*	*Hz*
joule	*J*	*milliequivalent*	*mEq*

5. Always capitalize genus name abbreviations when they are accompanied by the species name.

Examples:
H influenzae
E coli
C difficile

C. Punctuation.

1. Do not use periods within or at the end of most abbreviations, including acronyms, abbreviated units of measure, and brief forms. Use a period at the end of abbreviated English units of measure if they may be misread without the period (only in virgule and table construction).

Examples:

wbc	*WBC*	*mg*	*cm*
exam	*prep*	*mEq*	*mL*

inch preferred to *in.*
(Do not use *in* for *inch* without a period.)

2. Do not use periods with abbreviated academic degrees and professional credentials.

Examples:
John Smith, MD
Mary Jones, CMT
Robert Williams, PhD

3. Use periods in lowercase drug-related abbreviations derived from Latin terms.

   Examples:
   | *b.i.d.* | *t.i.d.* | *a.c.* |
   | *p.r.n.* | *p.o.* | *q.4 h.* |

   NOTE: AAMT continues to discourage dropping periods in lowercase abbreviations that might be misread as words (*bid* and *tid*). If you must drop the periods, use all capitals, but keep in mind that the overuse of capitals, particularly in relation to drug doses and dosages, would draw more attention to the capitalized abbreviations than to the drug names themselves.

4. Periods may be used with courtesy title abbreviations (e.g., *Mr., Mrs.*) and following *Jr.* and *Sr.*, although there is a trend toward dropping them. Either remains acceptable, but be consistent.

5. Use a lowercase *s* without an apostrophe to form the plural of a capitalized abbreviation, acronym, or brief form.

   Examples:
   | *EKGs* | *PVCs* | *exams* |
   | *labs* | *monos* | *CABGs* |

6. Use 's to form the plural of lowercase abbreviations.

   Examples:
   rbc's   *wbc's*

7. Use 's to form the plural of single-letter abbreviations.

   Examples:
   | *X's* | *K's* | *flipped T's* |

8. Add 's to most abbreviations or acronyms to show possession.

   Examples:
   The AMA's address is. . .
   AAMT's position paper on full disclosure states. . .

Ultimately, the application of these standards comes down to some fundamental, common sense principles. The objective, as stated initially, is to promote clarity in the healthcare record. An abbreviated form, when used, should meet this objective, and the application of capitalization or the use of punctuation to indicate plurality or possession should likewise promote clarity and be utilized consistently throughout the healthcare record. Of course, the overall goal of these standards is to encourage their consistent use across the entire healthcare delivery system.

REVIEW QUESTIONS

The goal of these questions is to test your knowledge of abbreviations and acronyms.

Directions: Select the correct answer for the multiple-choice questions provided below. *Answers are provided at the end of this chapter.*

1. Which of the following is an example of an ACRONYM?
   A. COPD
   B. t.i.d.
   C. CABG
   D. lymphs

2. Which of the following is an example of a BRIEF FORM?
   A. cath
   B. mmHg
   C. BKA
   D. all of the above

3. Which is correctly transcribed?
   A. TITLE OF OPERATION: ORIF, left radius.
   B. DIAGNOSIS: Pyelonephritis with elevated blood urea nitrogen (BUN).
   C. TITLE OF OPERATION: Transurethral resection of the prostate (TURP).
   D. DIAGNOSIS: IDDM.

4. A measurement would be correctly indicated by which of the following?
   A. 2 cm
   B. 3 inches
   C. a few centimeters
   D. all of the above

5. Which would represent the incorrect transcription of a measurement?
   A. 4.5 cm
   B. 3 in
   C. 4 feet
   D. all of the above

6. The Latin abbreviation referring to "twice per day" would be correctly transcribed as:
   A. bid
   B. B.I.D.
   C. b.i.d.
   D. BID

7. Which represents the incorrect capitalization of an abbreviation?
   A. Differential showed 58 SEGs.
   B. WBC was 48.2.
   C. Urinalysis revealed 8–10 wbc's.
   D. none of the above

8. Which of the following is correctly pluralized?
   A. serial K's
   B. EKG's
   C. lymph's
   D. rbcs

9. Which of the following genus/species reference is correctly transcribed?
   A. staphylococcus aureus
   B. s. aureus
   C. S Aureus
   D. S aureus

10. Which of the following is correctly transcribed?
    A. The baby weighed 8 lbs 12 oz.
    B. She was instructed to return on a prn basis.
    C. We injected 10 mL of lidocaine.
    D. CBC showed WBC's of 9.2.

ANSWER KEY

REVIEW QUESTIONS ANSWER KEY

1. C	3. C	5. B	7. A	9. D
2. A	4. D	6. C	8. A	10. C

System Chapters

4

Cardiology/Cardiac Surgery/ Thoracic Surgery

OBJECTIVES CHECKLIST

A prepared exam candidate will know the:

- [ ] Combining forms, prefixes, and suffixes related to the body system.

- [ ] Basic structures of the heart and how they function together.

- [ ] Major vessels of the circulatory system as well as the difference in vessel types and functions.

- [ ] Flow of blood along its full circulatory path and the correct order of coronary structures through which blood flows during the oxygenation process.

- [ ] Electrophysiology of the heartbeat, from the role of the sinoatrial node to ventricular contraction.

- [ ] Fundamentals of blood pressure and the indications of elevated and depressed diastolic and systolic levels.

- [ ] Common signs and symptoms associated with coronary and/or circulatory dysfunction or disease.

- [ ] Major disease processes associated with the heart and vessels and the general treatment course for each.

- [ ] Diagnostic imaging and nuclear medicine studies used in the assessment and treatment of heart/vessel disease.

- [ ] Terminology related to an electrocardiogram (EKG), including the accurate transcription of leads and trace findings.

- [ ] Laboratory tests used in the diagnosis and ongoing evaluation of heart/vessel disease.

- [ ] Commonly prescribed medications, by type, for diseases and symptoms related to the heart, vessels, and circulation.

RESOURCES FOR STUDY

1. *Bates' Guide to Physical Examination and History Taking*
   Chapter 8: The Cardiovascular System, pp. 279–335.

2. *The Language of Medicine*
   Chapter 11: Cardiovascular System, pp. 383–439.

3. *Memmler's Structure and Function of the Human Body*
   Chapter 13: The Heart, pp. 231–246.
   Chapter 14: Blood Vessels and Blood Circulation, pp. 249–266.

4. *Memmler's The Human Body in Health and Disease*
   Chapter 14: The Heart and Heart Disease, pp. 283–305; Study Guide, pp. 221–234.
   Chapter 15: Blood Vessels and Blood Circulation, pp. 307–328; Study Guide, pp. 235–253.

5. *H&P: A Nonphysician's Guide to the Medical History and Physical Examination*
   Chapter 8: Review of Systems: Cardiovascular, pp. 71–81.
   Chapter 23: Examination of the Heart: pp. 217–221.

6. *Human Diseases*
   Chapter 8: Diseases of the Cardiovascular System, pp. 105–126.

7. *Laboratory Tests & Diagnostic Procedures in Medicine*
   Chapter 4: Measurement of Temperature, Rates, Pressures and Volumes (Cardiovascular Measurements, Noninvasive Cardiac Measurements, and Invasive Cardiovascular Procedures), pp. 42–48.
   Chapter 6: Electrocardiography, pp. 75–92.
   Chapter 20: Blood Chemistry (Electrolytes and Acid-Base Balance, Arterial Blood Gases, and Enzymes), pp. 355–400.

8. *A Manual of Laboratory and Diagnostic Tests*
   Chapter 2: Blood Studies: Hematology and Coagulation, pp. 38–162.
   Chapter 9: Nuclear Medicine Studies, pp. 652–704.
   Chapter 10: X-Ray Studies, pp. 705–759.
   Chapter 13: Ultrasound Studies, pp. 862–899.
   Chapter 16: Special Systems, Organ Functions, and Postmortem Studies, pp. 1012–1093.

9. *The AAMT Book of Style for Medical Transcription*
   Cardiology, pp. 57–63.

10. *Using Medical Terminology: A Practical Approach*
    Chapter 11: Cardiovascular System, pp. 463–523.

11. *Pharmacology for Health Professionals*
    Unit IV: Drugs That Affect the Cardiovascular System (Chapters 14-18), pp. 199–274

12. *Understanding Pharmacology for Health Professionals*
    Chapter 15: Cardiovascular Drugs, pp. 150–177.

13. *Medical Terminology: The Language of Health Care*
    Chapter 7: Cardiovascular System, pp. 192–240.

SAMPLE REPORTS

The following four reports are examples of reports you might encounter while transcribing cardiology, cardiac surgery, or thoracic surgery.

OPERATIVE REPORT

DATE OF OPERATION
05/01/2004

ATTENDING SURGEON
John Smith, MD.

PREOPERATIVE DIAGNOSIS
End-stage cardiomyopathy.

POSTOPERATIVE DIAGNOSIS
End-stage cardiomyopathy.

PROCEDURE PERFORMED
Heart transplantation.

ANESTHESIA
General endotracheal.

JUSTIFICATION FOR PROCEDURE
The patient is a 65-year-old man with ischemic cardiomyopathy. He had been evaluated for heart transplantation at this facility and placed on the national computer waiting list.

PROCEDURE IN DETAIL
On the night of this surgery, a suitable donor was identified. The patient had previous laryngeal cancer with radiation to the neck, and he was brought to the operating room somewhat early because difficulty with his airway was anticipated. For this reason, he underwent fiberoptic awake intubation which was accomplished without difficulty. A left subclavian Swan-Ganz catheter was placed, as was a radial arterial line and a Foley catheter. With notification from the donor site that the heart was acceptable, the anterior chest, abdomen, groin, and legs were prepped with Betadine and draped as a sterile field.

With notification from the donor site that the heart had been harvested, we began the operation by making a skin incision over the sternum. The sternum was then split in the midline with a saw. A self-retaining retractor was placed, and the pericardium was opened to the right side of the midline. Heparin was administered, and cannulation pursestrings were placed in the ascending aorta, high right superior vena cava, and low lateral right atrium. Cannulation was accomplished and the connection was made to the heart/lung machine.

With notification that the heart had arrived in town, cardiopulmonary bypass was instituted, and a vent was placed through the right superior pulmonary vein through a pursestring. With the heart in the hospital, we cross-clamped the aorta, snugged down on tapes which had been placed around the inferior vena cava and superior vena cava, and divided the superior vena cava, the

(continued)

ascending aorta after cross-clamping it, the pulmonary artery, the inferior vena cava, and then the left atrium. The heart was then removed and hemostasis was obtained at the left atrial cuff.

The donor heart was then brought into the room and prepared for implantation. There was no patent foramen ovale. The pulmonary artery was shortened appropriately, as was the left atrial cuff. The anastomosis was begun on the left side. We placed a 3-0 Prolene suture in a running fashion to accomplish the left atrial anastomosis. Just prior to completion of this anastomosis, the left ventricular vent was placed across the mitral valve and continued on gentle suction. A 4-0 Prolene suture was then used, interrupted in two places, to anastomose the inferior vena cava of the donor and the recipient. A 5-0 Prolene suture was then used to anastomose the pulmonary artery of the donor and recipient, again using interrupted technique at three different points. The ascending aorta was then anastomosed using a running 4-0 Prolene suture in two layers reinforced by pledgets. After completion of the inner layer, the left ventricular vent was turned off, the aortic root was allowed to fill with left ventricular blood, a vent was placed in the ascending aorta and placed on gentle suction, and the cross-clamp was removed. The outer layer was then accomplished using a second layer of running Prolene. The superior vena cava was then anastomosed using a running 6-0 Prolene, which was interrupted in four spots to prevent pursestringing.

The heart began to beat spontaneously, first with an idioventricular rhythm and then subsequently with a nice, normal sinus rhythm. We checked for bleeding and found one spot on the left atrium; this was oversewn with 3-0 Prolene. Pacing wires were placed on the surface of the atrium and the ventricle. The superior vena cava cannula was clamped and removed, and the cannulation site was repaired in longitudinal fashion using a running 6-0 Prolene. The heart was then reperfused for a total of one-half the ischemic interval, or 92 minutes. We then weaned from cardiopulmonary bypass without a great deal of difficulty. There was a significant amount of bleeding from the posterior wall of the aortic anastomosis, and this required several sutures to control. Ultimately, however, we were able to get it under control.

The patient then remained quite hemodynamically labile over the next several minutes, with blood pressures as high as 200 and as low as 90. He gradually stabilized and we were able to administer Protamine and remove the cannulas after reinfusion of all shed blood.

The pursestring sutures were secured and all suture lines were inspected and found to be hemostatic. Two chest tubes were then brought in through separate stab wounds in the mediastinum and secured with silk sutures. After a final check for hemostasis, we went ahead and closed the sternum using interrupted figure-of-8 stainless steel wires. The skin and subcutaneous layers were then closed with absorbable sutures. A dry sterile dressing was applied. The chest tubes were placed for Pleur-evac suction. Sponge, laparotomy pad, instrument, and needle counts were reported as correct at the end of the case.

TOTAL BYPASS TIME
146 minutes.

TOTAL ISCHEMIC TIME
148 minutes.

ADDENDUM
The patient was cooled to 28°C on cardiopulmonary bypass.

OPERATIVE REPORT

DATE OF OPERATION
05/01/2004

ATTENDING SURGEON
John Smith, MD.

PREOPERATIVE DIAGNOSIS
Ventricular tachycardia.

POSTOPERATIVE DIAGNOSIS
Ventricular tachycardia.

PROCEDURE PERFORMED
Placement of automatic implantable cardioverter-defibrillator (AICD).

ANESTHESIA
General endotracheal.

JUSTIFICATION FOR PROCEDURE
The patient is a 75-year-old man with a history of ventricular fibrillation and tachycardia.

PROCEDURE IN DETAIL
At the time of surgery, the patient was brought to the operating room and placed in the supine position where he underwent general endotracheal anesthesia without any difficulty. The patient was prepped with Betadine scrub and Betadine paint and draped in the usual sterile fashion.

An incision was then made in the left deltopectoral fold, and a pocket was made underneath the pectoralis major muscle. A percutaneous stick was then made into the left subclavian vein and attached to the guide wire. It should be noted that, during this, some air was retrieved, and the patient had a small pneumothorax for which a left chest tube was placed at the end of the procedure without difficulty.

Once the guide wire was in, the AICD lead was implanted. This was a Corpus model #1234, serial #123456, with threshold measurements of 1.1 milliampere, 600 ohms resistance, 16 millivolt R-wave, and a 0.6 volt threshold. The patient then had inducible ventricular fibrillation with a 15-joule shock and returned to normal sinus rhythm. This was done a second time, and he returned to normal sinus rhythm once again.

After this, the patient did well, and the wound was irrigated with antibiotic solution and closed with a 3-0 Vicryl subcutaneous layer and a 4-0 Vicryl subcuticular layer. The patient was transferred to the recovery room in stable condition.

ECHOCARDIOGRAM

M-MODE ECHOCARDIOGRAM

AORTIC VALVE LEVEL
The aortic valve opening is normal. The aortic root motion is normal. The left atrial intracavitary dimensions are increased.

MITRAL VALVE LEVEL
The mitral valve opening is normal. The DE and EF slopes are reduced. The E-point septal separation is increased. There is no pericardial effusion.

LEFT VENTRICULAR LEVEL
The left ventricular and septal wall thickness is increased. The left ventricular intracavitary dimensions are increased.

IMPRESSION
1. Mild concentric left ventricular hypertrophy.
2. Dilated left ventricle.
3. Reduced left ventricular function by increased E-point septal separation.
4. Dilated left atrium.

2-D ECHOCARDIOGRAM, DOPPLER AND COLOR FLOW
The 2-dimensional echocardiographic study revealed increased left ventricular and septal thickness. The left ventricular and septal wall motion and contractility revealed generalized diffuse hypokinesia. The intracavitary dimensions of the left ventricle are increased during systole and diastole. The left atrial intracavitary dimensions are increased. The aortic root motion is reduced. The aortic root and mitral anulus are thickened. There is no evidence of intracavitary mass, thrombus or pericardial effusion.

The right ventricular wall motion and contractility are normal.

DOPPLER STUDIES
The Doppler studies reveal a regurgitant jet across the mitral valve with a jet velocity of 4.25 m/s with a gradient of 72 mmHg. The E and A velocities appeared to be fairly normal with decreased deceleration time and evidence of increased left ventricular relaxation time. However, the E and the A velocities could not be sampled. Pulmonary studies were not obtained.

Transtricuspid Doppler interrogation revealed a regurgitant jet with a jet velocity of 3.2 m/s with a calculated right ventricular systolic pressure of 50 mmHg. The transaortic and pulmonic valve Doppler studies are unremarkable, with normal velocities.

IMPRESSION
1. Left ventricular and systolic and diastolic dysfunction.
2. Mild concentric left ventricular hypertrophy.
3. Dilated left ventricle and left atrium.
4. Thickening of the aortic root and mitral anulus.

MYOCARDIAL PERFUSION IMAGING

MYOCARDIAL PERFUSION IMAGING AT REST AND WITH EXERCISE

HISTORY
A 63-year-old female with known coronary artery disease and recurrent chest pain.

INDICATION
Chest pain.

PROCEDURE
The patient exercised on a treadmill for a total of 9 minutes, reaching stage IV of the Bruce protocol, achieving an estimated workload of 7 METs. The heart rate was 80 bpm at baseline and increased to 171 bpm at peak exercise, representing 109% of age-predicted maximal heart rate. The blood pressure response was normal.

The patient did not have chest pain during the procedure. The electrocardiogram showed ST changes which were inconclusive.

The patient's heart was tomographically imaged with 10 mCi of Myoview (^{99m}Tc-tetrofosmin) at rest and 29 mCi of Myoview before gated acquisition was performed.

FINDINGS
There was no evidence of significant motion artifact or extracardiac uptake. Left ventricular hypertrophy was noted with diastolic dysfunction. Anteroseptal wall motion abnormalities were noted. LVEF was calculated at 40%. There were anteroapical and anteroseptal perfusion defects on stress images that were partially reversible on the rest images.

IMPRESSION
1. Left ventricular hypertrophy.
2. Diastolic dysfunction.
3. Anteroapical and anteroseptal perfusion defects with stress.
4. Technically difficult test.

REVIEW QUESTIONS

The goal of these questions is to test your knowledge in the areas of cardiology, cardiac surgery, and thoracic surgery.

Directions: Select the correct answer for each of the multiple-choice questions provided below. *Answers are provided at the end of this chapter.*

1. The smooth layer of endothelial cells that lines the interior of the heart and the heart valves is called
   A. endocardium.
   B. interventricular septum.
   C. myocardium.
   D. pericardium.

2. The record used to detect electrical changes in the heart muscle as the heart is beating is called a (an)
   A. echocardiogram.
   B. electrocardiogram.
   C. electroencephalogram.
   D. sphygmomanometer.

3. Which of the following is given to treat acute attacks of angina by increasing coronary blood flow?
   A. an ACE inhibitor
   B. aspirin
   C. nitroglycerin
   D. a statin

4. Retrosternal pain is located
   A. above the sternum.
   B. behind the sternum.
   C. below the sternum.
   D. beside the sternum.

5. Which of the following types of medications has the primary function of preventing blood clots?
   A. ACE inhibitors
   B. angiotensin II receptor blockers
   C. antiplatelet drugs
   D. antiarrhythmic medications

6. A patient comes in with trouble breathing and swelling in the lower legs. The provider suspects
   A. congestive heart failure.
   B. a heart murmur.
   C. myocardial infarction.
   D. aneurysm.

7. Which of the following risk factors for cardiac disease can be modified?
   A. age
   B. diabetes mellitus
   C. family history
   D. gender

8. Which test, when elevated, is most indicative of heart failure?
   A. BMP
   B. BNP
   C. CMP
   D. INR

9. Which of the following is a type of heart murmur?
   A. cyanotic
   B. serophilic
   C. sessile
   D. systolic

10. What suffix combined with *cardio-* means enlarged heart?
    A. -megaly
    B. -metry
    C. -malacia
    D. -myotomy

11. In this procedure, a small flexible tube is guided into the heart via the femoral artery in order to detect pressures and patterns of blood flow in the heart.
    A. coronary artery bypass graft
    B. exercise tolerance test
    C. cardiac catheterization
    D. endarterectomy

12. Which of the following laboratory tests is used to diagnose a myocardial infarction?
    A. CEA and CA 19-9
    B. CK-MB and troponin
    C. MCH and MCV
    D. PSA and PTH

13. The contraction phase of the cardiac cycle is
    A. diastole.
    B. endocardium.
    C. systole.
    D. tachycardia.

14. Which of the following is the medical term for a heart attack?
    A. diphtheritic myocarditis
    B. myocardial hamartoma
    C. myocardial infarction
    D. septal myomectomy

15. Blood pressure measurement is expressed as
    A. diastolic pressure over systolic pressure.
    B. sacral pressure over diagonal pressure.
    C. systemic pressure over diaphragm pressure.
    D. systolic pressure over diastolic pressure.

16. The antiarrhythmic agent used to treat congestive heart failure and arrhythmias like atrial fibrillation is
    A. digoxin.
    B. doxepin.
    C. doxycycline.
    D. Doxidan.

17. Which of these terms means an abnormal bulge in the wall of an artery?
    A. aneuploidy
    B. aneurysm
    C. angionecrosis
    D. annulus

18. Premature heartbeat is also known as
    A. arrhythmia.
    B. bradycardia.
    C. extrasystole.
    D. tachycardia.

19. Pain, tension, and weakness in a leg after walking with absence of the pain at rest is called
    A. claudication.
    B. embolus.
    C. infarction.
    D. occlusion.

20. Which of the following tests is used to monitor a patient on Coumadin therapy?
    A. INR
    B. transferrin
    C. CBC
    D. platelet count

21. Which node is considered the dominant pacemaker?
    A. atrioventricular node
    B. coronary node
    C. sentinel node
    D. sinoatrial node

22. Which of the following is placed within a coronary artery to keep the artery patent?
    A. valve
    B. stint
    C. stent
    D. catheter

23. Which of the following are forms of cholesterol?
    A. homocysteine and fibrinogen
    B. creatinine and LH
    C. AST and ALT
    D. HDL and LDL

24. Which of the following is a surgical procedure used to restore blood flow to an area of the heart when an artery is occluded by atherosclerosis?
    A. echocardiogram
    B. pacemaker implantation
    C. AV node ablation
    D. CABG

25. How many leads are in a standard electrocardiogram?
    A. 9
    B. 11
    C. 12
    D. 13

26. Fainting is also referred to as
    A. a cerebrovascular accident.
    B. thrombosis.
    C. claudication.
    D. syncope.

27. Which are normal heart sounds?
    A. S1 and S2
    B. S1 and S4
    C. S2 and S3
    D. S3 and S4

28. Which of the following is a humming or buzzing sound caused by the passage of blood through an artery narrowed by arteriosclerosis?
    A. PMI
    B. rub
    C. click
    D. bruit

29. Which of the following is a diuretic that is often combined with antihypertensive medications?
    A. ibuprofen
    B. acetylsalicylic acid
    C. lovastatin
    D. hydrochlorothiazide

30. Sudden episodes of labored breathing that awaken the patient from sleep is referred to as
    A. P and D.
    B. PCP.
    C. PND.
    D. O and P.

Please see the accompanying CD for additional review materials for this section.

ANSWER KEY

REVIEW QUESTIONS ANSWER KEY

1. A	6. A	11. C	16. A	21. D	26. D
2. B	7. B	12. B	17. B	22. C	27. A
3. C	8. B	13. C	18. C	23. D	28. D
4. B	9. D	14. C	19. A	24. D	29. D
5. C	10. A	15. D	20. A	25. C	30. C

Emergency Medicine

OBJECTIVES CHECKLIST

A prepared exam candidate will know the:

☐ Basics of emergency medicine including assessment, triage, diagnostic intervention, and stabilization.

☐ Role of Advanced Cardiac Life Support (ACLS) protocol in resuscitation and critical cardiac intervention.

☐ ABCs (airway, breathing & circulation) of trauma evaluation as used on scene and in the emergency room.

☐ Fundamentals of the mental status exam as well as terminology unique to psychiatric assessment in the emergency setting.

☐ Typical first-line treatment course for most common presenting complaints in the emergency setting.

☐ Diagnostic imaging and laboratory studies related to emergency medicine.

☐ Interventional medications administered in critical treatment, particularly resuscitation, drug overdose, poisoning, envenomization, and acute trauma.

☐ Medications administered routinely for common presenting complaints.

RESOURCES FOR STUDY

1. *Bates' Guide to Physical Examination and History Taking*
   Chapter 1: Overview of Physical Examination and History Taking, pp. 3–21.
   Chapter 2: Interviewing and the Health History, pp. 23–63.
   Chapter 3: Clinical Reasoning, Assessment, and Plan, pp. 65–86.
   Chapter 4: Beginning the Physical Examination: General Survey and Vital Signs, pp. 89–120.
   Chapter 20: The Older Adult, pp. 839–873.

2. *H&P: A Nonphysician's Guide to the Medical History and Physical Examination*
   Chapter 1: General Remarks on the History, pp. 13–24.
   Chapter 2: Chief Complaint and History of Present Illness, pp. 25–34.
   Chapter 28: The Formal Mental Status Examination, pp. 273–280.

3. *Human Diseases*
   Chapter 6: Trauma and Poisoning, pp. 73–86.
   Chapter 20: Mental Disorders, pp. 315–332.

4. *Laboratory Tests & Diagnostic Procedures in Medicine*
   Chapter 4: Measurement of Temperature, Rates, Pressures and Volumes, pp. 39–60.
   Section VI (Chapters 19–24). *Note: Information in all of these chapters is pertinent to Emergency Medicine but will also be well covered in other chapters of this text.*

5. *A Manual of Laboratory and Diagnostic Tests*
   Chapter 7: Microbiologic Studies, pp. 456–529.
   Chapter 9: Nuclear Medicine Studies, pp. 652–704.
   Chapter 10: X-Ray Studies, pp. 705–759.
   Chapter 13: Ultrasound Studies, pp. 862–899.
   Chapter 16: Special Systems, Organ Functions, and Postmortem Studies, pp. 1012–1093.

6. *Pharmacology for Health Professionals*
   Unit II: Drugs That Affect the Neurologic System (Chapters 4–10), pp. 37–167.
   Unit III: Drugs That Affect the Respiratory System (Chapters 11–13), pp. 169–197.
   Unit IV: Drugs That Affect the Cardiovascular System (Chapters 14–18), pp. 199–274.
   Chapter 22: Antidiabetic Drugs, pp. 323–338.
   Chapter 32: Fluids and Electrolytes, pp. 542–554.

7. *Understanding Pharmacology for Health Professionals*
   Chapter 16: Emergency Drugs, pp. 178–191.
   Chapter 17: Anticoagulant and Thrombolytic Drugs, pp. 185–191.
   Chapter 26: Analgesic Drugs, pp. 296–310.
   Chapter 32: Intravenous Fluids and Blood Products, pp. 373–385.

8. *Medical Terminology: The Language of Health Care*
   Chapter 6: Musculoskeletal System, pp. 144–191.

The following four reports are examples of reports you might encounter while transcribing emergency medicine.

OPERATIVE NOTE

DATE OF OPERATION
02/21/2004

SURGEON OF RECORD
John Smith, MD.

PREOPERATIVE DIAGNOSIS
Left index finger cellulitis.

POSTOPERATIVE DIAGNOSIS
Left index finger cellulitis.

PROCEDURE PERFORMED
Hickman catheter placement.

ANESTHESIA
Monitored anesthesia care.

COMPLICATIONS
None noted.

ESTIMATED BLOOD LOSS
Minimal.

INTRAVENOUS FLUIDS
200 mL of Crystalloid.

INDICATIONS FOR PROCEDURE
The patient is a 33-year-old Haitian male who had a gunshot wound to his left index finger and subsequently underwent surgery by the orthopedic hand service. This included having a piece of hardware placed. The patient presented to the surgical emergency room today with purulent drainage from his finger and underwent incision and drainage of his left index finger. The patient will require long-term antibiotics and, for this reason, a Hickman catheter was requested by the orthopedic team.

PROCEDURE IN DETAIL
The patient was given intravenous sedation and then prepped and draped in the usual sterile fashion, still in the surgical emergency room. We then proceeded to cannulate the left subclavian vein and passed a guide wire through the needle.

Then we made a tunnel under the skin with an exit approximately 4 cm below our initial cannulation site. After that, we measured the Hickman catheter, making sure the cuff would be at the level of the skin of the lower incision and the tip would be at the level of the superior vena

(continued)

cava. After that, we proceeded, using the Seldinger technique, to introduce the dilator and introducer into the left subclavian vein. After removal of the dilator, good blood return was seen and we proceeded to introduce the Hickman catheter through the sheath, which was then removed. Good blood flow was obtained from the Hickman catheter.

At that time, an x-ray was obtained, noting the presence of no pneumothorax and the tip of the catheter at the level of the superior vena cava.

We then approximated the skin edges using 4-0 Vicryl in an inverted fashion, following which we applied a dry dressing.

OPERATIVE REPORT

DATE OF OPERATION
01/06/2004

SURGEON OF RECORD
John Jones, MD.

PREOPERATIVE DIAGNOSIS
Gunshot wound to the abdomen.

POSTOPERATIVE DIAGNOSES
1. Gunshot wound to the abdomen.
2. Laceration of the duodenum.
3. Injury to the head of the pancreas.
4. Injury to the inferior vena cava.
5. Injury to the right renal artery.

PROCEDURES PERFORMED
1. Closure of stomach laceration.
2. Closure of duodenal laceration.
3. Drainage of pancreas.
4. Repair of renal artery.
5. Repair of inferior vena cava.

ANESTHESIA
General endotracheal anesthesia.

JUSTIFICATION FOR PROCEDURE
This is an 18-year-old known gang member who presented to the trauma center with a gunshot wound to the abdomen.

PROCEDURE IN DETAIL
The patient was brought to the operating room in the trauma center, placed in the supine position, and prepped and draped in the usual sterile fashion. The abdomen was entered through a long midline incision. Upon entering the abdomen, the abdomen was packed to control bleeding.

Examination of the abdomen revealed the following injuries: There was a long laceration of the greater curvature of the stomach. There was a hole through-and-through on the head of the pancreas and a small laceration of the duodenum. The bullet projectile also caused a large right retroperitoneal hematoma. The right side of the colon was mobilized and the duodenum was kocherized. Kocherization of the duodenum revealed the through-and-through injury to the head of the pancreas and also revealed the small hole through the duodenum mentioned previously.

After the right side of the colon was mobilized, it was evident that the bullet had gone through the hilum of the right kidney, and exploration of that area revealed that the renal artery had been lacerated and there was also a small hole in the inferior vena cava. The small hole in the inferior vena cava was closed with figure-of-8 sutures of 5-0 Prolene. The renal artery was controlled proximally and distally and was completely divided and débrided. Following this, a primary anastomosis was performed with 6-0 Prolene interrupted stitches.

(continued)

The examination of the rest of the abdomen was normal, and the abdomen was thoroughly irrigated with normal saline, following which a Jackson-Pratt drain was placed over the head of the pancreas and the duodenum.

The patient tolerated the procedure well and was transferred to the postanesthesia recovery unit in good general condition.

EMERGENCY ROOM REPORT

CHIEF COMPLAINT/HISTORY OF PRESENT ILLNESS

The patient is a 40-year-old black male who was, unfortunately, shot by his brother this evening. The patient was shot in both legs. The patient then dove down the stairs. The patient was brought to the emergency room by EMS with stable vital signs, complaining of pain in both legs. The patient denies injuries elsewhere. The patient admits to abusing cocaine and alcohol today as well.

ALLERGIES

The patient is ALLERGIC to HALDOL, PROLIXIN, and THORAZINE.

MEDICATIONS

Valium and Tylenol No. 3.

PAST MEDICAL HISTORY

His medical problems include a history of schizophrenia.

SOCIAL HISTORY

The patient admits to polysubstance abuse as well as alcohol abuse. The patient also smokes cigarettes.

PAST SURGICAL HISTORY

Positive for a gunshot wound to the abdomen in the past with intraoperative repair.

PHYSICAL EXAMINATION

GENERAL: The patient is well-developed, well-nourished black male in moderate, nonrespiratory distress, presenting on a backboard with C-collar immobilization.

VITAL SIGNS: The patient's initial vital signs include an oral temperature of 97, pulse 70, respiratory rate 20, with a blood pressure of 91/50. At the time of transfer, his blood pressure was 115/61 (sitting) and his saturation was 100% on 100% oxygen via face mask.

SKIN: Revealed gunshot wounds to the right midthigh and to the left midshin with no exit wounds.

HEENT: Extraocular movements are intact and pupils are equally round and reactive to light. ENT examination was negative.

NECK: Supple.

CHEST: Lungs are clear anteriorly.

HEART: Regular rate and rhythm.

ABDOMEN: Reveals good bowel sounds, soft, nontender, nondistended, and otherwise negative.

GENITALIA: Normal.

EXTREMITIES: He has a gunshot wound to the right midthigh with no exit wound and a gunshot wound to the left midtibia and fibula with no exit wound. There are good femoral pulses, dorsalis pedis, and 2+ posterior tibialis pulses bilaterally and full range of motion at the toes except for decreased sensation to the left 5th toe. Otherwise, there is normal sensation.

NEUROLOGICAL: The patient is somewhat lethargic but he has a Glasgow coma scale of 15, and he is oriented x3 and otherwise nonfocal.

(continued)

DIAGNOSTIC STUDIES

His labs reveal a pH of 7.3, pCO_2 of 38, a pO_2 of 202, a HCO_3 of 18, and this is on 100% oxygen by mask. Coagulation studies reveal a PT of 12, an INR of 1.2, and a PTT of 26.4. The patient's urine is essentially negative but it does reveal a small amount of hematuria, and the patient's ABO/Rh type is O positive. The patient's urine drug screen revealed benzodiazepines and cocaine metabolites. A CBC revealed a white count of 9.8, hemoglobin and hematocrit of 12 and 35.1, respectively, with platelets of 305 and an MCV of 80. The patient's Chem-12 revealed a BUN of 23, a creatinine of 1.3, sodium 138, and bicarbonate 17.8. Alcohol level is 210. EKG revealed normal sinus rhythm with left ventricular hypertrophy.

EMERGENCY DEPARTMENT COURSE

The patient was given a tetanus toxoid booster and 2 g of Ancef as well as 1 unit of blood secondary to the initial low blood pressure reading. The patient had a Foley catheter placed and a hard cervical collar placed with towels to bolster the head, and this was secured at the forehead and the chin. The patient's left lower extremity was splinted with a short leg splint and the right with a long leg splint. The patient was given morphine 4 mg IV for pain and also received 1 L of normal saline and 2 L of lactated Ringers with a resultant output of 350 mL of urine.

I did speak with Dr. Smith, who is the trauma surgeon at Johnson Hospital, and their emergency room physician has accepted the patient for transfer. The patient's x-rays have been copied, as were all records and lab studies. These records will accompany the patient on transfer to the other hospital.

FINAL DIAGNOSES

1. Status post gunshot wounds to lower extremities; right femur fracture and left tibia fracture.
2. Polysubstance illicit drug ingestion.

EMERGENCY ROOM REPORT

CHIEF COMPLAINT/HISTORY OF PRESENT ILLNESS
The patient is a 30-year-old female who does not have a doctor at this hospital. She was brought to the emergency room by the paramedics. It seems that she was found "down" in the street, unconscious, with labored breathing.

ALLERGIES
No information is available at this time.

CURRENT MEDICATIONS
Her tetanus immunization status is unknown.

PHYSICAL EXAMINATION
VITAL SIGNS: Blood pressure 90/50, pulse 120, respirations 10, temperature 99.
GENERAL: The patient is unconscious, not responding, and incoherent. She smells of alcohol.
HEENT: Pupils are equal, round, and sluggishly reactive to light. The patient has multiple abrasions of the face with swelling of her upper lip. The patient also has multiple superficial avulsive lacerations, particularly involving the left periorbital area.
NECK: A C-collar is in place, and she is in full spinal precautions.
CHEST: Auscultation reveals rales and rhonchi.
HEART: Tachycardia is present.
ABDOMEN: No distention, feels soft, bowel sounds are difficult to hear.
EXTREMITIES: Upper extremities have no swelling, no deformities, and she moves all joints normally. Lower extremities have no swelling, no deformities, and she moves all joints normally.
NEUROLOGICAL: Cranial nerves intact. No motor or sensory deficits.

DIAGNOSTIC STUDIES
The patient had a CT of the head done which was negative. A CT of the C-spine was also negative, as were the chest and pelvic CTs. Among the laboratory work, the alcohol level is 409, glucose 85, BUN 9, creatinine 0.6, sodium 143, potassium 3.8, chloride 111. The WBC count is 4.4, hemoglobin is 13.7 with a hematocrit of 40, neutrophils of 31, lymphocytes of 43, and monocytes of 8.4.

EMERGENCY DEPARTMENT COURSE
The patient was started on normal saline wide open followed by D5 normal saline at 125 mL/h. She received thiamine 100 mg IV and also Ancef 2 grams IV piggyback and a tetanus shot. The laceration of the left orbital area was sutured with 5-0 nylon. We notified the trauma surgeon on call, and the patient is being admitted to his service for further evaluation and management.

FINAL DIAGNOSES
1. Head and facial trauma.
2. Alcohol abuse/alcohol intoxication.

REVIEW QUESTIONS

The goal of these questions is to test your knowledge in the area of emergency medicine.

Directions: Select the correct answer for each of the multiple-choice questions provided below. *Answers are provided at the end of this chapter.*

1. A female presents to the emergency room complaining of burning with urination. The ER physician will likely first order a (an)
   A. CBC.
   B. BNP.
   C. hCG.
   D. UA.

2. A patient comes to the ER with changes in mental status, fever, and nuchal rigidity. A possible diagnosis would be
   A. bacterial meningitis.
   B. bacterial sinusitis.
   C. stroke.
   D. transient ischemic attack.

3. The ABCs of trauma evaluation refer to
   A. abbreviated blood count.
   B. apnea, bradycardia, and cyanosis.
   C. airway, breathing, and circulation.
   D. assess, brace, console.

4. DNR means
   A. do not resuscitate.
   B. does not rebound.
   C. does not remember.
   D. do not recommend.

5. The definition of hypoxia is
   A. below normal levels of carbon dioxide.
   B. below normal levels of carbon monoxide.
   C. below normal levels of oxygen.
   D. above normal levels of oxygen.

6. A widely used scoring system to assess impaired consciousness following traumatic brain injury is called
   A. adaptive behavior scale.
   B. Karnofsky scale.
   C. French scale.
   D. Glasgow coma scale.

7. Which of the following would be the treatment of choice for a severe allergic reaction?
   A. epinephrine
   B. penicillin
   C. pseudoephedrine
   D. sulfasalazine

8. Blood in the pleural cavity is called
   A. hemothorax.
   B. pneumothorax.
   C. hemoptysis.
   D. pneumoperitoneum.

9. Which of the following is indicative of appendicitis?
   A. Tinel sign
   B. McBurney sign
   C. Murphy sign
   D. Phalen sign

10. Sudden onset of excruciating pain in the left lower abdomen and blood in the urine would be indicative of
    A. appendicitis.
    B. kidney stone.
    C. herniated disk.
    D. UTI.

11. The physician dictates a positive Battle sign in a patient who has been in a motor vehicle accident. Under which heading would you place this finding?
    A. Chest
    B. HEENT
    C. Abdomen
    D. Extremities

12. Severe back pain after lifting an extremely heavy object may be diagnosed as a
    A. spinal deformity.
    B. herniated nucleus pulposus.
    C. torn ACL.
    D. lordosis lumbalis.

13. Which of the following tests would be performed on a patient presenting with chest pain?
    A. electrocardiogram
    B. electroencephalogram
    C. myelogram
    D. esophagogram

14. Following a motor vehicle accident, a patient's neck would be immobilized in case of
    A. cervical injury.
    B. malleolar injury.
    C. navicular injury.
    D. ulnar injury.

15. Which of the following would be used to treat a burn caused by scalding water?
    A. Centrum Silver
    B. Skelaxin
    C. Sensodyne
    D. Silvadene

16. Triage means
    A. treat the sickest person first.
    B. 3-stage treatment.
    C. wash with copious fluid.
    D. 3-dose treatment.

17. Which class of drug might be used to treat ingestion of a toxin?
    A. statin
    B. emetic
    C. antacid
    D. antiemetic

18. A collection of air or gas in the pleural space is a
    A. hemothorax.
    B. pericardial effusion.
    C. pleural effusion.
    D. pneumothorax.

19. A patient is diagnosed with a sprained ankle and the provider has written orders for RICE, which is an acronym for
    A. rest, ice, compression, and elevation.
    B. rest, ibuprofen, contraction, and elevation.
    C. rest, ice, contraction, and elevation.
    D. rest, ibuprofen, compression, and elevation.

20. Activated charcoal would be given to treat
    A. heartburn.
    B. poisoning.
    C. stroke.
    D. sunburn.

21. This tube is inserted through the nasal passages and into the stomach.
    A. nasolabial
    B. nasogastric
    C. nasopharyngeal
    D. nasotracheal

22. Which over-the-counter medication should be given immediately for patients with acute coronary syndrome?
    A. aspirin
    B. Colace
    C. milk of magnesia
    D. ibuprofen

23. Absence of a heartbeat is also known as
    A. diastole.
    B. ectopy.
    C. asystole.
    D. atopy.

24. Another term for nosebleed is
    A. hematemesis.
    B. hemoptysis.
    C. hematochezia.
    D. epistaxis.

25. A patient presents in the middle of the night with severe right upper quadrant pain radiating to the shoulder, diaphoresis, nausea, and a positive Murphy sign. The differential diagnosis would include
    A. pancreatitis.
    B. acute cholecystitis.
    C. myocardial ischemia.
    D. diverticulitis.

26. Which of the following would be given to a patient with angina pectoris?
    A. nitroglycerin
    B. Ativan
    C. Zantac
    D. acetaminophen

27. A patient is brought to the ER following a motor vehicle accident, and the physician orders 2 units of pRBCs in order to
    A. relieve the patient's pain.
    B. replace lost blood.
    C. sedate the patient before surgery.
    D. restore coagulation factors.

28. The above patient is also given FFP which stands for
    A. fresh frozen plasma.
    B. fibrinopeptide.
    C. frozen factor IX.
    D. fexofenadine and pseudoephedrine.

29. Which of the following causes a serious respiratory infection primarily affecting infants and the elderly?
    A. EBV
    B. COPD
    C. RSV
    D. HSV

30. A patient arrives in the ER after a motor vehicle accident and is found to have a severely deviated septum. What part of the body was injured?
    A. eye
    B. throat
    C. nose
    D. knee

 Please see the accompanying CD for additional review materials for this section.

ANSWER KEY

REVIEW QUESTIONS ANSWER KEY

1. D	6. D	11. B	16. A	21. B	26. A
2. A	7. A	12. B	17. B	22. A	27. B
3. C	8. A	13. A	18. D	23. C	28. A
4. A	9. B	14. A	19. A	24. D	29. C
5. C	10. B	15. D	20. B	25. B	30. C

6

Hematology/Oncology

OBJECTIVES CHECKLIST

A prepared exam candidate will know:

☐ All combining forms, prefixes, and suffixes related to the blood system and to oncology.

☐ Composition and formation of the blood.

☐ Stages of blood cell development from stem cell to full differentiation.

☐ Role and function of each blood component, including the breakdown of each leukocyte type and its percentage in the blood.

☐ Physiology of clot formation.

☐ Different blood groups that identify human blood and the role of antigens and antibodies in determining blood type and preventing hemagglutination.

☐ Characteristics of tumors and the differences between benign and malignant neoplasms.

☐ Physiology of carcinogenesis and the role of DNA/RNA in cellular malignancy.

☐ Different environmental agents and hereditary factors that contribute to the development of cancer.

☐ Differences among carcinomas, sarcomas, and mixed-tissue tumors, as well as the tissues from which they derive.

☐ Diseases and disorders of each type of blood cell, of clotting, and of the bone marrow.

☐ Laboratory studies used in the identification and treatment of hematologic disorders and diseases.

☐ Grading and staging systems used to classify neoplasms.

☐ Four major approaches to cancer treatment (surgery, radiation therapy, chemotherapy, and biological therapy) and the terminology related to each.

☐ Common medications prescribed for blood disorders and diseases and for the side effects and symptoms associated with radiation and chemotherapy.

RESOURCES FOR STUDY

1. *The Language of Medicine*
   Chapter 13: Blood System, pp. 488–528.
   Chapter 19: Cancer Medicine (Oncology), pp. 770–816.

2. *Memmler's Structure and Function of the Human Body*
   Chapter 3: Cells and Their Functions, pp. 35–54.
   Chapter 12: The Blood, pp. 213–228.
   Chapter 15: The Lymphatic System and Body Defenses, pp. 269–285.

3. *Memmler's The Human Body in Health and Disease*
   Chapter 4: Tissues, Glands, and Membranes, pp. 56–74; Study Guide, pp. 53–67.
   Chapter 13: Blood, pp. 262–280; Study Guide, pp. 205–220.

4. *Human Diseases*
   Chapter 5: Neoplasia, pp. 57–72.
   Chapter 16: Disorders of Blood Cells, Blood-forming Tissues, and Blood Coagulation, pp. 241–258.

5. *Laboratory Tests & Diagnostic Procedures in Medicine*
   Section V: Anatomic Pathology, pp. 223–314.
   Chapter 19: Hematology, Coagulation and Blood Typing, pp. 323–354.

6. *A Manual of Laboratory and Diagnostic Tests*
   Chapter 2: Blood Studies: Hematology and Coagulation, pp. 38–162.
   Chapter 9: Nuclear Medicine Studies, pp. 652–704.
   Chapter 11: Cytologic, Histologic, and Genetic Studies, pp. 760–818.

7. *The AAMT Book of Style for Medical Transcription*
   Blood counts and Blood groups, pp. 39–40.
   Blood types, p. 41.
   Cancer classifications, pp. 50–56.
   Laboratory data and values: hemoglobin and hematocrit, p. 232.
   Laboratory data and values: tumor cell markers, p. 233.

8. *Using Medical Terminology: A Practical Approach*
   Chapter 10: Blood, pp. 417–461.

9. *Pharmacology for Health Professionals*
   Chapter 28: Antineoplastic Drugs, pp. 475–493.

10. *Understanding Pharmacology for Health Professionals*
    Chapter 17: Anticoagulant and Thrombolytic Drugs, pp. 139–142.
    Chapter 30: Chemotherapy Drugs, pp. 337–364.

SAMPLE REPORTS

The following four reports are examples of reports you might encounter while transcribing hematology and oncology.

FOLLOWUP

HISTORY
The patient is a 25-year-old woman, G3, P2, A0, who is being followed for idiopathic thrombocytopenic purpura developed during her third pregnancy. She was started on prednisone at 1 mg/kg/d when she came in with a platelet count of 40,000, easy bruising, and marked petechiae. Her platelet count responded to prednisone. Although she has not come in as scheduled because she was too busy, her platelet count had increased to 161,000 on March 22. At that time, I decreased the dose to 60 mg/d. The patient comes in today for reevaluation.

REVIEW OF SYSTEMS
She has had no fever. She has had the normal weight change expected from her pregnancy. No malaise, no dizziness. SKIN: No ulcers, spots, bleeding, changes in color or texture. HEENT: No headaches, sinus problems, hoarseness, visual or hearing problems. CARDIORESPIRATORY: No cough, sputum production, hemoptysis, dyspnea, paroxysmal nocturnal dyspnea, orthopnea, chest pain, palpitations, or cyanosis. GASTROINTESTINAL: Mild heartburn. No dysphagia, odynophagia, abdominal pain, tenesmus, bleeding, or change in bowel habits. GENITOURINARY: Negative. MUSCULOSKELETAL: Basically negative. NERVOUS: Negative. LYMPHATIC: Negative.

PHYSICAL EXAMINATION
HEENT: Intact external ocular movements, no nystagmus, oropharynx clear. NECK: Supple. No JVD, no lymph nodes. HEART: Regular rhythm, no murmurs. LUNGS: Clear. ABDOMEN: Soft, bowel sounds positive. Gravid uterus, normal size.

LABORATORY
CBC done today shows a platelet count of 139,000.

IMPRESSION
1. Pregnancy.
2. Idiopathic thrombocytopenic purpura.

PLAN
1. Will decrease prednisone to 40 mg p.o. daily.
2. CBC and differential in 2 weeks.
3. Office visit in 4 weeks.

FOLLOWUP

The patient is a 75-year-old gentleman with stage IIIB non-small cell lung cancer who received his first cycle of chemotherapy with carboplatin and Taxol on 4/27. The dosage is 225 mg/m^2 of Taxol and carboplatin to an AUC of 6. However, the patient's BSA was capped at 2 m^2 and the initial dose was reduced by 20%. The patient comes in today for reevaluation. He is feeling very well and has had no major complaints. He is breathing better than he has in a long time.

REVIEW OF SYSTEMS
The rest of the review of systems is per questionnaire.

PHYSICAL EXAMINATION
On physical examination, his height is 6 feet, weight is 200 pounds, BSA 2.08 m^2, blood pressure 150/70, pulse 80, temperature 97.9. HEENT: Intact external ocular movements, no nystagmus, oropharynx clear. NECK: Supple. No JVD, no lymph nodes. His face is not as swollen as on prior evaluations. HEART: Regular rhythm. LUNGS: Clear. ABDOMEN: Soft, bowel sounds positive. No liver or spleen enlargement. EXTREMITIES: No edema or cyanosis. NEUROLOGICAL: Nonfocal.

IMPRESSION
1. Non-small cell lung cancer stage IIIB (T4 N2 M0).
2. Superior vena cava syndrome, much improved.
3. Syndrome of inappropriate antidiuretic hormone secretion, so far not evaluated.

PLAN
1. Will do CBC and differential today.
2. Office visit on May 19 with chest x-ray, PA and lateral, and CBC and differential for possible chemotherapy.

CONSULTATION

The patient is a 76-year-old lady with no prior history of systemic disease who is referred by Dr. Smith for evaluation of lymphoma. She presented approximately 1 year ago with a mass in the right side of her neck which has increased in size. She has also developed other nodules in the opposite side of the neck. I am told the lymph nodes showed low-grade lymphoma with gene-rearrangement status and negative flow cytometry. Final pathology is still pending. I am consulted for recommendations for further treatment.

PAST MEDICAL HISTORY
Gastroesophageal reflux and occasional wheezing. Osteoarthritis.

PAST SURGICAL HISTORY
Cholecystectomy, appendectomy, and bladder resection.

MEDICATIONS
Prevacid and Vioxx.

ALLERGIES
None.

FAMILY HISTORY
Positive for COPD in most of her 10 siblings and in her father. There is also a history of lung cancer in a few of her siblings who were smokers.

SOCIAL HISTORY
She is married with 2 children. She does not work. She has never used alcohol, drugs, or cigarettes.

REVIEW OF SYSTEMS
Occasional shortness of breath, usually in the morning and related to postnasal drip, none on exercise. Otherwise, negative as per questionnaire.

PHYSICAL EXAMINATION
On physical examination, her weight is 203 pounds, height 5 feet 3-1/2 inches, BSA 1.95 m^2, blood pressure 110/70, pulse 80. She is conscious, oriented, and alert. HEENT: Intact external ocular movements, no nystagmus, oropharynx clear. Patient is edentulous. NECK: Supple. No thyromegaly. Trachea is midline. There are lymph nodes palpable measuring about 3 × 3 cm in the submandibular area as well as smaller lymph nodes along the cervical areas on both sides. Also, there are lymph nodes in the supraclavicular region. They are non-matted. Cranial nerves are intact. No JVD. HEART: Regular rhythm, no murmurs. LUNGS: Clear. ABDOMEN: Soft, bowel sounds positive. No liver or spleen enlargement. NEUROLOGICAL: Nonfocal. SKIN: No petechiae or eruptions.

I performed a bone marrow aspirate and biopsy on the right iliac crest. Patient was prepped with Betadine and infiltrated with 1% lidocaine. The procedure was indicated for staging of her lymphoma. She did not have any complications.

(continued)

IMPRESSION

Non-Hodgkin lymphoma, currently being staged, but at least stage II. By preliminary report, it looks like a low-grade lymphoma. I discussed with the patient, her daughter, and husband for more than 90 minutes the characteristics of low-grade lymphomas and her expected prognosis. In general, low-grade lymphomas are characterized by indolent clinical behavior and comparatively long survival with a median survival between 6 and 10 years. Most patients have advanced stage disease at diagnosis and only about 10%–20% have stage I or II. There is a very low potential for cure when the disease presents in the more advanced stages and the treatment is usually palliative. Since the patient is having some discomfort, she would be a candidate for treatment.

ADDENDUM

Basically, her CT scan of the chest was negative as well as her bone marrow biopsy. The CT scan of the abdomen shows mild retroperitoneal adenopathy in the infrarenal region as well as near the obturator muscle. She also has lymphadenopathy around the right common femoral vein and inguinal adenopathy, most measuring between 1 and 2 cm. This would definitely convert her from stage II to stage III. This has further implications for her prognosis. In general, for localized, low-grade non-Hodgkin lymphoma of the head and neck, the treatment of choice is involved-field radiation therapy with or without adjuvant chemotherapy. This results in 5-year survival of over 50%. However, if she has stage III disease, she is not a candidate for radiation at all and would have to have chemotherapy. After explaining this, we have decided to do a PET scan as well as MUGA scan, since the patient would be receiving CHOP chemotherapy which has Adriamycin. We will see again after the PET scan to evaluate whether she needs chemotherapy only or chemotherapy with radiation.

EVALUATION

The patient is a 46-year-old woman, with no prior history of systemic illness, who about 6 years ago was evaluated for enlarged submandibular lymph nodes. The patient is quite apprehensive, but after several questions, she tells me it was diagnosed as hypertrophic adenopathy. She was told to follow them regularly because it might change. She was scared and did not want to get a bone marrow biopsy, which was offered at that time. One to 2 years ago, she started to develop axillary lymph nodes and finally she went to see Dr. Smith who did a biopsy of a cervical lymph node, which showed lymphocytic lymphoma/CLL. She is referred for recommendations on further management.

PAST MEDICAL HISTORY
As above.

PAST SURGICAL HISTORY
Laparoscopic cholecystectomy due to gallstones in February of 2000.

FAMILY HISTORY
Father is alive, with diabetes. Her mother died, but she does not know the cause of her death. She has 2 brothers in good health and a sister in good health.

TOXIC HABITS
She quit smoking cigarettes several years ago.

SOCIAL HISTORY
She has been married for 27 years and has 2 children, ages 15 and 25.

REVIEW OF SYSTEMS
Remarkably negative. She does not have fever, chills, or weight loss. She only notices the lymph nodes when she looks in the mirror. She gets shortness of breath with exercise, but she has no chest pain. She occasionally has nausea and heartburn. The rest of the review of systems is per questionnaire.

PHYSICAL EXAMINATION
On physical examination, her weight is 150 pounds, height 5 feet 4 inches, blood pressure 158/89, pulse 98. She is conscious, oriented, and alert. HEENT: Intact external ocular movements, no nystagmus, oropharynx clear. NECK: Supple. No JVD. No thyromegaly. She has extensive shotty adenopathy bilaterally in the submandibular, cervical, and supraclavicular regions, some of them as large as 4 cm. HEART: Regular rhythm, no murmurs. LUNGS: Clear. ABDOMEN: Soft, bowel sounds positive. No liver or spleen enlargement. EXTREMITIES: She does have bilateral axillary lymphadenopathy, large and shotty. No inguinal lymphadenopathy.

LABORATORY DATA
Biopsy of the lymph nodes as described. CBC drawn on 3/29 shows a WBC of 10,200 with 25% lymphocytes, hemoglobin of 10.4 with hematocrit of 31.8, MCV of 74, and RDW of 18, which is quite suggestive of iron-deficiency anemia.

CT scan of the chest shows evidence of supraclavicular and axillary lymph nodes, and CT scan of the abdomen shows several intraabdominal mesenteric nodes and periaortic nodes.

(continued)

IMPRESSION

Small lymphocytic lymphoma/CLL, currently asymptomatic except for shotty adenopathy. I would like to try a low-dose regimen with low toxicity, such as CVP. Another option would be Fludara, but the schedule would be daily for 5 days and she cannot work under those conditions. Patient will not even consider a bone marrow biopsy at this time. Actually, except for bulky disease, she does not have other known bad prognostic features, although I have not done a bone marrow biopsy. My plan for now is to start chemotherapy with Cytoxan, vincristine, and prednisone and watch closely to see if we can induce remission. Side effects were explained to the patient and she was given written information about chemotherapy.

PLAN

1. Cytoxan 400 mg/m^2 plus vincristine 2 mg/m^2 plus prednisone 60 mg IV on day 1 for 3 weeks.
2. Bone marrow aspirate and biopsy. Patient is quite reluctant to have this done.
3. Iron sulfate 300 mg p.o. t.i.d.
4. CBC and differential today and then in 10 days for nadir counts.
5. Metabolic panel, LDH, beta-2-microglobulin, SPEP and immunofixation, iron, TIBC, and ferritin.
6. Office visit next week.

REVIEW QUESTIONS

The goal of these questions is to test your knowledge in the areas of hematology and oncology.

Directions: Select the correct answer for each of the multiple-choice questions provided below. *Answers are provided at the end of this chapter.*

1. Which of the following radiation therapy modalities uses radioactive seeds implanted directly into the tumor?
   A. electron beam
   B. fractionation
   C. linear accelerator
   D. brachytherapy

2. Which of the following are types of skin cancer?
   A. adrenocortical carcinoma and neuroma
   B. basal cell carcinoma and melanoma
   C. cholangiocarcinoma and teratoma
   D. ductal carcinoma and retinoma

3. A mass that arises from normal tissue, proliferates more rapidly, and ceases to behave the same as the original tissue is called a
   A. mutation.
   B. neoplasm.
   C. polyposis.
   D. gene.

4. Which of the following is characterized by prolonged bleeding due to decreased or missing clotting factors?
   A. hemophilia
   B. thrombocytopenia
   C. leukopenia
   D. polycythemia

5. The original site of a tumor is called the
   A. primary.
   B. metastasis.
   C. node.
   D. biopsy.

6. Adjuvant therapy is defined as
   A. chemotherapy given in addition to surgery.
   B. chemotherapy only.
   C. radiation therapy.
   D. surgical excision.

7. Movement of cancer cells from one part of the body to another is called
   A. metastasis.
   B. carcinogenesis.
   C. oncogenesis.
   D. stasis.

8. Environmental agents such as chemicals, drugs, tobacco smoke, and radiation that can cause damage to DNA and produce cancer are called
   A. oncogenes.
   B. carcinogens.
   C. hydrocarbons.
   D. viruses.

9. Treatment for painful mouth sores resulting from chemotherapy includes
   A. Pepto-Bismol.
   B. viscous lidocaine.
   C. Betadine.
   D. Listerine.

10. Basophils are a type of
    A. leukocyte.
    B. erythrocyte.
    C. platelet.
    D. agranulocyte.

11. The outer lining of organs and body cavities of the abdomen and chest is called the
    A. fibrosa.
    B. mucosa.
    C. nodosa.
    D. serosa.

12. Small cell carcinoma is associated with the
    A. skin.
    B. colon.
    C. lung.
    D. prostate.

13. The term peau d'orange would be used in the physical exam under which heading?
    A. Eyes
    B. Abdomen
    C. Lungs
    D. Skin

14. Which of the following is a chemotherapy regimen?
    A. clindamycin, doxorubicin, vincristine
    B. cyclophosphamide, daptomycin, vincristine
    C. cyclophosphamide, doxorubicin, vincristine
    D. cyclophosphamide, doxorubicin, vancomycin

15. Which of the following would be prescribed for iron-deficiency anemia?
    A. furosemide
    B. ferrous sulfate
    C. folic acid
    D. fibrinogen

16. Which of the following is a hemoglobinopathy that affects primarily African Americans?
    A. polycythemia
    B. aplastic anemia
    C. idiopathic thrombocytopenic purpura
    D. sickle cell anemia

17. PSA is a screening test for
    A. prostate cancer.
    B. ovarian cancer.
    C. colon cancer.
    D. skin cancer.

18. The lymph node that is the first to receive lymphatic drainage from a malignant tumor and tested for the spread of cancerous cells is called the
    A. Virchow node.
    B. obturator node.
    C. sentinel node.
    D. submental node.

19. The cancer commonly associated with full-blown AIDS is
    A. Kaposi sarcoma.
    B. leukemia.
    C. Hodgkin lymphoma.
    D. esophageal cancer.

20. The term used for measurement of the unit of absorbed radiation dose is
    A. centiliter.
    B. centigray.
    C. millimole.
    D. picogram.

21. Thrombocytopenia is
    A. a decreased platelet count.
    B. a decreased white count.
    C. a decreased red cell count.
    D. decreased plasma volume.

22. A "CBC with diff" would include
    A. a Gram stain.
    B. a reticulocyte count.
    C. the percentage of each type of white cell.
    D. cytology.

23. A marked increase in white cells circulating in the peripheral blood is called
    A. leukocytosis.
    B. thrombocytosis.
    C. polycythemia.
    D. leukopenia.

24. Which classification system is used for colon cancer?
    A. Clark
    B. Dukes
    C. Gleason
    D. Jewett

25. The genes BRCA1 and BRCA2 relate to which type of cancer?
    A. bladder
    B. breast
    C. endometrial
    D. bone

26. Blood cell formation is called
    A. hematopoiesis.
    B. hematemesis.
    C. hemostasis.
    D. hematochezia.

27. A glioma would be found in the
    A. brain.
    B. lung.
    C. bone.
    D. liver.

28. X-ray examination of the breast used in the detection breast cancer is known as
    A. radionuclide scan.
    B. mammography.
    C. bone scan.
    D. PET scan.

29. Which of the following terms is used to describe a growth that possesses a stem or stalk?
    A. sessile
    B. serous
    C. anaplastic
    D. pedunculated

30. Anemia is a deficiency of
    A. angiogenic cells.
    B. plasma.
    C. red blood cells.
    D. white blood cells.

 Please see the accompanying CD for additional review materials for this section.

ANSWER KEY

REVIEW QUESTIONS ANSWER KEY

1. D	6. A	11. D	16. D	21. A	26. A
2. B	7. A	12. C	17. A	22. C	27. A
3. B	8. B	13. D	18. C	23. A	28. B
4. A	9. B	14. C	19. A	24. B	29. D
5. A	10. A	15. B	20. B	25. B	30. C

Allergy/Immunology/ Rheumatology

OBJECTIVES CHECKLIST

A prepared exam candidate will know:

- ❑ All combining forms, prefixes, and suffixes related to the immune system.
- ❑ Signs, symptoms, and diseases related to the lymphatic and immune systems.
- ❑ Imaging and diagnostic studies used in the identification and treatment planning of lymphatic and immunologic disorders.
- ❑ Laboratory studies related to the diagnosis and treatment of lymphatic and immunologic disorders.
- ❑ Common medications prescribed for lymphatic and immunologic disorders.
- ❑ Transcription standards pertaining to allergies and lymphocytes.
- ❑ Fundamentals of rheumatic disease and the common disorders associated with rheumatology.
- ❑ Laboratory studies related to rheumatic conditions.
- ❑ Medications commonly prescribed for rheumatic disorders, symptoms, and diseases.

RESOURCES FOR STUDY

1. *The Language of Medicine*
   Chapter 14: Lymphatic and Immune Systems, pp. 529–558.
   Chapter 15: Musculoskeletal System, Pathological Conditions, pp. 587–591.

2. *Memmler's Structure and Function of the Human Body*
   Chapter 8: The Skeleton: Bones and Joints, pp. 85–109.
   Chapter 15: The Lymphatic System and Body Defenses, pp. 269–285.

3. *Memmler's The Human Body in Health and Disease*
   Chapter 17: Body Defenses, Immunity, and Vaccines, pp. 345–359; Study Guide, pp. 267–276.

4. *H&P: A Nonphysician's Guide to the Medical History and Physical Examination*
   Chapter 14: Review of Systems: Skin, pp. 125–130.

5. *Human Diseases*
   Chapter 4: The Immune System, pp. 43–56.

6. *Laboratory Tests & Diagnostic Procedures in Medicine*
   Chapter 16: Normal Anatomy and Histology, pp. 225–250.
   Chapter 17: Procedures and Practice in Anatomic Pathology, pp. 251–278.
   Chapter 18: Pathologic Change and Pathologic Diagnosis (Inflammation, Allergy, and Infection), pp. 283–288.

7. *A Manual of Laboratory and Diagnostic Tests*
   Chapter 7: Microbiologic Studies, pp. 456–529.
   Chapter 8: Immunodiagnostic Studies, pp. 530–651.

8. *The AAMT Book of Style for Medical Transcription*
   Allergies, p. 19.
   Lymphocytes, pp. 245–246.

9. *Using Medical Terminology: A Practical Approach*
   Chapter 6: Articulations, pp. 243–277.
   Chapter 12: Lymphatic System and Immunity, pp. 525–569.

10. *Pharmacology for Health Professionals*
    Unit III: Drugs That Affect the Respiratory System (Chapters 11–13), pp. 169–197.
    Unit VII: Drugs That Affect the Immune System (Chapters 25–28), pp. 389–493.

11. *Understanding Pharmacology for Health Professionals*
    Chapter 19: Ear, Nose and Throat, pp. 205–216.
    *Note: Chapter 18 (Pulmonary Drugs) also contains medications given for allergy and should be reviewed in this section.

12. *Medical Terminology: The Language of Health Care*
    Chapter 5: Integumentary System, pp. 107–143.
    Chapter 8: Blood and Lymph Systems, pp. 241–268.

SAMPLE REPORTS

The following five reports are examples of reports you might encounter while transcribing allergy, immunology, and rheumatology.

HISTORY & PHYSICAL

HISTORY
The patient presents for followup of a cough. She did see the allergist and was found to be allergic to grass, dust mites, and molds. She is currently taking Claritin-D daily; Flovent 110 mcg/dose, 2 puffs b.i.d.; Serevent 2 puffs b.i.d.; and Rhinocort 2 sprays each nostril b.i.d.; as well as albuterol p.r.n. She does not have any shortness of breath. Her cough is much improved. She is taking some measures around the house to help with her allergies; however, she has not been very aggressive about this. Her only remaining complaint is hoarseness, which occurs toward the end of the day.

PHYSICAL EXAMINATION
GENERAL: On exam, she is alert and in no acute distress.
VITAL SIGNS: Respirations were 20, blood pressure 130/90, and saturation 96%.
LUNGS: The lungs are clear with good air movement bilaterally.
HEENT: The throat is clear; there may be a slight amount of mucus.
NECK: Supple.
CHEST: Respirations are clear with good air movement.
CARDIOVASCULAR: Regular.
ABDOMEN: Soft and nontender.
EXTREMITIES: No edema.

IMPRESSION
Mild asthma with ongoing cough secondary to allergies and postnasal drip. She seems fairly well controlled on the current regimen. I am not sure that she is not having some ongoing, low-grade postnasal drip that accounts for her hoarseness; however, it may also be secondary to the Flovent.

PLAN
The plan at this time is to switch the Flovent to 44 mcg so she can get the same antiinflammatory effect with less hoarseness. I advised the patient once again to gargle well after use, which she states she is doing. I have advised her that after a couple of months she can come off the Flovent and see if just controlling her sinuses will be enough to stop the cough from recurring, and I did talk to her in more detail about trying to control her environment for the allergies.

HISTORY & PHYSICAL

HISTORY

I had the pleasure of seeing this woman, who is self-referred, for an evaluation of dyspnea. She has had a diagnosis of asthma since 1986 when she acquired 2 cats. Subsequent evaluation demonstrated significant extrinsic asthma with allergies to cats, feathers, and cottonwood. When she avoids these triggers, she very rarely has asthma symptoms and equally rarely has to use her albuterol metered-dose inhaler. She subsequently remodeled her house and has hardwood and tile flooring.

She was well until the last month when she noticed an increase in her dyspnea. She walks for exercise and noticed more dyspnea when walking at the moderate pace of 3 miles per hour. This occurs when she walks indoors and outdoors, although it seems to be worse inside. Parenthetically, her dyspnea seems better when breathing cold air. She has also noticed a significant amount of coughing in the last month, especially nocturnally. This has caused her husband to sleep in an adjacent room. She also noticed worsening of these symptoms over the Thanksgiving weekend when exposed to burning leaves and last summer when she was in Santa Fe and exposed to particulate matter from a nearby forest fire. Her typical asthma symptoms are chest tightness, shortness of breath, wheezing, and coughing.

PAST MEDICAL HISTORY

1. Gastroesophageal reflux symptoms. She has a chronic H pylori infection and has received 3 treatment regimens of antibiotics without success. As long as she avoids tomatoes, citrus, caffeine, and chocolate and sleeps on 4 pillows, she has reflux symptoms only 1-2 times a month.
2. Hysterectomy for fibroids.
3. Benign cystic disease of her breasts with lumps removed in 1988 and 2001.
4. Right oophorectomy in 1998.

ALLERGIES

Sulfa, latex, and Ceclor, which all cause blotchiness and predominantly skin manifestations. Also allergic to iodine dye, which causes shortness of breath and an increase in blood pressure, and bee stings.

MEDICATIONS

1. Tums as needed for GERD symptoms.
2. Albuterol metered-dose inhaler.
3. Multivitamins.
4. Vitamin E.
5. EpiPen.

FAMILY HISTORY

Notable for her mother having breast cancer, bladder cancer, and metastatic colon cancer, although she is still alive at age 78. Her maternal grandmother had breast cancer and colon cancer.

SOCIAL HISTORY

Notable for 1/2-pack-a-day habit for 12 years, which she quit when she became pregnant at age 30. She is currently a housewife, having sold her business 2 years ago, and has been successfully participating in a Weight Watchers program, with weight loss from 177 to 150 pounds.

(continued)

REVIEW OF SYSTEMS

Notable for the absence of constitutional symptoms, fevers, chills, night sweats, myalgias, arthralgias, nasal congestion, painful or watery eyes, nausea, vomiting, constipation, diarrhea, or paresthesias. The remainder of her systems review is negative.

PHYSICAL EXAMINATION

VITAL SIGNS: Her heart rate is 108, blood pressure 136/78, weight is 150, and respiratory rate is 18.

HEENT: Notable for nasal mucosal erythema with mild congestion. Pharynx is normal. Mouth shows normal dentition.

NECK: Supple without thyromegaly or lymphadenopathy.

LUNGS: Clear to auscultation and percussion bilaterally.

CARDIOVASCULAR: Exam demonstrates a normal S1 and S2 without an S3, S4, murmurs, rubs, or clicks.

ABDOMEN: Exam demonstrates normal bowel sounds without tenderness, masses, or palpable organomegaly.

EXTREMITIES: Without clubbing, cyanosis, or edema.

NEUROLOGIC: Exam is nonfocal, and her affect is rather anxious.

IMPRESSION

She is a woman with a 16-year history of asthma who presents with progressive dyspnea on exertion and worsening cough of 1 month's duration. First on the differential diagnosis is a worsening of her asthma. Gastroesophageal reflux disease or other respiratory diseases are other considerations, although are less likely at this time.

PLAN

In conjunction with the patient, we have decided on an empiric trial of an inhaled corticosteroid. I have given her a sample of Advair 250/50 and asked her to use 1 puff b.i.d. I have also refilled her albuterol metered-dose inhaler and given her a prescription for a peak flow meter at her request. I will obtain baseline spirometry and, at the patient's request, obtain a PA and lateral chest x-ray to exclude other potential etiologies for her dyspnea.

She will call me in a couple of weeks to let me know of any progress with the treatment of these symptoms. Otherwise, I will plan to see her again in followup after the new year.

FOLLOWUP REPORT

The patient was seen on July 1, 2004. The patient comes in today after being off methotrexate since I saw her in the office back in May. She has been off methotrexate since that time and has noticed increasing swelling and tenderness in her joints. She has had a marked increase in pain and swelling in her MCPs, PIPs, feet, and ankles. We had to hold the methotrexate because of elevated liver function tests. I did repeat the LFTs on November 5, 2002, and she had an elevated gamma-GT of 218, an elevated alkaline phosphatase of 194, and the isoenzymes revealed predominantly hepatobiliary fraction. Her other liver function tests were normal.

The patient's physical exam revealed marked synovitis in MCPs, PIPs, wrists, elbows, ankles, and MTPs. Her chest was clear to percussion and auscultation.

The patient is having an active flare of rheumatoid arthritis. We needed to stop the methotrexate because of her elevated liver function tests. I am also having her hold the Celebrex at the present time so that we can evaluate the etiology of her liver function elevation. I did suggest that she be evaluated, and an appointment has been made. We will repeat the liver function tests off the Celebrex in 2 weeks, however.

I am concerned about the patient's heavy workload. She is doing a great deal of heavy lifting at work, which is of great concern. Her x-rays revealed an erosion in her right hand at the radial base of the proximal phalanx, and the patient is going to need more therapy for remission. I did discuss Enbrel with the patient and her daughter and gave them one of the pamphlets about biologic therapy. In the meantime, I did have her increase her prednisone, with warnings, to 10 mg a day for a week and then tapering to 7.5 mg a day.

I did express concern over the fact that her swelling may inhibit her ability to get off her left fourth finger wedding ring. I told them to try to soap it off after the swelling goes down with the prednisone, but to call me if they are not able to do so.

In this patient with active rheumatoid arthritis, we will need to increase her therapy, probably with Enbrel, but we will need to keep her off methotrexate while evaluating her liver function tests.

FOLLOWUP REPORT

HISTORY

It was my pleasure to see this delightful woman in rheumatologic followup. I saw her at my new office and have not yet received the copy of her records. The patient has been taking Mobic 15 mg a day, along with nortriptyline, femhrt, Synthroid, Combivent, and Pulmicort.

As you know, the patient has had a history of a positive ANA that was felt to be possibly drug-induced. She has, over the last several months, experienced much less knee pain and has had no rash. In general, she is doing well on the Mobic with good relief.

With respect to the patient's previous history of fibromyalgia, she states that she has had some increased stiffness and diffuse pain but that it "comes and goes."

The patient has noted some increased bilateral hand pain and stiffness, as well as some slight increase in her heel pain.

The patient is followed by you for her hypothyroidism and states that she has a followup planned next month with you for her thyroid.

The patient states that she recently saw you for her increasing exercise intolerance. She was prescribed Pulmicort, which seems to be helping. She does state, however, that her pulmonary function tests revealed a worsening in her diffusion capacity. The patient has had followup for an abnormality in her chest CT and has a planned followup in the near future.

The patient is postmenopausal and has been taking Femhrt. She will be discussing with you the issue of hormone replacement at her followup appointment.

PHYSICAL EXAM

The patient's physical exam was remarkable for a mild, erythematous, maculopapular rash on her anterior chest. Her blood pressure was 150/80. She had patellofemoral crepitus in her knees and hallux valgus in her feet, without any active synovitis in her other joints. Her chest was clear to percussion and auscultation.

PLAN

I did ask the patient to obtain labs, including anti-DNA, C3, C4, and sedimentation rate, as well as her other connective tissue blood workup.

Certainly, if her diffusion capacity is decreasing and there is any consideration of interstitial lung disease, we may have to pursue a high-resolution CT scan to evaluate her, with possible further workup if there is concern about connective tissue disease involving her lungs. I will forward a copy of this letter, and we will discuss this after her labs are back. I did tell the patient about her slightly elevated blood pressure, which she will be following up with you as well. I will be discussing the patient's results with her next week, but I told her to call if she has any questions or concerns. We did plan a followup appointment in 3 months, but I told her to call me if she has any exacerbation of her symptomatology before that time.

It is my pleasure to provide rheumatologic followup on this delightful woman.

HISTORY & PHYSICAL

HISTORY

The patient is a 53-year-old female with a past medical history of systemic lupus erythematosus that was complicated with vasculitis of her temporal arteries. She had a stroke and also had a partial loss of her vision. She comes in today for a followup visit and stated that, in general, she is doing better, but she is very concerned that, since she has been on a high dose of prednisone, she is having significant weight gain. Occasionally, she has some headaches, but she does not have any other complaints.

CURRENT MEDICATIONS

CellCept 1 g p.o. b.i.d., prednisone 60 mg a day, calcium with vitamin D, and antihypertensive medications.

PHYSICAL EXAMINATION

Weight 228 pounds, height is 63-3/4 inches, blood pressure 150/92, pulse 90, and respiratory rate 20. Her temperature is 97.8 degrees. She is well developed and not in acute distress. She does not have any oral ulcers. Her neck is supple. The lungs are clear to auscultation bilaterally. The heart was regular without murmurs. The musculoskeletal exam is negative for synovitis. There is no edema.

IMPRESSION

This is a patient with systemic lupus erythematosus complicated with vasculitis of the temporal arteries.

RECOMMENDATIONS

Because she is having significant side effects with the prednisone, I am going to increase the CellCept to 1.5 g p.o. b.i.d., and I am going to start a slow tapering of the prednisone by 5 mg every other day. To evaluate activity of her lupus, I ordered complement levels, CBC, double-stranded DNA, and urinalysis. I will follow up with the patient in 6 weeks.

REVIEW QUESTIONS

The goal of these questions is to test your knowledge in the areas of allergy, immunology, and rheumatology.

Directions: Select the correct answer for each of the multiple-choice questions provided below. *Answers are provided at the end of this chapter.*

1. An allergic reaction that occurs at certain times of the year is
   A. atopic allergy.
   B. seasonal rhinitis.
   C. otitis media.
   D. chronic rhinitis.

2. An autoimmune disease involving the connective tissues that is progressive and may lead to disability is
   A. rheumatoid arthritis.
   B. osteoarthritis.
   C. septic arthritis.
   D. gonococcal arthritis.

3. Which of the following tests would be performed in suspected rheumatoid arthritis?
   A. rheumatoid factor, VDRL
   B. C-reactive protein, CBC
   C. sedimentation rate, CBC
   D. rheumatoid factor, sedimentation rate

4. A chronic condition that affects lacrimal and salivary glands, causing dry mucous membranes and affecting primarily post-menopausal women is
   A. Acosta disease.
   B. DiGeorge syndrome.
   C. Wiskott-Aldrich syndrome.
   D. Sjögren syndrome.

5. Which of the following would be used to treat gout?
   A. colchicine
   B. alendronate
   C. Plaquenil
   D. cytarabine

6. A common long-term treatment for generalized arthritis is
   A. Lexapro.
   B. Vicodin.
   C. Naprosyn.
   D. Ambien.

7. A characteristic wiping or rubbing of the nose with an upward movement of the hand, especially in children with chronic rhinitis, is called
   A. an allergic salute.
   B. anatripsis.
   C. an R wave.
   D. bruxism.

8. Which of the following affects children?
   A. arthritis deformans
   B. Jaccoud
   C. juvenile arthritis
   D. polymyalgia rheumatica

9. Which of the following is caused by uric acid crystals in the joints?
   A. psoriatic arthritis
   B. reactive arthritis
   C. gout
   D. degenerative arthritis

10. Which form of arthritis is triggered by an infection?
    A. degenerative arthritis
    B. rheumatoid arthritis
    C. reactive arthritis
    D. juvenile arthritis

11. Which of the following is a skin condition characterized by silvery white scale?

    A. eczema
    B. psoriasis
    C. dermatitis
    D. seborrhea

12. Which is a treatment for seasonal allergies?

    A. Xopenex
    B. Zyprexa
    C. Zyrtec
    D. Zestril

13. This common, chronic disorder is characterized by muscle pain, fatigue, and multiple trigger points.
    A. gout
    B. lupus
    C. malaria
    D. fibromyalgia

14. Ankylosing spondylitis affects the
    A. spine.
    B. hip.
    C. finger.
    D. knee.

15. Low serum antibodies caused by an inherited B lymphocyte dysfunction is called
    A. agammaglobulinemia.
    B. Job syndrome.
    C. macroglobulinemia.
    D. hyperglobulinemia.

16. An inherited disease characterized by failure of both B and T lymphocyte function with severely heightened risk of infection is called
    A. AIDS (acquired immunodeficiency syndrome).
    B. SCID (severe combined immunodeficiency disease).
    C. CMV (cytomegalovirus).
    D. SLE (systemic lupus erythematosus).

17. Which of the following is transcribed correctly?
    A. She denied any nodules, molar rash, photosensitivity, oral ulcers, or ray nod symptoms. C-reactive protein and ANA studies were negative.
    B. She denied any nodules, malar rash, photosensitivity, oral ulcers, or Raynaud symptoms. T-reactive protein and ANA studies were negative.
    C. She denied any nodules, malar rash, photosensitivity, oral ulcers, or ray nod symptoms. C-reactive protein and ANA studies were negative.
    D. She denied any nodules, malar rash, photosensitivity, oral ulcers, or Raynaud symptoms. C-reactive protein and ANA studies were negative.

18. Which of the following is an autoimmune disease, often accompanying polymyalgia rheumatica, which causes headache, scalp tenderness, jaw pain, and visual symptoms?
    A. Graves disease
    B. temporal arteritis
    C. migraine headaches
    D. Still disease

19. Which of the following is a class of antiinflammatory medications?
    A. SERMs
    B. COX-2 inhibitors
    C. mydriatics
    D. SSRIs

20. IgG, IgM, and IgE are examples of
    A. lymphocytes.
    B. macrophages.
    C. vaccines.
    D. immunoglobulins.

21. The prefix *arthr/o* refers to
    A. artery.
    B. cartilage.
    C. joint.
    D. tendon.

22. Which of the following medications is used in the treatment of rheumatoid arthritis?
    A. methicillin
    B. methotrexate
    C. Lotensin
    D. Celexa

23. Side effects of prednisone include
    A. anorexia, fluid retention, hypotension.
    B. fluid retention, delayed wound healing, increased blood pressure.
    C. increased urine output, joint swelling, hypotension.
    D. seizure, atrial fibrillation, stroke.

24. This disorder is characterized by achy joints, fever, prolonged fatigue, photosensitivity, and characteristic butterfly rash on the face.
    A. rheumatoid arthritis
    B. Lyme disease
    C. systemic lupus erythematosus
    D. Reye syndrome

25. This over-the-counter ophthalmologic treatment is used for allergy relief of itchy, watery eyes.
    A. Flovent
    B. Naphcon-A
    C. Timoptic
    D. Advair

26. Raynaud phenomenon affects
    A. blood vessels in the face.
    B. blood vessels in the temporoparietal area.
    C. blood vessels in the calves.
    D. arteries in the fingers and toes.

27. Which of the following is transcribed correctly?
    A. This patient is a 22-year-old male with a history of brachial asthma. He has been wheezing and using excess muscles of respiration.
    B. This patient is a 22-year-old male with a history of bronchial asthma. He has been wheezing and using excess muscles of respiration.
    C. This patient is a 22-year-old male with a history of bronchial asthma. He has been wheezing and using accessory muscles of respiration.
    D. This patient is a 22-year-old male with a history of brachial asthma. He has been wheezing and using accessory muscles of respiration.

28. Another term for asthma is
    A. reactive airway disease.
    B. chronic obstructive pulmonary disease.
    C. seasonal allergy.
    D. bronchitis.

29. Inguinal lymph nodes are located
    A. in the arms.
    B. in the chest.
    C. in the groin.
    D. in the neck.

30. Zyrtec, Claritin, and Allegra are examples of
    A. antihistamines.
    B. steroids.
    C. salicylates.
    D. decongestants.

 Please see the accompanying CD for additional review materials for this section.

ANSWER KEY

REVIEW QUESTIONS ANSWER KEY

1. B	6. C	11. B	16. B	21. C	26. D
2. A	7. A	12. C	17. D	22. B	27. C
3. D	8. C	13. D	18. B	23. B	28. A
4. D	9. C	14. A	19. B	24. C	29. C
5. A	10. C	15. A	20. D	25. B	30. A

Infectious Disease

OBJECTIVES CHECKLIST

A prepared exam candidate will know:

❑ Combining forms, prefixes, and suffixes related to the study of microbiology.

❑ Imaging and diagnostic studies used in the identification and treatment of infectious diseases.

❑ Laboratory studies related to the diagnosis and treatment of infectious diseases.

❑ Modes of transmission related to the spread of infectious disease.

❑ Common medications indicated and prescribed for infectious diseases.

❑ Transcription standards pertaining to infectious agents (genus and species) and infectious diseases.

RESOURCES FOR STUDY

1. *The Language of Medicine*
   Chapter 14: Lymphatic and Immune Systems (immunity, antigens, and antibodies), pp. 529–558.

2. *Memmler's Structure and Function of the Human Body*
   Chapter 3: Cells and Their Functions, pp. 35–54.
   Chapter 15: The Lymphatic System and Body Defenses, pp. 269–285.

3. *Memmler's The Human Body in Health and Disease*
   Chapter 5: Disease and Disease-Producing Organisms, pp. 76–98; Study Guide, pp. 69–82.

4. *Disease: Identification, Prevention, and Control*
   Unit 2: Infectious Diseases.

5. *Human Diseases*
   Chapter 3: Infectious Diseases, pp. 27–42.

6. *Laboratory Tests & Diagnostic Procedures in Medicine*
   Chapter 21: Microbiology, pp. 401–410.

7. *A Manual of Laboratory and Diagnostic Tests*
   Chapter 5: Cerebrospinal Fluid Studies, pp. 289–315.
   Chapter 7: Microbiologic Studies, pp. 456–529.
   Chapter 8: Immunodiagnostic Studies, pp. 530–651.
   Chapter 11: Cytologic, Histologic, and Genetic Studies, pp. 760–816.

8. *The AAMT Book of Style for Medical Transcription*
   Blood counts, differential, p. 39.
   Genus names, pp. 188–190.
   Gram stain, p. 195.
   Hepatitis nomenclature, pp. 201–202.
   Lymphocytes, pp. 245–246.
   Virus names, pp. 419–420.

9. *Pharmacology for Health Professionals*
   Unit VII: Drugs That Affect the Immune System (Chapters 25–28), pp. 389–493.

10. *Understanding Pharmacology for Health Professionals*
    Chapter 27: Anti-Infective Drugs, pp. 311–322.
    Chapter 28: AIDS Drugs and Antiviral Drugs, pp. 323–333.
    Chapter 29: Anti-Fungal Drugs, pp. 334–336.

11. *Medical Terminology: The Language of Health Care*
    Chapter 5: Integumentary System, pp. 107–143.
    Chapter 8: Blood and Lymph Systems, pp. 241–268.

SAMPLE REPORTS

The following five reports are examples of reports you might encounter while transcribing reports involving infectious diseases.

HISTORY & PHYSICAL

HISTORY OF PRESENT ILLNESS
This is a 30-year-old female with a history of HIV infection diagnosed 5 years ago, with an unknown CD4 count and viral load, and a history of opportunistic infections. The patient presented with fever of 102.2 degrees of 5 days' duration. She also had abdominal pain and vomiting. She has developed a large mass lesion in the right submandibular area that, according to her own report, comes and goes.

The patient was placed on IV ceftriaxone and then clindamycin by Dr. Smith. The patient denies cough, sputum production, or shortness of breath. There are no other concomitant symptoms.

ALLERGIES
No known allergies.

MEDICATIONS
Her current medications include cefepime, fluconazole, Lasix, clindamycin, Demerol, and Ambien.

PHYSICAL EXAMINATION
GENERAL: Examination reveals a chronically ill appearing female, lying in bed in no apparent distress.
HEENT: Pupils are reactive to light and accommodation. Mouth is moist. Throat has evidence of erythema.
NECK: Supple. There are at least 2 rounded lesions in the right submandibular area that are mildly tender to palpation. They may correspond to lymphadenopathy.
LUNGS: Clear to auscultation and percussion.
CARDIOVASCULAR: Normal S1 and S2. Regular rate and rhythm.
ABDOMEN: Soft and nontender. Good bowel sounds.
EXTREMITIES: No clubbing, cyanosis, or edema.
NEUROLOGIC: Grossly nonfocal.

DIAGNOSTIC STUDIES
She had a V/Q scan that showed no evidence of pulmonary embolism. She had a chest x-ray that showed no evidence of acute pulmonary disease.

LABORATORY DATA
Her initial white count was 8900 and currently is 4900, with 63% neutrophils, 5% bands, 20% lymphocytes, and 11% monocytes. Creatinine was 1.8 and now is 1.4.

MICROBIOLOGY DATA
Remarkable for a urine culture collected on 08/11/04 that showed 100,000 CFU of E coli. She had 90 wbc's on urinalysis. Blood culture showed no growth after 24 hours.

(continued)

IMPRESSION

1. Neck mass, likely secondary to lymphadenopathy. Differential diagnosis includes:
   a. Bacterial infectious process.
   b. Mycobacterial disease such as mycobacterial tuberculosis versus atypical mycobacteria.
   c. Neoplastic process such as lymphoma.
   d. Other unusual infections cannot be excluded. I did not think that this patient had parotitis; however, a CT scan of the neck clearly indicates same. An ENT consultation was advised.
2. Urinary tract infection.
3. HIV/AIDS.
4. Renal insufficiency, improving.
5. Anemia.

PLAN

1. Obtain a CT scan.
2. Schedule lymph node biopsy, based on review of CT scan.
3. Give a PPD.
4. Agree with current antibiotics.

CONSULTATION

HISTORY OF PRESENT ILLNESS
This is a 74-year-old black female who was recently admitted for pneumonia and hypertension. Apparently, the patient came to the emergency department with a 1-day history of shortness of breath. She had a minimal cough. She did admit to chest pain, stomach pain, and back pain. She described the chest pain as being along the rib area, perhaps related to coughing. No diaphoresis, nausea, vomiting, or diarrhea. No other concomitant symptoms.

On initial evaluation, the patient was found to have bilateral infiltrates in both lung bases, for which she was placed on empiric antibiotics, including IV vancomycin and levofloxacin. Currently, the patient is alert and interactive. She does not look toxic. She has been afebrile since admission.

ALLERGIES
No known allergies.

CURRENT MEDICATIONS
Ferrous sulfate, docusate sodium, Lasix, Nitro-Dur, Lovenox, Ecotrin, Protonix, Zithromax, Catapres, albuterol, vancomycin, and levofloxacin.

PHYSICAL EXAMINATION
GENERAL: Elderly female in no apparent distress.
HEENT: Pupils are reactive to light and accommodation. Mouth is moist.
NECK: Supple. No JVD or bruits.
CARDIOVASCULAR: Normal S1 and S2. Regular rate and rhythm.
LUNGS: Bibasilar crackles.
ABDOMEN: Soft and nontender. Positive bowel sounds.
EXTREMITIES: No cyanosis, clubbing, or edema.
NEUROLOGICAL: Grossly nonfocal.

LABORATORY DATA
Chest x-ray shows bibasilar crackles. White count is 22,800. Her BNP was 928 on 08/10/04. In addition, 2 out of 2 blood cultures grew out gram-positive cocci in pairs on the second day after blood culture collection.

IMPRESSION
1. Bibasilar pneumonia adequately treated with Levaquin.
2. Gram-positive organisms in blood cultures growing 2 days after collection, which may suggest contamination rather than infection. The patient had been treated with IV vancomycin, which should cover for possible bacteremia. I will request another 2 sets of blood cultures. We will formulate further recommendations once bacteriology is finalized.
3. Congestive heart failure.
4. Respiratory insufficiency.
5. Status post myocardial infarction.

PLAN
1. We will be following along with you.
2. Continue current therapy.

CONSULTATION

HISTORY OF PRESENT ILLNESS

This is a 63-year-old male with multiple medical problems including hypertension, diabetes mellitus, and end-stage renal disease, on hemodialysis. The patient apparently was referred from home with an acute change in his mental status.

On initial evaluation in the ER, he was very agitated. It was initially reported that the patient was throwing things at home. His initial vital signs were remarkable for a temperature of 95.6, respiratory rate of 18, pulse of 94, and a blood pressure of 170/87. The patient was admitted to intensive care with a working diagnosis of sepsis syndrome, rule out acute myocardial infarction, and end-stage renal disease on dialysis.

Currently, the patient is lethargic but can be aroused. He mumbles some words. He is unable to provide any further history. The patient has a dialysis catheter in the right side of his neck. He states that there is no tenderness. There is a complaint of shaking chills.

ALLERGIES

No known allergies.

PAST MEDICAL HISTORY

This is reflected in the first paragraph.

PHYSICAL EXAMINATION

GENERAL: Elderly male, chronically and acutely ill appearing and lying in bed in no apparent distress.
HEENT: Pupils are reactive to light and accommodation. Mouth is slightly dry.
NECK: Supple; no JVD or bruits.
CARDIOVASCULAR: Normal S1 and S2; regular rate and rhythm.
CHEST: Normal expansion. There is a dialysis catheter on the right side. There is no evidence of erythema or tenderness.
ABDOMEN: Soft and nontender; positive bowel sounds.
EXTREMITIES: No clubbing, cyanosis, or edema.
NEUROLOGIC: The patient is alert and able to be aroused but lethargic, and he moves all 4 extremities.

RADIOLOGICAL DATA

Initial chest x-ray is consistent with CHF changes. A CT scan of the brain was reportedly negative.

LABORATORY DATA

Remarkable for blood cultures collected on August 14 that are negative so far. Creatinine 7.6. Initial white count 11,900, with 76% neutrophils, 2% bands, and 5% lymphocytes. PT 13, INR 1.07, and D-dimer 1.1.

(continued)

IMPRESSION

1. Patient with altered mental status and multiple medical problems. Admitted to the intensive care unit. Working diagnosis is sepsis. The patient does not have fever or an elevated white count on initial evaluation. He does not have hypotension or any other features of sepsis. However, being immunosuppressed from dialysis, some of these features may be masked and develop in subsequent days. Therefore, I would support empiric antibiotics until further diagnostic testing is completed. Cefepime seems to be adequate coverage. Since there is no evidence of gram-positive cocci in the blood cultures, I do not see a need for methicillin-resistant Staphylococcus aureus coverage with vancomycin or other antibiotics.

2. Encephalopathy, likely multifactorial.

3. End-stage renal disease, on dialysis.

4. Rule out acute myocardial infarction. Management as per Dr. Smith.

5. Uncontrolled hypertension.

6. Anemia.

RECOMMENDATION

The patient is critically ill. I agree with ICU monitoring. For the time being I would recommend continuation of his current antibiotics.

CONSULTATION

REASON FOR CONSULTATION
Fungemia history.

HISTORY OF PRESENT ILLNESS
The patient is a 59-year-old African American male recently diagnosed with a squamous cell carcinoma of the piriform sinus, status post tracheostomy, who has now developed complications including colocutaneous and enterocutaneous fistulae. He has been in the hospital since his original initiation of treatment. He was transferred back here with increasing abdominal pain and evidence of feculent drainage from his abdominal wound, and he was started on ertapenem. Antibiotics were discontinued yesterday, but last night he spiked a temperature and was placed back on Primaxin. Blood cultures were drawn and are already positive for yeast. He has been receiving TPN for about a week and bowel rest for treatment of his enterocutaneous fistula, which was demonstrated on fistulogram. He has now been transferred to the step-down unit, and Infectious Disease is consulted regarding management of fungemia. He is currently awake and does answer some questions, but he is lethargic and somewhat uncooperative. He denies significant pain and states his pain is well controlled. No shortness of breath or chest pain.

PAST MEDICAL HISTORY
1. Metastatic squamous cell carcinoma of the piriform sinus, diagnosed 1 month ago. He was admitted with stridor and had an emergent tracheostomy. Workup revealed metastatic carcinoma, and he had a gastrostomy tube placed. His postoperative course was complicated by development of a colocutaneous fistula, which was repaired, but he has now developed an enterocutaneous fistula, as per history of present illness. He has been receiving radiation therapy and chemotherapy over at Kindred.
2. Hypertension.
3. Benign prostatic hypertrophy.
4. Tracheostomy.
5. Gastrostomy.
6. Enterocutaneous fistula repair.

MEDICATIONS
1. Epoetin.
2. Protonix.
3. Primaxin 1 g IV q.8 h.
4. Caspofungin 50 mg IV daily.
5. Morphine.
6. Zofran.

ALLERGIES
PENICILLIN causes a rash.

REVIEW OF SYSTEMS
Limited due to communication issues and mental status.

FAMILY HISTORY
Noncontributory.

(continued)

SOCIAL HISTORY

He is an ex-smoker.

PHYSICAL EXAMINATION

T-max 103.5, blood pressure 84/60, respiratory rate 18, and heart rate 84. In general, he is a lethargic, uncomfortable-appearing African American male. He is thin and appears chronically ill. HEENT exam is unremarkable other than tracheostomy site, which is clean. Neck is supple. Heart exam with normal S1 and S2. No murmurs, clicks, or rubs. Regular rate and rhythm. Lungs are clear. Abdomen is soft with mild tenderness. He has an open wound, which is covered by an ostomy bag. Extremities without edema or rash. He has intact distal pulses.

LABORATORY DATA

White count 3.23, with 79% polys. Hematocrit 33.4, platelets 114. Creatinine 0.6. Electrolytes unremarkable. AST 13, ALT 27. Blood cultures from 10/29/2004 show no growth. Blood cultures from 11/08/2004 have 1 out of 2 sets with budding yeast at 24 hours. Urine culture with greater than 10,000 colonies of yeast as well.

RADIOLOGY

Chest x-ray with no focal consolidation.

IMPRESSION

A 59-year-old African American male with metastatic squamous cell carcinoma of the piriform sinus. Now re-admitted with enterocutaneous fistula. New blood cultures are showing fungemia quickly.

RECOMMENDATIONS

I think we have an explanation for the fever spike yesterday. Caspofungin is an appropriate choice for empiric antifungal therapy in this case. He could certainly have a non-albicans candida. I do not have adequate records to tell if he has received Diflucan, but if he did, that would increase his chance of having an azole-resistant organism. Regardless, the main benefit of using an azole is to use oral therapy, and he is not a candidate right now for oral fluconazole, so caspofungin is most appropriate. He should have his port removed. He will need an ophthalmologic exam to rule out an ophthalmitis at some point. There is no evidence on cardiac exam of endocarditis. If he rapidly clears this fungemia, and the port is removed, then 2 weeks of antifungal therapy should be appropriate. He should have his LFTs checked within the first few days of starting caspofungin.

CONSULTATION

HISTORY OF PRESENT ILLNESS
This is a 48-year-old male, without any past medical history, who presented with a 2-day history of fevers and headaches. The patient is a poor historian. Apparently, he has been experiencing a cough that is nonproductive. He has nausea and vomiting as well. He is fairly weak but has no other symptoms. In the ER, he was noted to have a temperature of 101.2, pulse of 94, blood pressure 94/53, and respiratory rate 18.

ALLERGIES
No known allergies.

PAST MEDICAL HISTORY
Negative.

PAST SURGICAL HISTORY
Tonsillectomy.

REVIEW OF SYSTEMS
Weakness, myalgias, cough, wheezing, nausea, vomiting, occasional confusion, and headaches.

PHYSICAL EXAMINATION
GENERAL: The patient is a middle-aged man, lying in bed in no apparent distress.
HEENT: Pupils are equal, round, reactive to light and accommodation. Mouth is moist.
NECK: Supple. There is no JVD.
LUNGS: No wheezing. Clear to auscultation and percussion.
HEART: Normal S1 and S2. Regular rate and rhythm.
ABDOMEN: Soft, nontender. Positive bowel sounds.
EXTREMITIES: No clubbing, cyanosis, or edema.
NEUROLOGIC: Grossly nonfocal.

RADIOLOGICAL DATA
Chest x-ray changes are consistent with COPD. There are no infiltrates.

DIAGNOSTIC DATA
A CT scan of the brain was negative.

LABORATORY DATA
White count 8800, lymphocytes 21, monocytes 9, and eosinophils 2. Normal PT/PTT and INR. LDH 243 and creatinine 1. Liver function tests were within normal limits. CSF showed negative agglutination for bacteria or pathogens. Gram stain showed no white blood cells. No organisms were seen. CSF revealed 12 wbc's, 2 rbc's, 0% segmented neutrophils, 100% lymphocytes, glucose 50, and protein 87. The urine culture was negative.

(continued)

IMPRESSION

1. Aseptic meningitis. The differential diagnosis would include viral pathogens such as enterovirus and St. Louis encephalitis, and West Nile virus needs to be excluded in the end, since Florida has become an endemic area.
2. Rule out HIV.
3. A parameningeal infection cannot be excluded.
4. The patient has already received 2 g of Rocephin that would provide coverage for the next 24 hours. My suspicion for bacterial meningitis is very low. The patient is to be ruled out for HIV.

RECOMMENDATION

I recommend sending serologies for all the above-mentioned pathogens. Specimens should be sent to the health department for further testing.

REVIEW QUESTIONS

The goal of these questions is to test your knowledge in the area of infectious disease.

Directions: Select the correct answer for each of the multiple-choice questions provided below. *Answers are provided at the end of this chapter.*

1. Infectious agents transmitted by blood transfusion, contaminated surgical or dental instruments, shared needles, or intimate contact are
   A. congenital pathogens.
   B. bloodborne pathogens.
   C. fomite pathogens.
   D. airborne pathogens.

2. Which of the following is a class of antiinfective drugs?
   A. cephalosporin
   B. statin
   C. analgesic
   D. steroid

3. Another name for a spinal tap is
   A. lumbar biopsy.
   B. lumbar puncture.
   C. pleurocentesis.
   D. pleurodesis.

4. The medical term for "flesh-eating disease" is
   A. necrotizing fasciitis.
   B. nodular vasculitis.
   C. nonparalytic poliomyelitis.
   D. nutritional steatitis.

5. Bacteria that do not require oxygen are called
   A. anaerobes.
   B. gram-negative organisms.
   C. aerobes.
   D. acid-fast bacilli.

6. Which of the following is a virus which is spread via mosquito bites?
   A. cytomegalovirus
   B. Norwalk virus
   C. parvovirus
   D. West Nile virus

7. Shingles is caused by
   A. Varicella zoster.
   B. Herpes simplex 1 virus.
   C. Epstein-Barr virus.
   D. Herpes simplex 2 virus.

8. The medical term for chickenpox is
   A. adenovirus.
   B. varicella.
   C. mononucleosis.
   D. toxoplasmosis.

9. The body's ability to protect itself against an infection is called
   A. autoimmunity.
   B. hypersensitivity.
   C. immunity.
   D. immunodeficiency.

10. Which of the following suffixes denotes a class of antibiotics?
   A. *-azapam*
   B. *-olol*
   C. *-cillin*
   D. *-caine*

11. Which of the following tests is used to classify bacteria by their morphological characteristics?
    A. Wright stain
    B. Sedimentation rate
    C. Gram stain
    D. CBC

12. Which of the following is an opportunistic infection that occurs predominantly in patients with HIV/AIDS?
    A. Pneumocystis jiroveci (P. carinii)
    B. Mycoplasma pneumoniae
    C. Helicobacter pylori
    D. Legionella pneumophila

13. Microorganisms grown in a medium in a laboratory for a specific length of time is called a (an)
    A. serology test.
    B. Gram stain.
    C. ANA.
    D. culture.

14. Which of the following is known to cause stomach ulcers?
    A. Helicobacter pylori
    B. Escherichia coli
    C. Clostridium difficile
    D. Varicella zoster

15. The class of drugs used to kill or inhibit bacterial pathogens is called
    A. antivirals.
    B. antiemetics.
    C. antibiotics.
    D. antifungals.

16. The range of organisms against which a particular antibiotic can be used is called a (an)
    A. spectrum.
    B. CBC.
    C. portfolio.
    D. antibiotic sensitivity test.

17. Prophylactic antibiotics are given
    A. during an infection.
    B. after the resolution of an infection.
    C. to prevent infection.
    D. to see if an antibiotic will work.

18. Examples of immunoglobulins include
    A. IgA, IgG.
    B. monocytes.
    C. lymphocytes.
    D. hepatocytes.

19. Which of the following describes a slight increase in the number of lymphocytes?
    A. lymphocytosis
    B. lymphopoiesis
    C. lymphedema
    D. lymphocytopenia

20. An antifungal agent would be effective against
    A. gonorrhea.
    B. herpes.
    C. candida.
    D. HIV.

21. HIV is the
    A. virus that causes AIDS.
    B. virus that causes genital warts.
    C. virus that causes shingles.
    D. virus that causes mumps.

22. Which of the following is transcribed correctly?
    A. Patient was found to have an elevated white count at 14,000 with 80% polys and 30% lymphocytes.
    B. Patient was found to have an elevated white count at 4,000 with 80% polys and 10% lymphocytes.
    C. Patient was found to have a depressed white count at 14,000 with 80% polys and 10% lymphocytes.
    D. Patient was found to have an elevated white count at 14,000 with 80% polys and 10% lymphocytes.

23. Which of the following is transcribed correctly?
    A. The patient was found to have S aureus.
    B. The patient was found to have Staphylococcus a.
    C. The patient was found to have s. aureus.
    D. The patient was found to have strep aureus.

24. A physician aspirates fluid from a swollen and painful knee and orders a "see-en-ess." What laboratory test(s) is the physician requesting?
    A. CNS fluid analysis
    B. culture and serology
    C. calcium and sodium
    D. culture and sensitivity

25. CD4 counts are used to
    A. monitor patients with meningitis.
    B. grade the severity of varicella infection.
    C. assess immune response to vaccination.
    D. monitor AIDS patients.

26. Mycology is the study of
    A. fungi.
    B. muscle.
    C. viruses.
    D. tissue.

27. A common tick-borne illness in the United States is
    A. diphtheria.
    B. Lyme disease.
    C. tuberculosis.
    D. sporotrichosis.

28. Which of the following classes of drugs are antibiotics?
    A. anxiolytics and antivirals
    B. beta agonists and anthelmintics
    C. cephalosporins and sulfonamides
    D. diuretics and anticholinergics

29. Serology tests help to diagnose disease by
    A. detecting specific antigens or antibodies in the patient's blood.
    B. isolating the infectious agent.
    C. visualizing the infectious agent using stains.
    D. culturing the infectious agent.

30. A severe bacterial infection may cause
    A. a increase in eosinophils.
    B. an increase in neutrophils ("polys").
    C. an increase in monocytes.
    D. a decrease in red cells.

 Please see the accompanying CD for additional review materials for this section.

ANSWER KEY

REVIEW QUESTIONS ANSWER KEY

1. B	6. D	11. A	16. A	21. A	26. A
2. A	7. A	12. A	17. C	22. D	27. B
3. B	8. B	13. D	18. A	23. A	28. C
4. A	9. C	14. A	19. A	24. D	29. A
5. A	10. C	15. C	20. C	25. D	30. B

Otorhinolaryngology

OBJECTIVES CHECKLIST

A prepared exam candidate will know the:

- ❏ Combining forms, prefixes, and suffixes related to the body system.

- ❏ Anatomical structures of the outer, middle, and inner ear.

- ❏ Anatomical structures of the nose and throat.

- ❏ Abnormal and pathologic conditions related to the ear, nose, and throat.

- ❏ Clinical procedures utilized to identify and treat diseases and abnormalities of the ear, nose, and throat.

- ❏ Common medications used to treat diseases and abnormalities of the ear, nose, and throat.

- ❏ Imaging studies related to the diagnosis and treatment of ear, nose, and throat disorders.

- ❏ Laboratory studies related to diagnosis and treatment of ear, nose, and throat disorders.

RESOURCES FOR STUDY

1. *Bates' Guide to Physical Examination and History Taking*
   Chapter 6: The Head and Neck, pp. 153–239.

2. *The Language of Medicine*
   Chapter 5: Digestive System, Pharynx, pp. 143–144.
   Chapter 12: Respiratory System, Section II. Anatomy and Physiology of Respiration, pp. 442–443; 446–452.
   Chapter 17: Sense Organs: The Eye and the Ear, pp. 689–698, 705–707.

3. *Memmler's Structure and Function of the Human Body*
   Chapter 10: The Sensory System, pp. 177–194.

4. *Memmler's The Human Body in Health and Disease*
   Chapter 11: The Sensory System, pp. 222–243; Study Guide, pp. 174–191.

5. *H&P: A Nonphysician's Guide to the Medical History and Physical Examination*
   Chapter 7: Review of Systems: Head, Eyes, Ears, Nose, Throat, Mouth, Teeth, pp. 59–70.
   Chapter 20: Examination of the Ears, pp. 189–198.
   Chapter 21: Examination of the Nose, Throat, Mouth, and Teeth, pp. 199–208.

6. *Human Diseases*
   Chapter 9: Diseases of the Ear, Nose and Throat, pp. 127–140.

7. *Laboratory Tests & Diagnostic Procedures in Medicine*
   Chapter 3: Measurement of Vision and Hearing, pp. 29–38.
   Chapter 7: Endoscopy: Visual Examination of the Eyes, Ears, Nose, and Respiratory Tract, pp. 95–106.

8. *A Manual of Laboratory and Diagnostic Tests*
   Chapter 7: Microbiologic Studies, pp. 456–529.
   Chapter 10: X-Ray Studies, pp. 705–759.
   Chapter 12: Endoscopic Studies, pp. 819–861.
   Chapter 16: Special Systems, Organ Functions, and Postmortem Studies, pp. 1012–1093.

9. *Using Medical Terminology: A Practical Approach*
   Chapter 8: Nervous System and Special Senses, pp. 313–377.

10. *Pharmacology for Health Professionals*
    Unit III: Drugs That Affect the Respiratory System (Chapters 11–13), pp. 169–197.
    Chapter 31: Otic and Ophthalmic Preparations, pp. 526–541.

11. *Understanding Pharmacology for Health Professionals*
    Chapter 19: Ear, Nose and Throat Drugs, pp. 205–216.

12. *Medical Terminology: The Language of Health Care*
    Chapter 13: Ear, pp. 415–436.

SAMPLE REPORTS

The following four reports are examples of reports you might encounter while transcribing otorhinolaryngology.

HISTORY AND PHYSICAL

HISTORY

The patient presents with a chronic history of nasion pressure, frequent upper respiratory infections, occasional bronchitis, cough, sneezing, and possible incipient asthma. For many years, she has also had a postnasal drip. Her nasal obstruction is noted to be bilateral and equal and is associated with sneezing and a clear rhinorrhea. She has no abnormal sensation of smell but breathes through her mouth and nose. There has been no nasal trauma, and she is aware of pressure in the nasion area. She also snores. There is itching of the throat, occasional postnasal drip, and clearing of her throat. It was felt that she had a possible reflux problem. She was given information on reflux and placed on Nexium, which does help her. She also has a history of significant heartburn and gastritis with a history of ulcer disease, for which she takes Librax.

The patient wears glasses for reading and distance but notes itching and tearing of her eyes when her nasal symptoms are active. There is no significant hearing loss. She does occasionally have balance and tinnitus problems. When she has respiratory symptoms, she notes pressure in her ear, but otherwise her hearing is unremarkable. As noted, for the past year, she has had occasional wheezing. One year ago, she had pneumonia. She has had episodes of bronchitis but has never been diagnosed as an asthmatic. She smokes and drinks alcohol on a social basis only. Headaches, as described above, are treated with over-the-counter medication such as ibuprofen and Aleve. There are no cardiovascular disorders. The patient has no history of thyroid disease, diabetes, or anemia. There is no osteoporosis.

Head and neck surgery is limited to a tonsillectomy in New Jersey in 1978. There are no specific drug allergies. Her mother and sister both have sinus problems. The patient was given Astelin by Dr. Jones, which seems to have helped her. She has not used any of the newer antihistamines on a regular basis. Three or 4 years ago, she was tested in Florida for inhalant allergies and told that no significant findings were uncovered. The patient has no pets and notes no reactions from animals. She is aware that her symptoms increase with weather changes, and dust causes significant nasal symptoms, including sneezing and rhinorrhea.

A CT scan of the sinuses was ordered and was completely normal, only showing a left septal deviation. A culture of the nose at the time was negative as well.

PHYSICAL EXAMINATION

Examination reveals a comfortable lady in no distress with multiple upper respiratory complaints. The oropharyngeal examination is unremarkable. The teeth are in a good state of repair. The oral mucosa is well hydrated. There are large, residual tonsil tags despite the history of a tonsillectomy. The intranasal inspection shows hypertrophy of the turbinates with a purplish appearance and bilateral septal spurs widening the septum and resulting in a decreased nasal airway. There is no evidence of rhinorrhea or polyps. There is no sinus percussive tenderness. It is noted that the patient has prominent allergic shiners and Dennie lines. She is breathing through her nose and

(continued)

mouth. The otoscopic visualization shows intact tympanic membranes and auditory canals. There is no cerumen accumulation. There is no evidence of middle ear disease. Palpation of the neck elicits no tenderness or adenopathy. The carotid pulses are full and equal. The thyroid is not palpable. There is normal laryngeal crepitus, and the salivary glands are unremarkable. The patient's facial movements are normal. There are no temporomandibular joint findings.

The patient's history and examination are strongly suggestive of an underlying allergic diathesis, especially with a normal CT scan of the sinuses and culture of the nasal mucus. She notes some relief with the Astelin spray and will continue this. I have added Zyrtec-D and Zyrtec tablets to the regimen. I have scheduled her for intradermal allergy testing. She is very interested in possibly having septum and turbinate surgery to improve her nasal airway. This will be addressed after the completion of the allergy testing and the trial of medications.

OPERATIVE REPORT

PREOPERATIVE DIAGNOSES
1. Obstructive sleep apnea.
2. Tonsillar hypertrophy.
3. Oropharyngeal obstruction.
4. Tongue base hypertrophy.

POSTOPERATIVE DIAGNOSES
1. Obstructive sleep apnea.
2. Tonsillar hypertrophy.
3. Oropharyngeal obstruction.
4. Tongue base hypertrophy.

PROCEDURES PERFORMED
1. Uvulopalatopharyngoplasty.
2. Partial resection of the tongue base by radiofrequency.
3. Tonsillectomy.

SURGEON
John Smith, MD.

ANESTHESIA
General anesthesia.

HISTORY
This is a 33-year-old who has a history of obstructive sleep apnea, intolerant to CPAP, with tonsillar hypertrophy, redundant uvula and soft palate, and prominent tongue base.

PROCEDURE
The patient was taken to the operating room and placed on the table in the supine position. Satisfactory general anesthesia was administered via endotracheal tube. The patient was placed in the Rose tonsil position. The Crowe-Davis mouth gag was introduced into the patient's mouth and suspended from the Mayo stand. The soft palate was elevated with a red rubber catheter.

The tonsils were dissected from the tonsillar fossae bilaterally, along with resection of a small cuff of anterior tonsillar pillar mucosa using the suction cautery. The posterior tonsillar pillars were then rotated laterally and anteriorly and sutured to the anterior tonsillar pillar mucosa with interrupted 3-0 Vicryl sutures. This was performed bilaterally.

Incision was then made across the soft palate, resecting the musculus uvuli and a small cuff of anterior mucosa of the margin of the soft palate. The posterior mucosa was preserved, and bilateral diagonal relaxing incisions were made at the junction of the soft palate and the superior tonsillar pole. Flaps were rotated laterally and superiorly and secured with 3-0 Vicryl, and the posterior mucosa of the soft palate was rotated anteriorly and secured to the anterior mucosa using 3-0 Vicryl interrupted sutures. Adequate soft palate length was preserved for velopharyngeal competence, and then the mouth gag was removed.

(continued)

A side-biting mouth gag was introduced into the patient's mouth. The mouth was irrigated with Betadine and then the tongue was brought forward. The tongue base was visualized using the Somnos 2-channel tongue base probe. Four passes at the tongue base at 1500 joules per pass were then performed, 2 on the right and 2 on the left, anterior and posterior to the circumvallate papillae. Prior to each lesion, approximately 4 mL of normal saline was injected into the site. A total of 6000 joules was delivered to the tongue base.

The patient was awakened, extubated, and taken to the recovery room in satisfactory condition.

OPERATIVE REPORT

PREOPERATIVE DIAGNOSES
1. Nasal airway obstruction.
2. Nasal septal deformity.
3. Inferior turbinate hypertrophy.

POSTOPERATIVE DIAGNOSES
1. Nasal airway obstruction.
2. Nasal septal deformity.
3. Inferior turbinate hypertrophy.

OPERATION
1. Septoplasty.
2. Bilateral submucous resection of the inferior turbinates.

SURGEON
John Smith, MD.

ANESTHESIA
General via endotracheal tube.

PROCEDURE
The patient was taken to the operating room and placed on the table in the supine position. Satisfactory general anesthesia was administered via endotracheal tube. The nose was cocainized and injected with 1% Xylocaine with epinephrine for local anesthesia.

Following adequate prepping and draping, a right hemitransfixion incision was made. A left mucoperichondrial tunnel was elevated over the cartilage to the bony cartilaginous junction. The cartilage was separated from the bone. Bilateral posterior tunnels were elevated. Severely deviated bony septum was resected. The cartilage was freed up off the maxillary crest, and a large maxillary crest spur was resected. The maxillary crest was then fractured back to the midline. The cartilage was shortened inferiorly to fit back on the maxillary crest, and the hemitransfixion incision was closed with 4-0 chromic.

The inferior turbinate was injected with 1% Xylocaine with epinephrine. Then, using the turbinate microdebrider blade through an anterior stab incision, bilateral submucosal resection of the inferior turbinates was performed bilaterally and remaining turbinate tissue was out-fractured.

The nose was then packed with hydrocolloid gel packs. The patient was awakened and taken to the recovery room in satisfactory condition.

CONSULTATION

CHIEF COMPLAINT
Vertigo and questionable sleep apnea.

HISTORY OF PRESENT ILLNESS
This is a 43-year-old Caucasian female who came down with rotational vertigo in January. This occurred over the course of the day and was severe for about 3 days. She presented to Dr. Smith and had blood work performed which was reportedly normal. She had questionable blood pressure elevation at that time and was followed up by Dr. Jones, at which time she states her blood pressure was 160/115, and she was placed on Tiazac. She continued to have a feeling of rotational vertigo, worse with eyes closed, and accompanied by nausea but no vomiting. The acute symptoms lasted for approximately 8 days, and she did as much activity as she could. She had significant improvement at that point, just noting that her symptoms return when she is tired or while watching TV. She has avoided skiing or other athletic activity for fear it would aggravate her symptoms again. She had a prior episode of vertigo 3 years ago which lasted for 4 days, rotational, continuous, with nausea and vomiting. Two years ago, she had a similar episode, although it was of less magnitude and resulted in minimal debility. She has never had any significant fluctuation in hearing or tinnitus. She denies any vision problems. Did have mild blurring initially. No recent upper respiratory symptoms. She is also concerned about possible apnea, as on several occasions she has been told by friends and family that she has a peculiar breathing pattern in which she will suddenly stop, and they are afraid she is not going to start breathing again. She has some daytime fatigue but does not nap and is functioning well. She has recently started a new business in addition to her real estate business, which is taking a lot of time. Moderate stress but nothing that she feels is unusual. She has had a 20-pound weight gain in the last year. Always wakes in the morning with a dry mouth. No history of head injury or chronic medical illness.

PAST MEDICAL HISTORY
Nausea with codeine and other pain medications. Hospitalized for a broken wrist in 1996 and nasal fracture in 1979.

CURRENT MEDICATIONS
Paxil 20 mg daily and Tiazac 180 mg p.o. daily for hypertension, still in her first week of treatment.

SOCIAL HISTORY
She has smoked a 1/2 pack of cigarettes a day for the past 27 years. She drinks 2–4 glasses of wine a day.

FAMILY HISTORY
Parents in good health. Father with heart disease and multiple family members are hypertensive.

REVIEW OF SYSTEMS
Positive for cervical degenerative joint disease and recent hypertension and depression. No cardiac disease, GI or GU problems, easy bleeding or bruising, diabetes, endocrine or metabolic disease, or neurologic illness.

(continued)

PHYSICAL EXAMINATION

Alert, Caucasian female. Blood pressure 156/88, pulse 77. No cervical adenopathy or masses. Well-defined cervical triangle. Thyroid is normal, trachea midline. External ears, canals, and tympanic membranes unremarkable. Deviated nasal septum to the left, mild. No polyps, drainage, or inflammation. Lips and teeth unremarkable. Palate, tongue, floor of mouth normal. Grade 2 soft palate ptosis. Atrophic tonsils. Nasopharynx and hypopharynx clear. Pupils round and reactive to light, extraocular muscles are intact. No nystagmus. In 3-inch heels, patient performs Romberg, tandem gait, and stands on 1 foot, all without any difficulty. Cranial nerves II through XII grossly intact.

Audiogram shows normal hearing bilaterally with 5 dB SRT on the right with 96% discrimination, 5 dB SRT on the left with 100% discrimination. Impedance testing and reflex are normal.

IMPRESSION

1. Vestibular neuronitis, symptomatically resolved.
2. Erratic nocturnal respiratory pattern. Rule out obstructive sleep apnea.

PLAN

1. Polysomnography.
2. Maximize visual and environmental clues to optimize balance.
3. Continue antihypertensive. Follow up with Dr. Jones. Recheck after polysomnography.

REVIEW QUESTIONS

The goal of these questions is to test your knowledge in the area of otorhinolaryngology.

Directions: Select the correct answer for each of the multiple-choice questions provided below. *Answers are provided at the end of this chapter.*

1. An accumulation of fluid behind the eardrum is called
   A. malignant otitis externa.
   B. labyrinthitis.
   C. serous otitis media.
   D. serous otitis externa.

2. A surgical procedure to repair or reshape the nose is called
   A. rhinoplasty.
   B. rhinotomy.
   C. rhytidoplasty.
   D. rhizotomy.

3. A yellowish brown, waxy substance that lubricates and protects the ear is called
   A. perilymph.
   B. endolymph.
   C. cerumen.
   D. mucus.

4. Which of the following closes the larynx during swallowing to prevent choking?
   A. epiglottis
   B. lingula
   C. malleus
   D. uvula

5. The sensation of ringing, buzzing, or whistling in the ear is known as
   A. vertigo.
   B. otosclerosis.
   C. tinnitus.
   D. myringitis.

6. Which of the following is a blood test to detect allergies?
   A. RAST
   B. ELIZA
   C. PPD test
   D. patch test

7. The vestibulum auris is located in the
   A. ear.
   B. mouth.
   C. nose.
   D. throat.

8. The anterior opening to the nasal cavity is called the
   A. naris.
   B. auricle.
   C. ossis.
   D. meatus.

9. Which of the following is transcribed correctly?
   A. The patient will be referred to speech therapy for dysphagia and will undergo a swallowing test for aphasia.
   B. The patient will be referred to speech therapy for dysphasia and will undergo a swallowing test for dysphagia.
   C. The patient will be referred to speech therapy for aphagia and will undergo a swallowing test for dysphagia.
   D. The patient will be referred to speech therapy for dysphasia and will undergo a swallowing test for aphasia.

10. The bony and muscular area at the roof of the mouth is called the
    A. palate.
    B. bucca.
    C. mandible.
    D. maxilla.

11. A patient has a chronically stuffy nose. Which of the following could be diseased?
    A. turbinates
    B. mastoid
    C. cochlea
    D. semicircular canals

12. Antitussive medications are used to treat
    A. congestion.
    B. motion sickness.
    C. cough.
    D. postnasal drip.

13. Which of the following is transcribed correctly?
    A. The patient was diagnosed with labial herpes and labile hypertension.
    B. The patient was diagnosed with labile herpes and labial hypertension.
    C. The patient was diagnosed with labial herpes and labial hypertension.
    D. The patient was diagnosed with labile herpes and labile hypertension.

14. This disorder is characterized by recurrent interruptions of breathing during sleep due to temporary blockage of the airway.
    A. hypoxia
    B. deglutition apnea
    C. obstructive sleep apnea
    D. sleep-induced apnea

15. Monitoring of relevant normal and abnormal activity during sleep is called
    A. polytomography.
    B. electroencephalography.
    C. tympanography.
    D. polysomnography.

16. Which of the following is transcribed correctly?
    A. HEENT: Mucus membranes are erythematous with excess mucous in the nasopharynx.
    B. HEENT: Mucous membranes are erythematous with excess mucus in the nasal pharynx.
    C. HEENT: Mucous membranes are erythematous with excess mucus in the nasopharynx.
    D. HEENT: Mucous membranes are erythematous with excess mucous in the nasopharynx.

17. Hearing loss due to obstruction of the outer ear is called
    A. neural hearing loss.
    B. conductive hearing loss.
    C. sensory hearing loss.
    D. permanent hearing loss.

18. The back of the throat is called the
    A. larynx.
    B. phalanx.
    C. pharynx.
    D. syrinx.

19. Which of the following disorders is characterized by dizziness and loss of balance?
    A. ossicular
    B. dysthymic
    C. cochlear
    D. vestibular

20. The prefix *presby-* means
    A. old age.
    B. elevated pressure.
    C. nearby.
    D. early age.

21. Which of the following are hearing tests?
    A. Rinne and Webster
    B. Tine and Weber
    C. Rinne and Weber
    D. Webster and Tine

22. Dysgeusia is
    A. abnormal taste.
    B. abnormal smell.
    C. abnormal hearing.
    D. abnormal sight.

23. The suffix -*osmia* pertains to
    A. smell.
    B. hearing.
    C. sight.
    D. taste.

24. Which diagnostic procedure inspects the external auditory meatus and tympanic membrane with an instrument that directs light into the ear through a speculum?
    A. Weber test
    B. Rinne test
    C. otoscopy
    D. tympanostomy

25. An audiometer is used to test
    A. sight.
    B. hearing.
    C. speech.
    D. the vocal cords.

26. A collection of skin cells and cholesterol in a sac within the middle ear that is also associated with perforation of the tympanic membrane is called a (an)
    A. acoustic neuroma.
    B. ceruminous impaction.
    C. cholesteatoma.
    D. cauliflower ear.

27. The small cartilaginous projection anterior to the external opening of the ear is called the
    A. concha.
    B. helix.
    C. pinna.
    D. tragus.

28. The suffix -*o/scopy* refers to an
    A. instrument used in suturing.
    B. instrument used in cutting.
    C. instrument used in viewing.
    D. instrument used in surgery.

29. A surgical incision in the tympanic membrane is called a
    A. myringotomy.
    B. alveolotomy.
    C. cordotomy.
    D. thyrotomy.

30. Which of the following is found in the inner ear?
    A. cochlea
    B. hyoid
    C. trachea
    D. uvula

 Please see the accompanying CD for additional review materials for this section.

ANSWER KEY

REVIEW QUESTIONS ANSWER KEY

1. C	6. A	11. A	16. C	21. C	26. C
2. A	7. A	12. C	17. B	22. A	27. D
3. C	8. A	13. A	18. C	23. A	28. C
4. A	9. B	14. C	19. D	24. C	29. A
5. C	10. A	15. D	20. A	25. B	30. A

10

Dermatology

OBJECTIVES CHECKLIST

A prepared exam candidate will know:

- ❏ All combining forms, prefixes, and suffixes related to dermatology.
- ❏ Layers of the skin and the role/function of each.
- ❏ Anatomy and function of the accessory organs of the skin (hair, nails, and glands).
- ❏ Definitions and attributes of all lesion types.
- ❏ Signs, symptoms, and diseases related to the skin and accessory organs.
- ❏ Laboratory studies related to the diagnosis and treatment of dermatologic dysfunction and disease.
- ❏ Common medications prescribed for dermatologic symptoms and diseases.
- ❏ Transcription standards pertaining to allergies, immunologic disorders, and lymphocytes.

RESOURCES FOR STUDY

1. *Bates' Guide to Physical Examination and History Taking*
   Chapter 5: The Skin, Hair, and Nails, pp. 121–151.

2. *The Language of Medicine*
   Chapter 16: Skin, pp. 629–668.

3. *Memmler's Structure and Function of the Human Body*
   Chapter 4: Tissues, Glands, and Membranes, pp. 57–70.
   Chapter 5: The Integumentary System, pp. 73–82.

4. *Memmler's The Human Body in Health and Disease*
   Chapter 6: The Skin in Health and Disease, pp. 100–117; pp. 83–94.

5. *H&P: A Nonphysician's Guide to the Medical History and Physical Examination*
   Chapter 14: Review of Systems: Skin, pp. 125–130.
   Chapter 17: Examination of the Skin, pp. 157–168.

6. *Human Diseases*
   Chapter 7: Diseases of the Skin, pp. 87–104.

7. *Laboratory Tests & Diagnostic Procedures in Medicine*
   Chapter 16: Normal Anatomy and Histology, pp. 225–250.
   Chapter 17: Procedures and Practice in Anatomic Pathology, pp. 251–278.

8. *A Manual of Laboratory and Diagnostic Tests*
   Chapter 7: Microbiologic Studies, pp. 456–529.
   Chapter 11: Cytologic, Histologic, and Genetic Studies, pp. 760–816.

9. *The AAMT Book of Style for Medical Transcription*
   Clark level, pp. 51–52.

10. *Using Medical Terminology: A Practical Approach*
    Chapter 4: Integumentary System, pp. 133–187.

11. *Pharmacology for Health Professionals*
    Chapter 30: Topical Drugs Used in the Treatment of Skin Disorders, pp. 510–525.

12. *Understanding Pharmacology for Health Professionals*
    Chapter 11: Dermatologic Drugs, pp. 82–101.

13. *Medical Terminology: The Language of Health Care*
    Chapter 5: Integumentary System, pp. 107–143.

SAMPLE REPORTS

The following four reports are examples of reports you might encounter while transcribing dermatology.

OFFICE NOTE

HISTORY
This is a 68-year-old man who has a 10-month history of an intermittent, itchy rash on his right thigh. This settles with a topical steroid, and between episodes the skin is normal. He occasionally has a similar eruption on his left chest but has had no rashes anywhere else.

SOCIAL HISTORY
He works part-time as a bookmaker's assistant. He smokes a pipe, but his personal and family history is otherwise noncontributory.

PHYSICAL EXAMINATION
Shows eczematous rash with redness, weeping, scaling, and vesiculation on the anterior thighs. Some lichenification is present. There are no abnormal findings elsewhere on general examination.

Patch test was performed and was positive for acrylates.

ASSESSMENT
Allergic contact dermatitis. He does not have a history of joint replacement to account for his exposure to acrylates, and after extensive interviewing, we suspect the causative agent is from his work environment. He often carries bank notes in his pants pockets and sometimes in his shirt pocket.

PLAN
1. Avoid carrying papers in pockets.
2. Return p.r.n.

OFFICE NOTE

HISTORY

The patient presents for assessment of pigmented lesions developing on the trunk and extremities. The patient has no previous history of skin cancer. She states she has had previous nevi excised. She has had significant sun exposure in the past and likes to tan using indoor tanning beds.

PAST MEDICAL HISTORY

Hypothyroidism, on replacement; otherwise, no health problems.

CURRENT MEDICATIONS

Synthroid.

PHYSICAL EXAMINATION

Revealed several seborrheic keratoses and lentigines on the trunk and upper extremities. A small actinic keratosis was seen on the right forehead. Erythematous lichenoid keratoses were present on the left lower leg.

ASSESSMENT

1. Actinic keratosis of right forehead.
2. Lichenoid keratoses of left lower leg.

PLAN

1. Liquid nitrogen cryotherapy.
2. Return p.r.n.

HISTORY AND PHYSICAL

HISTORY OF PRESENT ILLNESS
The patient is seen today for an initial evaluation. She is a very pleasant 50-year-old female with a history of anxiety, hypercholesterolemia, and recent skin loss on her arms and legs as well as a recurring lesion on the lower back area. She also has multiple general complaints.

CURRENT MEDICATIONS
She is on Paxil, Ambien, Lopid, Premarin, and another medicine that I cannot read.

ALLERGIES
She is allergic to ASPIRIN.

PAST MEDICAL HISTORY
There is no diabetes, hepatitis, heart disease, or recent blood transfusion. She is a nonsmoker.

DIAGNOSES
1. Skin loss areas on the arms and legs consistent with idiopathic guttate hypomelanosis.
2. A recurring eruption on the lower back, upper buttock area. She has post-inflammatory changes as well, but no active rash is seen. We have to consider herpes simplex.

PLAN
She will return to the office right away the next time the rash occurs.

OFFICE NOTE

HISTORY
The patient presents for assessment of acne symptoms. She develops papules and pustules as well as inflammatory nodules. She has taken systemic antibiotic therapy, including erythromycin, which she took for 2 months. She has also used Retin-A but found this to be too irritating. Her menstrual cycles are regular and she is on birth control pills. She also gives a history of easy flushing and blushing of the face.

PHYSICAL EXAMINATION
Revealed papules and pustules distributed on the forehead, cheeks, and chin. Only a slight comedone component was present.

ASSESSMENT
Combination of both rosacea and acne vulgaris.

PLAN
1. Doxycycline 100 mg daily.
2. Hydrocortisone 1%, clindamycin 1%, and metronidazole 1% in Complex 15 lotion, applied twice a day.

REVIEW QUESTIONS

The goal of these questions is to test your knowledge in the area of dermatology.

Directions: Select the correct answer for each of the multiple-choice questions provided below. *Answers are provided at the end of this chapter.*

1. The skin, hair, nails, and glands all make up this system of the body.
   A. integumentary system
   B. lymphatic system
   C. musculoskeletal system
   D. nervous system

2. Of the three layers of the skin, which is the thick, fat-containing layer?
   A. dermis
   B. epidermis
   C. epithelium
   D. subcutaneous tissue

3. The brown-black pigment of the skin that is transferred to other epidermal cells and gives the skin its color is called
   A. albumin.
   B. collagen.
   C. keratin.
   D. melanin.

4. The half-moon shaped, white area located at the base of a fingernail is called the
   A. basal layer.
   B. cuticle.
   C. lunula.
   D. stratum.

5. Which of the following is transcribed correctly?
   A. The patient was given metronidazole for rosacea and Lamisil for onychomycosis.
   B. The patient was given metronidazole for roseola and Lamisil for onychomycosis.
   C. The patient was given metronidazole for roseola and Lamisil for onychomycosis.
   D. The patient was given metoprolol for rosacea and Lamisil for onychomycosis.

6. This type of cyst contains yellowish sebum and is commonly found on the scalp, vulva, and scrotum.
   A. papule
   B. sebaceous cyst
   C. ulcer
   D. vesicle

7. A groove or a crack-like sore is called a (an)
   A. fissure.
   B. nodule
   C. polyp.
   D. ulcer.

8. Death of tissue associated with loss of blood supply to the affected area is called
   A. cellulitis.
   B. eczema.
   C. gangrene.
   D. psoriasis.

9. Which skin neoplasm is associated with an increase in the growth of cells in the keratin layer of the epidermis caused by pressure or friction?
   A. callus
   B. keloid
   C. keratosis
   D. leukoplakia

10. An epidermal growth caused by a virus (wart) is called a
    A. impetigo.
    B. melanoma.
    C. nevus.
    D. verruca.

11. In this condition, there is a scaly dermatitis affecting parts of the skin that are supplied by oil glands.
    A. chronic dermatitis
    B. contact dermatitis
    C. eczema
    D. seborrheic dermatitis

12. Which of following infections is also known as ringworm?
    A. folliculitis
    B. herpes simplex
    C. impetigo
    D. tinea corporis

13. An acute eruption of intensely itchy papules or wheals is called
    A. acne vulgaris.
    B. pityriasis rosea.
    C. psoriasis.
    D. urticaria (hives).

14. The outermost layer of skin is the
    A. dermis.
    B. endodermis.
    C. epidermis.
    D. hypodermis.

15. The vascular layer of skin is the
    A. dermis.
    B. epidermis.
    C. stratum corneum unguis.
    D. hypodermis.

16. Apocrine glands produce
    A. mucus.
    B. sebum.
    C. sweat.
    D. keratin.

17. Which of the following is transcribed correctly?
    A. This 58-year-old woman had a biopsy proven melanoma, Clarks level 1, on the left cheek.
    B. This 58-year-old woman had a biopsy-proven melanoma, Clark's level 1, on the left cheek.
    C. This 58-year-old woman had a biopsy proven melena, Clark level 1, on the left cheek
    D. This 58-year-old woman had a biopsy-proven melanoma, Clark level 1, on the left cheek.

18. Follicular dilatation involving the nose and portions of the cheeks, erythema, papules, and pustules are classic signs of this dermatologic disorder.
    A. acne cosmetica
    B. acne pustulosa
    C. acne rosacea
    D. acne vulgaris

19. A skin disorder most often caused by the herpes virus and consisting of red lesions that look like targets is
    A. candidiasis.
    B. erythema multiforme.
    C. hirsutism.
    D. keratosis pilaris.

20. Which of the following would be prescribed for acne?
    A. Actiq
    B. Actonel
    C. Accu-Chek
    D. Accutane

21. A burn which involves 2 layers of the skin and destroys the nerves and blood vessels, but does not go down to muscle or bone is a
    A. first-degree burn.
    B. second-degree burn.
    C. third-degree burn.
    D. full-thickness burn.

22. Yellowing of the skin is indicative of
    A. hyperbilirubinemia.
    B. hyperuricemia.
    C. hyperkalemia.
    D. hyporeninemia.

23. Clotrimazole and nystatin are both
    A. topical antifungals.
    B. anti-itch creams.
    C. topical antibiotics.
    D. used to treat eczema.

24. Which of the following is a combining form meaning skin?
    A. *adip/o*
    B. *cutane/o*
    C. *pachy/o*
    D. *xanth/o*

25. Which of the following is a fungal infection?
    A. lichen planus
    B. keratosis
    C. seborrhea
    D. tinea capitis

26. Moles with the potential to develop into malignant melanoma are
    A. intradermal nevi.
    B. dysplastic nevi.
    C. giant nevi.
    D. verrucae.

27. An absence of pigment in the skin is called
    A. acanthosis nigricans.
    B. albinism.
    C. melanism.
    D. xanthoderma.

28. Another term for itching is
    A. dermatitis.
    B. keratosis.
    C. petechiae.
    D. pruritus.

29. A chronic dermatitis of unknown etiology in patients with a history of allergy is called
    A. actinic dermatitis.
    B. atopic dermatitis.
    C. stasis dermatitis.
    D. seborrheic dermatitis.

30. Excessive hair on the face or body, especially in women, is called:
    A. albinism.
    B. atrichia.
    C. alopecia.
    D. hirsutism.

Please see the accompanying CD for additional review materials for this section.

ANSWER KEY

REVIEW QUESTIONS ANSWER KEY

1. A	6. B	11. D	16. C	21. B	26. B
2. D	7. A	12. D	17. D	22. A	27. B
3. D	8. C	13. D	18. C	23. A	28. D
4. C	9. A	14. C	19. B	24. B	29. B
5. A	10. D	15. A	20. D	25. D	30. D

11

General Surgery/Plastic Surgery

OBJECTIVES CHECKLIST

A prepared exam candidate will know:

- ☐ Common terminology related to surgical intervention and fundamentals of the surgical process.

- ☐ Fundamental terminology related to muscular and skeletal anatomy.

- ☐ Fundamental terminology related to all dermatologic, subcutaneous, and fascial layers for the purposes of surgical entry, repair, and closure.

- ☐ Procedures associated with surgical incisions, hemostasis, and wound closure, including bandages and dressings.

- ☐ Risk management issues pertaining to the documentation of surgical treatment, including blood loss and material counts.

- ☐ Common terminology related to surgical instrumentation, including but not limited to: catheters, forceps, blades, elevators, drains, curettes, tubes, tenaculums, scopes, sutures, stents, screws, wires, pins, scissors, rongeurs, rasps, rods, retractors, needles, lasers, clamps, knives, and guides.

- ☐ Medications administered before, during, and after surgical intervention for sedation, pain control, nausea, etc.

RESOURCES FOR STUDY

1. *The Language of Medicine*
   Chapter 5: Digestive System, pp. 145–169.
   Chapter 6: Additional Suffixes and Digestive System Terminology, pp. 185–196.
   Chapter 7: Urinary Anatomy, p. 215–227.
   Chapter 8: Female Reproductive Anatomy, pp. 254–261, 273–274.
   Chapter 9: Male Reproductive Anatomy, pp. 306–311.
   Chapter 15: Musculoskeletal System Anatomy, pp. 563–573, 593–594.
   Chapter 16: Skin, pp. 630–632.

2. *Memmler's Structure and Function of the Human Body*
   Chapter 1: Organization of the Human Body, pp. 3–16.
   Chapter 5: The Integumentary System, pp. 73–82.
   Chapter 6: The Skeleton: Bones and Joints, pp. 85–109.
   Chapter 7: The Muscular System, pp. 111–133.

3. *Laboratory Tests & Diagnostic Procedures in Medicine*
   Chapter 16: Normal Anatomy and Histology, pp. 225–250.

4. *The AAMT Book of Style for Medical Transcription*
   Sutures, pp. 380–381.

5. *Pharmacology for Health Professionals*
   Chapter 9: Anesthetic Drugs, pp. 132–139.

6. *Understanding Pharmacology for Health Professionals*
   Chapter 31: Anesthetics, pp. 365–372.
   Chapter 32: Intravenous Fluids and Blood Products, pp. 373–380.

7. *Prentice Hall Health's Complete Review of Surgery Technology.*

8. *Introduction to Surgery.*

9. *Berry & Kohn's Operating Room Technique.*

SAMPLE REPORTS

The following three reports are examples of reports you might encounter while transcribing general and plastic surgery.

OPERATIVE REPORT

DATE OF PROCEDURE
04/08/05

PREOPERATIVE DIAGNOSIS
Recurrent pregnancy loss.

POSTOPERATIVE DIAGNOSES
Recurrent pregnancy loss; small, septate uterus; and partial right hydrosalpinx.

SURGEON
John Cutem, MD.

PROCEDURE
1. Hysteroscopy.
2. Incision of uterine septum (septoplasty).
3. Hysterosalpingogram.
4. Endometrial biopsy with cultures.

COMPLICATIONS
None.

ESTIMATED BLOOD LOSS
Minimal.

ANESTHESIA
IV sedation.

FINDINGS AT SURGERY
On hysteroscopy, the patient had a small septate uterus, which was incised. This was a small to moderate-sized septum. The uterine cavity itself otherwise was within normal limits without any evidence of any indentations from fibroids, and she did not have any polyps. She does have intramural fibroids, but they do not appear to be impinging on the uterine cavity. Endometrial biopsy was taken for cultures. Hysterosalpingogram was performed that showed the uterus to have an arcuate shape. The left tube was patent with some delay of dye coming out the distal end of the tube. The right tube was dilated. There was some dye extruding from the tube; therefore it was not completely occluded. However, it is a partial hydrosalpinx.

DETAILS OF PROCEDURE
The patient was prepped and draped in sterile fashion and placed in dorsal lithotomy position. Next, a speculum was placed in the vagina, and the anterior lip of the cervix was grasped with a single-toothed tenaculum. Cervix was gently dilated and hysteroscope was introduced into the endometrial cavity. Using saline as distention media, the endometrial cavity was inspected. A small

(continued)

septum was visualized, and scissors were used to excise it. The remainder of the cavity was within normal limits. After this, the hysteroscope was removed, and a curette was placed. A small specimen of the endometrium was removed and sent for anaerobic and aerobic cultures. Next, a balloon catheter was placed in the endometrial cavity, and hysterosalpingogram was performed.

The uterus appeared to be of approximately normal contour and shape, with small arcuate configuration at the fundal aspect of the uterus. The left tube was first filled with a moderate amount of dye and spill was visualized. Rugae were not clearly visualized. There appeared to be some delay of spill of the tube after 5 minutes. The right tube was with some delayed fill. After a fair amount of dye was placed in the tube, there was some extrusion of dye. She had a slight hydrosalpinx of the right side based on 5-minute film. The dye was delayed in the right fallopian tube. At 5 minutes, there was no dye left in the uterus.

The patient tolerated the procedure well. All instruments and sponge counts were correct. The patient was sent to recovery room in stable condition.

OPERATIVE REPORT

PREOPERATIVE DIAGNOSIS
Left inguinal hernia.

POSTOPERATIVE DIAGNOSIS
Left direct inguinal hernia.

SURGEON
John Cutem, MD.

PROCEDURE
Cooper ligament repair of left direct inguinal hernia with Marlex mesh.

ANESTHESIA
General.

DETAILS OF PROCEDURE
The patient was placed in the supine position and his left groin was prepped and draped. An oblique incision was made in the left groin and carried down through the external oblique fascia. The spermatic cord was mobilized and the floor of the canal was cleaned out. The ilioinguinal and iliohypogastric nerves were mobilized and resected out of the field. The cremasteric fibers were divided and ligated with silk ties, and the cord was skeletonized. A cord lipoma was also removed. There was no indirect hernia, but there was a moderately large direct hernia coming out medial to the epigastric vessels. I then incised the transversalis fascia from the pubic tubercle out to the internal ring without dividing the inferior epigastric vessels. The Cooper ligament was cleaned off from the pubic tubercle, out to and including the medial wall of the femoral vein. The conjoined tendon was cleaned off above and mobilized with a relaxing incision in the usual place. A Cooper ligament repair was then done with interrupted 0 silk sutures, bringing the conjoined tendon down to the Cooper ligament out to the femoral space. Two transition stitches were placed from the Cooper ligament up to the anterior femoral sheath to close off the femoral space. The conjoined tendon did come down to the Cooper ligament with a minimal amount of tension. The remainder of the stitch brought the conjoined tendon down to the shelving edge of the Cooper ligament out to the internal ring. After tying and cutting all the stitches, I could place only a Kelly clamp on the internal ring. A piece of Marlex mesh was soaked in antibiotic solution, cut to size, and sutured into the relaxing incision defect with a running Prolene stitch. The external oblique fascia was then closed over the cord with a running chromic stitch. The subcutaneous was irrigated and closed with interrupted chromic stitches. The wound was closed with staples and was injected with 10 mL of 0.5% Marcaine with epinephrine during closure.

A dressing was placed, and the patient was taken to recovery in stable condition.

OPERATIVE REPORT

PREOPERATIVE DIAGNOSES
Bilateral hypermastia, neck ache, backache, intertrigo, and breast asymmetry.

POSTOPERATIVE DIAGNOSES
Bilateral hypermastia, neck ache, backache, intertrigo, and breast asymmetry.

SURGEON
John Cutem, MD.

PROCEDURE
Bilateral reduction mammoplasties.

ANESTHESIA
General.

DRAINS
15-mm Blake.

ESTIMATED BLOOD LOSS
200 mL.

INDICATIONS
This is a 49-year-old female with worsening problems of backache and neck ache because of the size of her breasts. She tried nonoperative measures without success. Plan today was for bilateral breast reduction. I discussed with her the options that were available, the risks, the benefits, and alternatives, including no treatment, and possible consequences.

DETAILS OF PROCEDURE
After adequate anesthesia, the patient was prepped and draped in the usual sterile fashion. She had been marked in the sitting position. She had a modified inferomedial pedicle created with epithelialization. She then had resection of tissue, mostly laterally and minimal superiorly. Once this had been accomplished, the nipple-areola was on the pedicle and it was about 42–44 mm in diameter. Bleeders were controlled with an electrocoagulation unit. A couple of bleeders had to be ligated with 3-0 Vicryl suture.

After this had been completed, she was closed with inverted 2-0 PDS, inverted 3-0 Vicryl, and subcuticular pullout 4-0 Vicryl. She had a few interrupted 4-0 Prolene stitches. Nipple was inset with inverted using 3-0 Vicryl and subcuticular pullout 4-0 Monocryl. Each side had been irrigated with saline. She had 15-French round Blake drain placed. It was sutured in with 4-0 Prolene. Same was done on the contralateral side. On her left side, she had 965 g removed; on her right side, she had 761 g removed. She was placed in the upright position. She was about equal in size. She then had her chest dressed with Adaptic, 4 x 4, slough, soft Kling, and an Ace bandage. The patient tolerated the procedure well. She was taken to postanesthesia care area in satisfactory condition.

REVIEW QUESTIONS

The goal of these questions is to test your knowledge in the areas of general and plastic surgery.

Directions: Select the correct answer for each of the multiple-choice questions provided below. *Answers are provided at the end of this chapter.*

1. Which of the following terms means to cut off or remove?
   A. resect
   B. biopsy
   C. incise
   D. suture

2. Adipose tissue is composed of
   A. muscle.
   B. bone.
   C. fat.
   D. intestines.

3. Viscera refers to
   A. bones.
   B. joints.
   C. brain.
   D. organs.

4. Anesthesia obtained by means of injection of an anesthetic drug directly to the operative site or by topical application is called
   A. general.
   B. local.
   C. regional.
   D. spinal.

5. Which of the following terms refers to the belly or anterior of the body?
   A. ventral
   B. posterior
   C. abdominal
   D. thoracic

6. Which position would have the patient lying face down?
   A. dorsal
   B. supine
   C. prone
   D. Trendelenburg

7. An incision 15 cm caudal to T1 would be
   A. below T1 (toward the end of the spine).
   B. above T1 (toward the head).
   C. to the right of T1.
   D. to the left of T1.

8. Which of the following is commonly used to drain the urinary bladder during a surgical procedure?
   A. Hickman catheter
   B. Broviac catheter
   C. Swan-Ganz catheter
   D. Foley catheter

9. This is commonly used in surgery to temporarily arrest the flow of blood to or from a distal part by applying pressure.
   A. Ace wrap
   B. dry dressing
   C. Steri-Strips
   D. tourniquet

10. Which of the following is a common technique for inserting a catheter, especially during cardiac procedures?
    A. Mitrofanoff
    B. Pomeroy
    C. Seldinger
    D. Tzanck

11. Which of the following is an alternative way to provide nourishment to a patient who is unable to take food by mouth?
    A. through a T tube
    B. through an endotracheal tube
    C. through a PEG tube
    D. through an ileostomy

12. Removal of dead or necrotic tissue is called
    A. exsanguination.
    B. debridement.
    C. biopsy.
    D. resection.

13. Epidural anesthesia is a type of
    A. general anesthesia.
    B. local anesthesia.
    C. intravenous anesthesia.
    D. regional anesthesia.

14. Which of the following is a local anesthetic?
    A. Labetolol
    B. Lidocaine
    C. clonidine
    D. Trileptal

15. The suffix -rraphy means
    A. surgical suturing.
    B. surgical opening.
    C. flowing out.
    D. excessive discharge.

16. Anastomosis means
    A. surgical fixation.
    B. surgical removal.
    C. operative union of vessels or nerves.
    D. surgical excision.

17. The medical term for breast implant surgery is
    A. aggregation mammotomy.
    B. augmentation mammaplasty.
    C. inframammary amplification.
    D. intermammary expansion.

18. Approximating wound edges means
    A. bringing the edges together.
    B. trimming the edges.
    C. cauterizing to stop bleeding.
    D. bandaging the wound.

19. A surgical instrument that holds back the edges of a surgical incision is a
    A. catheter.
    B. retractor.
    C. dilator.
    D. trocar.

20. Removal of the voice box is called
    A. laryngectomy.
    B. pharyngotomy.
    C. pharyngectomy.
    D. tracheotomy.

21. Which of the following suffixes denotes a permanent surgical opening to the outside of the body?
    A. -ectomy
    B. -opsy
    C. -stomy
    D. -oma

22. Which of the following suffixes denotes a surgical repair or restoration?
    A. -centesis
    B. -cleisis
    C. -plasty
    D. -sect

23. A pedicle flap is also known as a (an)
    A. jump flap.
    B. island flap.
    C. skin flap.
    D. sliding flap.

24. Which of the following terms means removal of a kidney?
    A. nephrectomy
    B. cystectomy
    C. gastrectomy
    D. orchiectomy

25. Which of the following is a suffix that means surgical fixation?
    A. -clasis
    B. -pexy
    C. -tripsy
    D. -stenosis

26. A continuous suture is also known as a (an)
    A. approximation.
    B. figure-of-eight.
    C. purse-string.
    D. uninterrupted.

27. Which of the following is an instrument used to grasp a structure for compression or traction?
    A. forceps
    B. speculum
    C. retractor
    D. curette

28. Which of the following instruments is used for electrosurgical dissection and hemostasis?
    A. tenaculum
    B. Bovie
    C. sound
    D. rongeur

29. Which of the following is a sharply pointed surgical instrument contained in a cannula?
    A. biopsy needle
    B. columella forceps
    C. osteotome
    D. trocar

30. An incision made in the abdomen through the rectus muscle will reveal the
    A. peritoneum.
    B. chorion.
    C. perineum.
    D. dura mater.

 Please see the accompanying CD for additional review materials for this section.

ANSWER KEY

REVIEW QUESTIONS ANSWER KEY

1. A	6. C	11. C	16. C	21. C	26. D
2. C	7. A	12. B	17. B	22. C	27. A
3. D	8. D	13. D	18. A	23. C	28. B
4. B	9. D	14. B	19. B	24. A	29. D
5. A	10. C	15. A	20. A	25. B	30. A

12

Gastroenterology

OBJECTIVES CHECKLIST

A prepared exam candidate will know:

☐ All combining forms, prefixes, and suffixes related to the body system.

☐ Sequential structures of the digestive system, beginning with the mouth and ending with the anus.

☐ Primary function and role of those structures in the digestive process.

☐ Anatomy and function of the accessory organs, including the liver, gallbladder, and pancreas.

☐ Role and function of the hepatic portal system.

☐ Role and function of the primary digestive enzymes.

☐ Common gastrointestinal signs, symptoms, and disease processes.

☐ Imaging and diagnostic studies used in the identification and treatment of gastrointestinal disorders.

☐ Laboratory studies related to the diagnosis and treatment of gastrointestinal dysfunction and disease.

☐ Common medications indicated and prescribed for gastrointestinal symptoms and diseases.

RESOURCES FOR STUDY

1. *Bates' Guide to Physical Examination and History Taking*
   Chapter 10: The Abdomen, pp. 359–409.
   Chapter 13: The Anus, Rectum, and Prostate, pp. 459–471.

2. *The Language of Medicine*
   Chapter 5: Digestive System, pp. 139–184.
   Chapter 6: Additional Suffixes and Digestive System Terminology, pp. 185–211.

3. *Memmler's Structure and Function of the Human Body*
   Chapter 17: Digestion, pp. 305–320.

4. *Memmler's The Human Body in Health and Disease*
   Chapter 19: Digestion, pp. 384–405; Study Guide, pp. 292–311.

5. *H&P: A Nonphysician's Guide to the Medical History and Physical Examination*
   Chapter 10: Review of Systems: Gastrointestinal, pp. 89–96.
   Chapter 25: Examination of the Abdomen, pp. 235–248.

6. *Human Diseases*
   Chapter 11: Diseases of the Digestive System, pp. 153–172.

7. *Laboratory Tests & Diagnostic Procedures in Medicine*
   Chapter 8: Examination of the Digestive Tract and Genitourinary System, pp. 107–118.
   Chapter 20: Chemical Examination of the Blood, pp. 355–400.
   Chapter 21: Microbiology (Bacteriology, Mycology, Virology and Parasitology), pp. 401–409.
   Chapter 24: Examination of the Urine, Stool, and Other Fluids and Materials (Laboratory Examination of Stool), pp. 442–443.

8. *A Manual of Laboratory and Diagnostic Tests*
   Chapter 4: Stool Studies, pp. 264–288.
   Chapter 9: Nuclear Medicine Studies, pp. 652–704.
   Chapter 10: X-Ray Studies, pp. 705–759.
   Chapter 11: Cytologic, Histologic, and Genetic Studies, pp. 760–818.
   Chapter 12: Endoscopic Studies, pp. 819–861.
   Chapter 13: Ultrasound Studies, pp. 862–899.

9. *Using Medical Terminology: A Practical Approach*
   Chapter 14: Digestive System, pp. 633–706.

10. *Pharmacology for Health Professionals*
    Chapter 21: Drugs That Affect the Gastrointestinal System, pp. 299–321.

11. *Understanding Pharmacology for Health Professionals*
    Chapter 13: Gastrointestinal Drugs, p. 115–136.

12. *Medical Terminology: The Language of Health Care*
    Chapter 14: Gastrointestinal System, pp. 437–481.

SAMPLE REPORTS

The following five reports are examples of reports you might encounter while transcribing gastroenterology.

OPERATIVE REPORT

SURGEON
John Smith, MD.

PREOPERATIVE DIAGNOSIS
Biliary atresia.

POSTOPERATIVE DIAGNOSIS
Biliary atresia.

PROCEDURES PERFORMED
1. Kasai procedure (Roux-en-Y hepatic portoenterostomy).
2. Liver biopsy.

ANESTHESIA
General endotracheal.

ESTIMATED BLOOD LOSS
Approximately 10 mL.

SPECIMENS SUBMITTED
1. Wedge liver biopsy from segment IV of the liver.
2. Gallbladder with atretic extrahepatic biliary tree.

COMPLICATIONS
None apparent.

JUSTIFICATION FOR PROCEDURE
The patient is a 7-week-old male who presented to his pediatrician with jaundice. Evaluation, including right upper quadrant ultrasound and nuclear hepatobiliary scans, revealed evidence of biliary atresia. The patient is now being taken to the operating room for exploration with confirmation of the diagnosis and a Kasai procedure.

PROCEDURE IN DETAIL
In the operating room, general endotracheal anesthesia was induced. The abdomen and chest were prepped with Betadine and draped sterilely. The initial incision was a right upper quadrant subcostal incision. The abdominal wall was traversed using the Bovie electrocautery until the peritoneal cavity was entered. The falciform ligament was divided and ligated with silk suture. The liver appeared to be congested with bile. The liver was firm but was not hard or sclerotic as would be expected with cirrhosis. The gallbladder was noted to be atretic and, upon initial observation of the hepatoduodenal ligament, the extrahepatic biliary tree was not evident.

(continued)

We now performed a liver biopsy to evaluate for the presence or absence of bile ducts. Along the free edge of segment IV of the liver, two figure-of-8 Vicryl sutures were placed in a wedge configuration for hemostasis. The segment of liver isolated by these two sutures was sharply excised with a scalpel. This segment of liver was immediately sent to pathology for evaluation. Their initial report revealed evidence of microscopic biliary radicles. Thus, the patient had evidence of microscopic bile ducts and a Kasai procedure was now the procedure of choice.

Before performing the Kasai, we performed an intraoperative cholangiogram via the atretic gallbladder to further prove that there was no patent extrahepatic biliary tree. A small hole was made in the dome of the gallbladder into which a cholangiogram catheter was placed. This catheter was secured with suture. Now, using fluoroscopic assistance, a cholangiogram was obtained. This cholangiogram failed to demonstrate evidence of an extrahepatic or intrahepatic biliary tree. Upon entering the gallbladder, a small amount of white bile was encountered, further confirming the non-patency of the biliary tree. With pressure, the contrast extravasated from the gallbladder but still failed to fill a biliary tree. Thus, with the preoperative and intraoperative data, we were confident of the diagnosis of biliary atresia and proceeded with the Kasai procedure.

The next step was dissection of the gallbladder down from its peritoneal attachments at the undersurface of the liver. The entire atretic biliary tree was dissected out on the hepatoduodenal ligament, taking care to identify and preserve the vascular structures in the hepatoduodenal ligament, including the portal vein and its bifurcation as well as the hepatic artery and its bifurcation. The dissection was carried up to the porta hepatis where a disk of liver tissue was excised in continuity with the atretic biliary tree. This disk was carved out of the inner surface of the liver, the limits of which were on the left and right hepatic artery on either side. After removing this disk of liver and sending it to pathology for evaluation, close observation revealed bile emanating from the raw surface of the liver where the disk had been excised. The drainage from the atretic right hepatic duct was brisk and, with time, the drainage from the left side also appeared to be good. Hemostasis along the raw edge of the liver was obtained with Gelfoam and thrombin.

After gaining hemostasis, we turned our attention to the construction of a Roux-en-Y limb in order to perform our portoenterostomy. A window in the small bowel mesentery was made in the mid-jejunum. The bowel was transected at this point with an Endo GIA stapler, and 45 cm distal to this staple line the bowel was marked with a silk suture, thus noting the point of construction of the Roux-en-Y. The proximal end of the stapled bowel was now brought down to the point at which we placed our tag for construction of the Roux-en-Y limb.

Silk sutures of 5-0 were used to align the two segments of bowel. The anastomosis was constructed such that it was slightly larger than the lumen of each segment of bowel. A two-layer, hand-sewn anastomosis was now performed. The outside layer was constructed of interrupted 5-0 silk sutures and the inner layer was constructed of 5-0 Vicryl sutures, with a running, locking stitch for the back row and, after turning the corner, a Connell stitch for the top row. The order of the anastomosis proceeded with placement of the silk sutures for the back row, followed by the Vicryl sutures circumferentially, followed by completion of the anastomosis by Lembert suturing the front side with the 5-0 interrupted silk suture. The anastomosis was hemostatic and widely patent. Also, there were no kinks or twists in the anastomosis.

(continued)

The small bowel was now replaced into the peritoneal cavity, and the limb was brought up to the porta for construction of our biliary anastomosis. We removed the Gelfoam from the area and found it to be hemostatic. There was good bile drainage still, as manifested by saturation of the Gelfoam and gauze with biliary fluid. The liver surface was not as fibrotic as often seen in biliary atresia, and we were able to place our sutures in the liver and Glisson's capsule circumferentially in order to perform our anastomosis.

The biliary anastomosis was constructed as a hepatic portoenterostomy, suturing the side of the Roux to the porta. The anastomosis was constructed as a single-layer, hand-sewn anastomosis using 5-0 Prolene suture in an interrupted fashion. The limits of our anastomosis medially and laterally were the left and right hepatic arteries, respectively. Posteriorly, the limit of our anastomosis was the portal vein and anteriorly, the fibrotic edge of the liver and Glisson capsule. We proceeded first by placing the back row of interrupted sutures and then, after tying these down, the front row was constructed. The anastomosis was without kinks or evidence of a leak. In order to prevent kinking of the bowel just distal to the anastomosis, the limb was tacked to the undersurface of the liver a few centimeters from our anastomosis using silk suture.

The abdominal cavity was now copiously irrigated with warmed saline solution. Wound closure was carried out in the usual fashion, and the patient was transported to the pediatric surgery special care unit in stable condition, having tolerated the procedure well.

OPERATIVE REPORT

PREOPERATIVE DIAGNOSIS
Chronic cholecystitis and cholelithiasis.

POSTOPERATIVE DIAGNOSIS
Chronic cholecystitis and cholelithiasis.

OPERATION
Laparoscopic cholecystectomy and intraoperative cholangiogram.

ANESTHESIA
General endotracheal anesthesia.

PROCEDURE IN DETAIL
With the patient in the supine position, satisfactory general anesthesia was given. The patient had a Foley catheter and sequential compression devices were in place on both legs. The patient received 2 g of Ancef intravenously. The abdomen was then prepped with Betadine and draped in the usual manner.

The Hasson technique was utilized, making a small incision below the umbilicus. Bleeders were controlled with the electrocautery. The midline was grasped with a straight Kocher and lifted upwards. The midline was identified and entered with a small hemostat. I was able to introduce my index finger and there were no adhesions around the entrance. Two sutures of 0 Vicryl were placed in each corner, and then the Hasson trocar was introduced and secured to the opening.

The next step was to place the video camera. The patient was then placed in reverse Trendelenburg position, slightly tilted to the left. The patient presented the left lobe of the liver, which appeared to be covering the gallbladder area.

The next step was to make a small incision in the epigastric area, and under direct vision, a 10-mm trocar was introduced and advanced without difficulty. The gallbladder was identified and lifted in an upward position from the fundus with the help of the dolphin dissector.

Then 2 small openings were made in the lateral abdominal wall utilizing the 5-mm trocars. Then the tissue holder was utilized to pull the gallbladder by the fundus in an upward position, and the second one was at the infundibulum of the gallbladder with a small amount of lateral traction in order to expose Calot triangle. The anatomy was identified and dissected carefully with the dolphin dissector. The cystic duct at the junction of the gallbladder was identified, and also the cystic artery was identified, and then proximal and distal control was carried out with Ligaclips and transected.

Next, utilizing the peanut pusher for gallbladder surgery, I was able to expose very well the cystic duct, and also the junction with the common bile duct was identified. The cystic duct appeared to be going around the common bile duct. The next step was to place a Ligaclip at the junction of the gallbladder with the cystic duct, and then, with the Endoshears scissors, a small opening was made in the cystic duct. The next step was to place a #14 Cholangiocath into the abdominal wall, again under direct vision, and then the Reddick catheter for intraoperative cholangiogram was utilized. I was able to introduce the catheter into the cystic duct without difficulty. The small balloon was inflated, and then the patient underwent the intraoperative cholangiogram.

(continued)

The cholangiogram showed the dye going into the duodenum very well, with no evidence of filling defects, and the upper radicles, right and left, as well. The x-rays were interpreted by the radiologist and reported as normal. The Cholangiocath was deflated and removed, and then the cystic duct was controlled with a Ligaclip and transected. The gallbladder was then removed from the liver bed with the electrocautery and removed with an Endocatch through the epigastric area.

The liver bed was then inspected and a small area of oozing was controlled at the upper aspect of the liver edge. Another area down into the lower third, lateral aspect of the liver, was controlled with a small Ligaclip. A small piece of Surgicel was also left in the area. The abdominal cavity was irrigated with a copious amount of saline and aspirated. There was no evidence of any active bleeding from the operative area during this procedure. The epigastric port and the lateral port were removed. The next step was to remove the video camera. Then the infra-umbilical incision was approached, and the fascia was closed with figure-of-8 sutures of 0 Vicryl. The subcutaneous tissue was then approximated with 3-0 chromic catgut, and then a subcuticular suture was used for the incisions at the epigastric and infraumbilical areas.

The sponge, needle and instrument counts were given as correct. Blood loss was about 50 mL. The patient was then transferred to the recovery room in stable condition.

PROGRESS NOTE

PROBLEM
Hepatitis C, genotype 1a variant.

SUBJECTIVE
The patient returns for followup evaluation of hepatitis C on Pegasys and ribavirin therapy. The patient is doing much better on therapy. His mood is better. He has fewer physical symptoms. Anorexia is still a problem. He complains of itching. He was recently seen by Dr. Smith and was started on a Medrol Dosepak and has now almost completed therapy.

OBJECTIVE
VITAL SIGNS: Within normal limits. The patient is afebrile. Weight 160 pounds.
ABDOMEN: Soft, without masses, organomegaly, or ascites.

LABORATORY DATA
The patient's hemoglobin and hematocrit on 11/22/04 were 10 and 32, respectively. The liver function tests were normal. Hepatitis C RNA titer by PCR was less than 10 IU/mL.

ASSESSMENT
Normal liver function tests and low viral titer on Pegasys and ribavirin after 12 weeks of therapy; however, I could not find a pretreatment viral load. We will consider this an early virologic response.

PLAN
Continue treatment for another 3 months. CBC and CMP today. Follow up in 4 weeks. Will draw AFP titers to screen for hepatocellular carcinoma. I have advised the patient not to take prednisone in the future without consulting a gastroenterologist.

PROCEDURE

PROCEDURE PERFORMED
Esophagogastroduodenoscopy with gastrostomy tube placement.

INDICATIONS FOR PROCEDURE
The patient is a 79-year-old woman admitted to the hospital with generalized weakness. The patient has had very poor oral intake. Gastrostomy tube placement is requested to facilitate nutrition as well as the administration of medications.

MEDICATIONS GIVEN FOR THE PROCEDURE
Demerol 25 mg IV push plus Versed 1 mg IV push in incremental doses.

INSTRUMENT USED
Pentax EG-2901 upper endoscope.

PROCEDURE IN DETAIL
The patient was placed on her back and the above medications were given. When she appeared adequately sedated, the instrument was placed into the oral cavity and advanced beyond the upper esophageal sphincter into the stomach, into the pylorus, and into the second portion of the duodenum. The duodenal mucosa was unremarkable. The pylorus was symmetrical. The gastric body had scattered areas of erythema and old heme pigment. On retroflexion, no significant hiatal hernia was identified. The gastric mucosa was otherwise unremarkable.

GASTROSTOMY TUBE PLACEMENT
The site of the gastrostomy tube placement was determined by transillumination of the endoscope light through the anterior abdominal wall. A site was chosen in the left upper quadrant. This was confirmed by seeing an indentation of the gastric mucosa when external pressure was applied to the abdomen at that site. The area was then cleansed with Betadine and anesthetized with 1% Xylocaine. A small incision was made at the site, and then a Seldinger needle was introduced through the incision into the gastric lumen under endoscopic guidance.

A guide wire was threaded through the hub of the needle, grasped with a snare, and then pulled out through the endoscope, and the endoscope and guide wire were withdrawn from the patient. A 20-French Wilson-Cooke gastrostomy tube was then threaded over the guide wire, advanced into the oral cavity, into the stomach, and then out through the incision in the abdominal wall. When this was completed, the endoscope was reintroduced into the stomach and confirmed good placement of the inner bolster of the gastrostomy tube. The esophagus was examined as the endoscope was withdrawn, and this appeared unremarkable.

The patient tolerated the procedure well and no complications were encountered during the procedure.

IMPRESSION
1. Successful placement of a 20-French Wilson-Cooke gastrostomy tube.
2. Scattered areas of gastric mucosal erythema.

RECOMMENDATIONS
As per postprocedure orders.

PROCEDURE

PROCEDURES
Upper endoscopy and colonoscopy.

INDICATIONS FOR PROCEDURES
The patient is a 52-year-old man admitted to the hospital with anemia, diffuse abdominal pain, and diarrhea.

MEDICATIONS GIVEN FOR THE PROCEDURE
Demerol 100 mg IV push plus Versed 5 mg IV push in incremental doses.

INSTRUMENT USED
Pentax EG-2901 upper endoscope and EC-3801-L colonoscope.

PROCEDURE IN DETAIL
UPPER ENDOSCOPY: The patient was placed in the left lateral decubitus position. The above-noted medications were given. When he appeared adequately sedated, the instrument was placed into the oral cavity and advanced beyond the upper esophageal sphincter into the stomach, into the pylorus, and into the second portion of the duodenum. The duodenal mucosa was unremarkable. The pylorus was symmetrical. The gastric mucosa had a diffuse erythematous appearance with some suggestion of nodularity. This was seen primarily in the body, but the antrum and cardia were also involved. Biopsies were taken from the antrum for CLOtest and randomly from the gastric body for routine histology.

On retroflexion, a hiatal hernia was identified. The instrument was pulled back into the esophagus and the Z-line was distinct. The esophageal mucosa appeared unremarkable.

The patient tolerated the procedure well and no complications were encountered during the procedure.

IMPRESSION
1. Diffuse nodularity of upper gastric mucosa.
2. Otherwise normal upper endoscopy.

COLONOSCOPY: After the above, the patient was turned 180 degrees. The instrument was placed into the rectum and, utilizing the push-pull technique, advanced to the cecum. There was moderate tortuosity of the colonic wall.

The instrument was pulled back from the cecum with careful examination of the colonic mucosa. In the proximal portion of the colon, extending from the cecum to the proximal to midtransverse colon, the colonic mucosa was characterized by the presence of multiple, small nodular areas averaging from 3 to 5 mm in diameter. Some of these had central umbilication with focal mucosal erosion. Biopsies were taken for routine histology from some of these areas. The more distal portion of the colon had a much smaller number of these areas.

The instrument was retroflexed in the rectum and internal hemorrhoids were present.

The patient tolerated the procedure well and no complications were encountered during the procedure.

(continued)

IMPRESSION

1. Diffuse gastric mucosal erythema.
2. Hiatal hernia.
3. Proximal colonic mucosal lymphoid hyperplasia with central umbilication.
4. Internal hemorrhoids.
5. Tortuosity of colonic wall.

RECOMMENDATIONS

1. Check CLOtest and treat if this is positive.
2. Tagamet 400 mg b.i.d. for approximately 4 to 6 weeks.
3. Stool softeners as needed to avoid constipation.
4. Colonoscopy in 10 years.

REVIEW QUESTIONS

The goal of these questions is to test your knowledge in the area of gastroenterology.

Directions: Select the correct answer for each of the multiple-choice questions provided below. *Answers are provided at the end of this chapter.*

1. The small soft tissue projection that hangs from the soft palate and aids in the production of sound and speech is called the
   A. palate.
   B. papillae.
   C. tonsils.
   D. uvula.

2. Prevacid and Prilosec are used to treat
   A. GERD.
   B. diarrhea.
   C. constipation.
   D. nausea.

3. Which of the following terms is used to describe involuntary, progressive, and rhythmic contraction of the intestines that propels contents onward?
   A. intussusception
   B. osmosis
   C. diffusion
   D. peristalsis

4. The upper portion of the stomach is called the
   A. antrum.
   B. body.
   C. fundus.
   D. sphincter.

5. The folds contained within the mucous membrane lining the stomach are called
   A. diverticula.
   B. papillae.
   C. rugae.
   D. villi.

6. Which of the following is transcribed correctly?
   A. Colonoscopy was carried out to the cecum and terminal ileum. There were also small internal hemorrhoids and occasional diverticulum seen.
   B. Colonoscopy was carried out to the cecum and terminal ilium. There were also small internal hemorrhoids and occasional diverticula seen.
   C. Colonoscopy was carried out to the cecum and terminal ileum. There were also small internal hemorrhoids and occasional diverticula seen.
   D. Colonoscopy was carried out to the cecum and terminal ilium. There were also small internal hemorrhoids and occasional diverticulum seen.

7. Hepatitis B is caused by
   A. a bacterium.
   B. a virus.
   C. a drug.
   D. alcohol.

8. Phenergan and Reglan are used to treat
   A. nausea.
   B. jaundice.
   C. PUD.
   D. H. pylori.

9. ALT, AST, bilirubin, and alkaline phosphatase are
   A. tests to assess liver function.
   B. pancreatic enzymes.
   C. digestive enzymes.
   D. contained in bile.

10. Pedunculated and sessile describe
    A. villi.
    B. ulcers.
    C. polyps.
    D. hernias.

11. The combining form of *choledoch/o* refers to the
    A. cecum.
    B. colon.
    C. bile duct.
    D. intestines.

12. Which of the following is transcribed correctly?
    A. The patient presents to the ER status post motor vehicle accident with abominable injuries and possible fracture of the ilium.
    B. The patient presents to the ER status post motor vehicle accident with abdominal injuries and possible fracture of the ileum.
    C. The patient presents to the ER status post motor vehicle accident with abominable injuries and possible fracture of the ileum.
    D. The patient presents to the ER status post motor vehicle accident with abdominal injuries and possible fracture of the ilium.

13. A barium swallow is also known as a (an)
    A. upper GI series.
    B. ERCP.
    C. guaiac test.
    D. colonoscopy.

14. Epsom salt and milk of magnesia are used as
    A. antiemetics.
    B. contrast media.
    C. laxatives.
    D. antacids.

15. Which of the following is transcribed correctly?
    A. The patient presents today complaining of ascitic stomach, for which she has taken antacids, and colic in the left lower quadrant.
    B. The patient presents today complaining of acidic stomach, for which she has taken antacids, and colic in the left lower quadrant.
    C. The patient presents today complaining of ascitic stomach, for which she has taken antacids, and cholic in the left lower quadrant.
    D. The patient presents today complaining of acidic stomach, for which she has taken antacids, and cholic in the left lower quadrant.

16. The medical term for surgical removal of the gallbladder is
    A. cholecystectomy.
    B. enterostomy.
    C. colectomy.
    D. pylorotomy.

17. An abnormal twisting of the intestines resulting in intestinal blockage is a (an)
    A. intussusception.
    B. hernia.
    C. prolapse.
    D. volvulus.

18. A chronic, intermittent inflammatory bowel disease that causes bloody diarrhea with mucus and lesions in the lining of the large intestine is known as
    A. gastroenteritis.
    B. GERD.
    C. irritable bowel syndrome.
    D. ulcerative colitis.

19. Which of the following medications is used to treat diarrhea?
    A. Diuril
    B. senna
    C. Lomotil
    D. MiraLax

20. The part of the small intestine between the stomach and the jejunum is the
    A. cecum.
    B. duodenum.
    C. ileum.
    D. pylorus.

21. Steatorrhea is
    A. fat in the stool.
    B. bile in the stool.
    C. diarrhea caused by steroids.
    D. mucus in the stool.

22. Which of the following is transcribed correctly?
    A. The patient presents with a 5-day history of diarrhea and cramping after returning from Mexico. Stool will be sent for O&P.
    B. The patient presents with a 5 day history of diarrhea and cramping after returning from Mexico. Stool will be sent for ONP.
    C. The patient presents with a 5-day history of diarrhea and cramping after returning from Mexico. Stool will be sent for ONP.
    D. The patient presents with a 5 day history of diarrhea and cramping after returning from Mexico. Stool will be sent for O&P.

23. A tear in the mucosa at the gastroesophageal junction causing bleeding is known as
    A. ileus.
    B. achalasia.
    C. Mallory-Weiss syndrome.
    D. Prader-Willi syndrome.

24. Examination of the upper gastrointestinal tract with a fiberoptic instrument is called
    A. cystoscopy.
    B. esophagogastroduodenoscopy.
    C. nasopharyngoscopy.
    D. pharyngorhinoscopy.

25. Passage of bright red blood from the rectum is called
    A. hematochezia.
    B. melena.
    C. flatus.
    D. hematemesis.

26. The prefix *entero-* means
    A. abdomen.
    B. enamel.
    C. intestine.
    D. lining.

27. The word gastric relates to
    A. duct.
    B. flatus.
    C. gallbladder.
    D. stomach.

28. The name of the procedure that establishes an artificial connection between the lumen of the colon and the skin is called a
    A. calicotomy.
    B. cheilotomy.
    C. cicatrectomy.
    D. colostomy.

29. A bariatric procedure to reduce the size of the stomach is called
    A. gastric bypass.
    B. duodenectomy.
    C. anastomosis.
    D. ileostomy.

30. Amylase and lipase are
    A. hormones.
    B. components of bile acids.
    C. digestive enzymes.
    D. used to treat gallstones.

 Please see the accompanying CD for additional review materials for this section.

ANSWER KEY

REVIEW QUESTIONS ANSWER KEY

1. D	6. C	11. C	16. A	21. A	26. C
2. A	7. B	12. D	17. D	22. A	27. D
3. D	8. A	13. A	18. D	23. C	28. D
4. C	9. A	14. C	19. C	24. B	29. A
5. C	10. C	15. B	20. B	25. A	30. C

13

Neurology/Neurosurgery

OBJECTIVES CHECKLIST

A prepared exam candidate will know:

- ❏ Combining forms, prcfixcs, and suffixes related to the body system.
- ❏ Anatomical structures of the nervous system.
- ❏ Physiologic processes of the nervous system.
- ❏ Role of the nervous system as the communication network for the body.
- ❏ Imaging studies used in the identification and diagnosis of neurologic and neurosurgical diseases.
- ❏ Laboratory studies used in the diagnosis and treatment of neurologic symptoms, disorders, and diseases.
- ❏ Common medications prescribed for neurologic symptoms, disorders, and diseases.
- ❏ Transcription standards related to EEGs.

RESOURCES FOR STUDY

1. *Bates' Guide to Physical Examination and History Taking*
   Chapter 16: The Nervous System: Mental Status and Behavior, pp. 573–593.
   Chapter 17: The Nervous System: Cranial Nerves, Motor System, Sensory System, and Reflexes, pp. 595–667.

2. *The Language of Medicine*
   Chapter 10: Nervous System, pp. 333–382.

3. *Memmler's Structure and Function of the Human Body*
   Chapter 8: The Nervous System: The Spinal Cord and Spinal Nerves, pp. 137–156.
   Chapter 9: The Nervous System: The Brain and Cranial Nerves, pp. 159–175.

4. *Memmler's The Human Body in Health .and Disease*
   Chapter 9: The Nervous System: The Spinal Cord and Spinal Nerves, pp. 178–199; Study Guide, pp. 140–156.
   Chapter 10: The Nervous System: The Brain and Cranial Nerves, pp. 200–221; Study Guide, pp. 157–173.

5. *H&P: A Nonphysician's Guide to the Medical History and Physical Examination*
   Chapter 12: Review of Systems: Neuromuscular, pp. 107–116.
   Chapter 27: The Neurologic Examination, pp. 261–272.
   Chapter 28: The Formal Mental Status Examination, pp. 273–280.

6. *Human Diseases*
   Chapter 19: Diseases of the Nervous System, pp. 291–314.

7. *Laboratory Tests & Diagnostic Procedures in Medicine*
   Chapter 5: Electroencephalography, Electromyography, and Related Tests, pp. 61–62.

8. *A Manual of Laboratory and Diagnostic Tests*
   Chapter 5: Cerebrospinal Fluid Studies, pp. 289–315.
   Chapter 9: Nuclear Medicine Studies, pp. 652–704.
   Chapter 10: X-Ray Studies, pp. 705–759.
   Chapter 11: Cytologic, Histologic, and Genetic Studies, pp. 760–818.
   Chapter 16: Special Systems, Organ Functions, and Postmortem Studies, pp. 1012–1093.

9. *The AAMT Book of Style for Medical Transcription*
   Electroencephalographic Terms, pp. 159–160.

10. *Using Medical Terminology: A Practical Approach*
    Chapter 8: Nervous System and Special Senses, pp. 313–377.

11. *Pharmacology for Health Professionals*
    Unit II: Drugs That Affect the Neurologic System (Chapters 4–10), pp. 37–167.

12. *Understanding Pharmacology for Health Professionals*
    Chapter 24: Neurological Drugs, pp. 262–278.

13. *Medical Terminology: The Language of Health Care*
    Chapter 10: Nervous System, pp. 310–357.

SAMPLE REPORTS

The following five reports are examples of reports you might encounter while transcribing neurology and neurosurgery.

ELECTROENCEPHALOGRAM

HISTORY
The patient is an 82-year-old gentleman with a history of possible subclinical status epilepticus, given the persistent depressed neurological status.

DESCRIPTION OF PROCEDURE
Cerebral activity was grossly disorganized, with asynchrony between the two cerebral hemispheres. Cerebral activity over the left side consisted of medium- to high-amplitude, poorly sustained, 4-Hz to 5-Hz waveforms. Cerebral activity on the right hemisphere consisted of high-amplitude slow waves, often interspersed with spike and spike-and-wave complexes. Periods of attenuation of cerebral activity were noted to occur in the right cerebral hemisphere. At times, the spike and spike-and-wave complexes occurred in a periodic fashion. Superimposed low-amplitude beta activity was noted to occur over the left cerebral hemisphere.

The patient was reported to be obtunded throughout the tracing.

Simultaneous electrocardiogram recording revealed no cardiac arrhythmias.

Activation hyperventilation could not be performed; photic stimulation was not performed.

IMPRESSION
1. Periodic lateralizing epileptiform discharges over the right cerebral hemisphere, as may be seen following an ischemic insult.
2. Global disorganization and slowing of the cerebral activity signifying generalized encephalopathy.

ELECTROMYOGRAM

HISTORY
This is a 76-year-old right-handed gentleman who presents with a history of many months of worsening, intermittent burning, numbness, and tingling involving the hands, predominantly involving the thumbs, index, and middle fingers, somewhat more on the left than the right side. The symptoms lead to awakening around 4 a.m. He reports no significant weakness of the hands or tendency to drop objects, etc. There is no significant cervical pain. There is no history of pain involving the feet. There is a strong family history of carpal tunnel syndrome. There is no family history of diabetes.

EXAMINATION
Pertinent neurological examination shows weakness of the thenar muscles with slight atrophy, more on the left than the right side. There are sensory disturbances involving the palmar aspect of the hands. Positive Tinel sign. Negative median compression. Negative Phalen test bilaterally. Range of motion of the neck is painless though globally limited.

INTERPRETATION
1. Severe prolongation of the distal motor latencies, negligible compartment selection potentials, and reduction of motor conduction velocity in the right median nerve.
2. Marked prolongation of the resting motor latencies, reduction of compartment selection potentials, and normal conduction velocity in the left median nerve.
3. Prolongation of the distal motor latencies, reduction of the compartment selection potentials, and reduction of motor conduction velocities in both ulnar nerves.
4. Unobtainable F-wave latency of the right median nerve.
5. Prolongation of the F-wave latency in the left median nerve.
6. Marked prolongation of the distal motor latencies in both ulnar nerves.
7. Unobtainable NAP and SNAP amplitudes on the right median nerve.
8. Severe reduction of the NAP and SNAP amplitudes and moderate to severe reduction in sensory conduction velocity in the left median nerve.
9. Normal NAP and SNAP amplitudes and marked slowing of the sensory conduction velocity in both ulnar nerves.
10. Needle EMG of the muscles of the upper extremities reveals mild to moderate denervation changes involving the median-innervated hand muscles.

IMPRESSION
This study is consistent with bilateral sensorimotor median neuropathy at the wrists, as seen in association with carpal tunnel syndrome. This is of a severe degree on the right side and a moderate to severe degree on the left side. Surgical release is warranted to prevent ongoing axonal loss.

This study also reveals evidence of a mild bilateral sensory neuropathy. There is no evidence of lower cervical radiculopathy involving the upper extremities.

(continued)

RECOMMENDATIONS

1. Staged surgical release of the carpal tunnels, right followed by the left.
2. Staged steroid injections in the carpal tunnels while waiting for surgical release.
3. Cock-up wrist splints can be placed, properly fitting.
4. Avoidance of repetitive wrist movements and weightlifting.
5. Two-hour glucose tolerance test, CBC, Chem-25, ESR, ANA, RA, and TSH, if not already done.

OPERATIVE NOTE

DATE OF OPERATION
05/15/2004

ATTENDING SURGEON
John Smith, MD.

PREOPERATIVE DIAGNOSIS
Acquired cranial defect.

POSTOPERATIVE DIAGNOSIS
Acquired cranial defect.

PROCEDURE PERFORMED
Titanium bar and methyl methacrylate cranioplasty, left frontal, greater than 5 cm.

ANESTHESIA
General endotracheal.

INDICATIONS FOR PROCEDURE
The patient is a 33-year-old white male status post gunshot wound to the left frontal region. He has recovered well and presents now for replacement of the bone flap with a cranioplasty.

DESCRIPTION OF PROCEDURE
The patient was brought to the operating room and placed on the table in the supine position, intubated, and given general endotracheal anesthesia. The head was turned to the right side. The frontal portion of the skull was shaved and prepped with Betadine scrub and Betadine solution. The previous biparietal flap was identified, but it was opted to include our incision within the boundaries of the flap in order to minimize the amount of dissection.

A frontotemporal flap was then traced out and infiltrated with 0.5% lidocaine with 1:200,000 epinephrine, and a skin incision was made with a #10 blade. This incision was carried down through the pericranium. Raney clips were placed on the edges for hemostasis. The temporal muscle was left intact, and the flap was rotated anteriorly and held in place with towel clips. Using sharp dissection, we lifted the flap off the underlying dura. We revised the edges of the bone and then we placed several KLS Martin plates across the defect holding them in place with 5-mm screws.

With this being done, we mixed the methyl methacrylate and placed it over the cranial defect in order to approximate the shape and size of the defect. Once the plastic had cured adequately, and after copious amounts of antibiotic irrigation, we closed the galea with 2-0 Vicryl. The skin was closed with 3-0 Prolene, and we placed a sterile dressing over the area.

The patient was subsequently transferred to the recovery room in stable condition.

ESTIMATED BLOOD LOSS
Approximately 150 mL.

COMPLICATIONS
None.

OPERATIVE REPORT

OPERATIVE DATE
05/15/2004

ATTENDING SURGEON
John Smith, MD.

PREOPERATIVE DIAGNOSES
1. Open bitable frontal sinus fracture.
2. Cerebrospinal fluid leak.

POSTOPERATIVE DIAGNOSES
1. Open bitable frontal sinus fracture.
2. Cerebrospinal fluid leak.

PROCEDURES PERFORMED
1. Bifrontal craniotomy.
2. Exenteration of frontal sinuses.
3. Primary repair of dural tear and closure with pericranium of frontobasal dural tear.
4. Placement of lumbar drain.

ANESTHESIA
General endotracheal anesthesia.

COMPLICATIONS
None.

ESTIMATED BLOOD LOSS
Approximately 250 mL.

INDICATIONS FOR PROCEDURE
The patient is a 19-year-old female status post blunt head trauma to the right forehead and frontal region after she hit a tree during a boating accident. She lost consciousness but was initially a Glasgow coma score of 14 upon initial evaluation. She was subsequently intubated on the scene and transported to our facility for further management.

Her CT scan revealed a bitable frontal sinus fracture carrying down to the level of the cribriform plate and near the sella turcica. She also had cerebrospinal fluid emanating from the frontal skull fracture. She was awake and following commands at that time, although she was still intubated.

PROCEDURE IN DETAIL
After the patient was taken to the operating room and placed in the supine position, adequate general endotracheal anesthesia was induced. Her right bifrontal region was shaved and prepped in the usual sterile fashion.

(continued)

At this time, she was placed in the reflex position with the head up. The bifrontal skin flap was connected utilizing the existing laceration and carried down to approximately 1 cm above the zygoma bilaterally. The coronal skin flap was reflected anteriorly and, with the aid of the Bovie electrocautery, we carried the flap forward and undermined the temporalis muscle at the pericranium. This dissection was carried down to the level of the supraorbital ridge and also to the keyholes laterally.

Next, 1 bur hole each was placed on the keyhole sites as well as 2 parasagittal bur holes posteriorly, along with 1 midline bur hole near the midline over the sinus. After the underlying dura was dissected free with a #3 Penfield dissector, the craniotome was used to connect the bur holes. No dural tear was evident and the bone flap was elevated.

At this time, the exenteration of the frontal sinus was completed with the use of rongeurs as well as curettes. The posterior walls of the frontal sinus were bitten off with Leksell rongeurs. At this time, attention was turned to the frontal basilar dural tear, and the brain retractor was used to retract the frontal lobe backwards. The #1 Penfield dissector was used to dissect the dura away from the crista galli. A linear, anteroposterior, long dural tear, approximately 3 cm in length, was noted along the left basal frontal region over the cribriform plate. The area was irrigated and the anterior portion of the tear was closed primarily with a 5-0 Prolene suture.

Because of the depth of the injury and the possible injury that could be caused by further retraction and dissection, it was decided that a piece of pericranium would be used to cover the dural tear and a lumbar drain would be placed at the end of the procedure. The remainder of the dura was carefully inspected and no other dural tears were encountered. Dural tack-ups with 4-0 Prolene were next performed. Surgicel was placed over the bony edges as well as over the superior sagittal sinus. Adequate hemostasis was obtained with the above as well as with Gelfoam and bipolar electrocautery.

At this time, the procedure was turned over to the oral-maxillofacial surgery service for reconstruction of the frontal bone as well as the left orbital roof defect. A lumbar drain was placed at the end of this procedure.

Sponge, laparotomy pad, instrument, and needle counts were correct x2 at the end of our procedure. The patient tolerated this portion of the procedure well, remaining hemodynamically stable. She was given intravenous antibiotics as well as Dilantin.

HISTORY & PHYSICAL

This is a 23-year-old adult white male who was seen in neurological evaluation for a history of recurrent syncope. He reports his first episode took place in 1997, the second one in 2000, and the third one was in 2001. Each of these episodes was connected with drawing of blood, and right after that he passed out for a few seconds. There was no reported history of convulsant movements and no reported history of confusion following the episodes.

PAST MEDICAL HISTORY

He denies any injuries to his head. He has had some broken bones in his arms in the past. He denies any trouble seeing, hearing, or swallowing and has had no weakness, no numbness, no sphincter disturbances. He denies any chest pain, cough, nausea, vomiting, or urinary symptoms on review of systems.

SOCIAL HISTORY

He states that he is the only child in his family. His father used to have similar problems of passing out when blood was drawn in an office situation, but he does not pass out when blood is drawn in the home situation.

ALLERGIES

No known drug allergies.

PAST SURGICAL HISTORY

Positive for a tonsillectomy in the past.

PHYSICAL EXAMINATION

GENERAL: This is a well-built, tall male who appears to be in no acute distress.
HEAD: Normocephalic.
EENT: Extraocular movements are full, pupils are reactive to light, and disks are sharp. No apparent facial asymmetry seen. Facial sensations are preserved. Hearing is intact. Swallowing is intact. Tongue is midline on protrusion.
NECK: Supple, no bruit heard.
CHEST: Clear.
HEART: Normal sinus rhythm.
ABDOMEN: Soft, nontender with no organomegaly.
EXTREMITIES: Moves all 4 extremities.
NEUROLOGICAL EXAMINATION: Alert, mental status intact, cranial nerves intact, motor system intact for strength, tone, and bulk. Sensory examination intact to all modalities. Cerebellar functions are intact. Reflexes are 2+ to 3+ and symmetrical. Bilateral plantars are downgoing. Neurovascular examination is unremarkable.

IMPRESSION

Vasovagal syncope. Neurologically, no other significant abnormalities are noted. As he has never had an EEG, an EEG might be needed to exclude any possible seizure discharges. I doubt this, as his history does not indicate any evidence suggestive of seizures at this time.

REVIEW QUESTIONS

The goal of these questions is to test your knowledge in the areas of neurology and neurosurgery.

Directions: Select the correct answer for each of the multiple-choice questions provided below. *Answers are provided at the end of this chapter.*

1. How many pairs of cranial nerves are there in the nervous system?
   A. 10
   B. 12
   C. 14
   D. 16

2. Which of the following is the largest part of the brain?
   A. pons
   B. cerebrum
   C. cerebellum
   D. basal ganglia

3. The equally divided halves of brain are known as
   A. cerebral gyri.
   B. cerebral sulci.
   C. cerebral cortex.
   D. cerebral hemispheres.

4. Which of the following is a column of nervous tissue extending from the medulla oblongata to the second lumbar vertebra?
   A. brain stem
   B. cauda equine
   C. nerve root
   D. spinal cord

5. Which of the following procedures is used to withdraw cerebrospinal fluid?
   A. myelography
   B. cerebral angioplasty
   C. lumbar puncture
   D. MRA

6. The brain and the spinal cord make up the
   A. autonomic nervous system.
   B. brainstem.
   C. cerebral cortex.
   D. central nervous system.

7. The fluid-filled cavities in the brain containing CSF are called
   A. plexuses.
   B. sulci.
   C. synapses.
   D. ventricles.

8. The combining form *radicul/o* refers to a
   A. nerve cell.
   B. membrane.
   C. nerve root.
   D. sheath.

9. Which of the following is the term for an abnormal accumulation of CSF fluid in the brain?
   A. Huntington disease
   B. hydrocephalus
   C. multiple sclerosis
   D. spina bifida

10. A brain disorder marked by gradual deterioration of mental capacity, memory impairment, and confusion is known as
    A. Alzheimer disease.
    B. cerebral palsy.
    C. Tourette syndrome.
    D. myasthenia gravis.

11. Which of the following terms is associated with degeneration of nerves in the basal ganglia that leads to tremors, weakness of muscles, masklike facies, and slowness of movement?
    A. meningitis
    B. chorea
    C. Parkinson disease
    D. Tourette syndrome

12. Which of the following is caused by a thrombus which occludes an artery leading to or within the brain?
    A. aneurysm
    B. cerebrovascular accident
    C. cardiovascular accident
    D. ictal event

13. Which of the following is transcribed correctly?
    A. The patient presents with a history of progressive right hemiparesis. Skull films, EEG, and CSS analysis were all normal. MRA will be ordered to assess cerebral blood flow.
    B. The patient presents with a history of progressive right hemiparesis. Skull films, EEG, and CSF analysis were all normal. MRA will be ordered to assess cerebral blood flow.
    C. The patient presents with a history of progressive light hemiparesis. Skull films, EKG, and CSF analysis were all normal. MRH will be ordered to assess cerebral blood flow.
    D. The patient presents with a history of progressive right hemiparesis. Skull films, ECG, and ESF analysis were all normal. MRA will be ordered to assess cerebral blood flow.

14. Which of the following is transcribed correctly?
    A. Examination of the thumb shows weakness of the plantar muscles with slight atrophy. NCV shows decreased conduction velocity.
    B. Examination of the thumb shows weakness of the thenar muscles with slight atrophy. MCV shows decreased conduction velocity.
    C. Examination of the thumb shows weakness of the thenar muscles with slight atrophy. NCV shows decreased conduction velocity.
    D. Examination of the thumb shows weakness of the plantar muscles with slight atrophy. MCV shows decreased conduction velocity.

15. Diminished sensitivity to stimulation is called
    A. hypesthesia.
    B. anesthesia.
    C. bradykinesia.
    D. hyperesthesia.

16. Failure of muscle coordination, including unsteady movements and a staggering walk, due to disorders in the cerebellum is called
    A. anoxia.
    B. dyslexia.
    C. paraplegia.
    D. ataxia.

17. The inability to use or understand spoken or written language because of a brain lesion is known as
    A. anosmia.
    B. aphasia.
    C. dyslexia.
    D. dysphagia.

18. Which part of the brain regulates heartbeat, breathing, and other vital functions?
    A. brainstem
    B. gray matter
    C. occipital lobe
    D. white matter

19. A specialized cell which conducts nerve impulses is called a (an)
    A. glial cell.
    B. epithelial cell.
    C. neuron.
    D. proton.

20. A type of brain surgery that uses a system of three-dimensional coordinates to locate the operative site is called
    A. densitometric.
    B. microsurgery.
    C. stereotactic.
    D. laparoscopic.

21. A chronic disease characterized by a loss of the myelin sheath, causing paresthesias, muscle weakness, and unsteady gait is called
    A. multiple sclerosis.
    B. cerebral palsy.
    C. Huntington chorea.
    D. narcolepsy.

22. Which of the following is characterized a lack of muscular coordination caused by a loss of oxygen during pregnancy or the perinatal period?
    A. encephalopathy
    B. Bell palsy
    C. Cerebral palsy
    D. concussion

23. Serotonin and dopamine are
    A. neurotransmitters.
    B. components of CSF.
    C. only found in patients with neurological disorders.
    D. components of the myelin sheath.

24. The somatic nervous system
    A. is part of the central nervous system.
    B. regulates voluntary motor control.
    C. regulates involuntary motor control.
    D. transmits impulses to the cerebrum.

25. A sulcus is also known as a
    A. cortex.
    B. fissure.
    C. lobe.
    D. medulla.

26. Babinski and Hoffman are tests to evaluate
    A. response to pain.
    B. motor coordination.
    C. gait.
    D. reflexes.

27. This sign/reflex is used to diagnose meningitis.
    A. Homans
    B. Brudzinski
    C. anterior drawer
    D. startle

28. Demyelination is defined as
    A. loss of an axon in a neuron.
    B. loss of dendrites in a neuron.
    C. loss of protective sheath surrounding neurons.
    D. loss of the connective tissue between neurons.

29. The brainstem consists of the
    A. cerebellum, cerebrum, and spinal cord.
    B. dura mater and the pia mater.
    C. pons, midbrain, and medulla oblongata.
    D. thalamus and hypothalamus.

30. The cauda equina is located
    A. at the beginning of the spinal cord above the atlas.
    B. in the cerebellum.
    C. between vertebrae.
    D. at the end of the spinal cord below the first lumbar vertebra.

 Please see the accompanying CD for additional review materials for this section.

ANSWER KEY

REVIEW QUESTIONS ANSWER KEY

1. B	6. D	11. C	16. D	21. A	26. D
2. B	7. D	12. B	17. B	22. C	27. B
3. D	8. C	13. B	18. A	23. A	28. C
4. D	9. B	14. C	19. C	24. B	29. C
5. C	10. A	15. A	20. C	25. B	30. D

14

Obstetrics & Gynecology

OBJECTIVES CHECKLIST

A prepared exam candidate will know:

- ☐ Combining forms, prefixes, and suffixes related to the body system.
- ☐ Anatomy and structures of the female reproductive system.
- ☐ Physiology and function of the organs of the female reproductive system.
- ☐ Role of hormones in the reproductive process and reproductive health.
- ☐ Terminology related to gestation, labor, delivery, and neonatal care.
- ☐ Common imaging and diagnostic studies used in the treatment of obstetric and gynecologic diseases.
- ☐ Laboratory tests ordered to diagnose and monitor the symptoms and diseases related to reproductive medicine.
- ☐ Transcription standards pertaining to gestational terminology, labor, and delivery.

RESOURCES FOR STUDY

1. *Bates' Guide to Physical Examination and History Taking*
   Chapter 9: The Breasts and Axillae, pp. 337–357.
   Chapter 12: Female Genitalia, pp. 429–457.
   Chapter 19: The Pregnant Woman, pp. 817–838.

2. *The Language of Medicine*
   Chapter 8: Female Reproductive System, pp. 253–304.

3. *Memmler's Structure and Function of the Human Body*
   Chapter 11: The Endocrine System: Glands and Hormones, pp. 197–210.
   Chapter 20: The Male and Female Reproductive Systems, pp. 357–372.
   Chapter 21: Development and Heredity, pp. 375–390.

4. *Memmler's The Human Body in Health and Disease*
   Chapter 23: The Male and Female Reproductive Systems, pp. 454–475; Study Guide 350–365.
   Chapter 24: Development and Birth, pp. 476–490; Study Guide, pp. 366–376.

5. *H&P: A Nonphysician's Guide to the Medical History and Physical Examination*
   Chapter 11: Review of Systems: Genitourinary, pp. 97–106.
   Chapter 25: Examination of the Abdomen, Groins, Rectum, Anus, and Genitalia, pp. 235–248.

6. *Human Diseases*
   Chapter 13: Diseases of the Female Reproductive System, pp. 189–204.
   Chapter 14: Pregnancy and Childbirth, pp. 205–222.

7. *Laboratory Tests & Diagnostic Procedures in Medicine*
   Chapter 8: Examination of the Digestive Tract and Urinary System, pp. 107–118.
   Chapter 20: Chemical Examination of the Blood (Hormones), pp. 366–367.

8. *A Manual of Laboratory and Diagnostic Tests*
   Chapter 3: Urine Studies, pp. 163–263.
   Chapter 6: Chemistry Studies, pp. 316–455.
   Chapter 10: X-Ray Studies, pp. 705–759.
   Chapter 11: Cytologic, Histologic, and Genetic Studies, pp. 760–818.
   Chapter 12: Endoscopic Studies, pp. 819–861.
   Chapter 13: Ultrasound Studies, pp. 862–899.
   Chapter 15: Prenatal Diagnosis and Tests of Fetal Well-Being, pp. 973–1011.

9. *The AAMT Book of Style for Medical Transcription*
   Obstetrics, pp. 289–291.
   Genetics, pp. 183–186.
   Genes, pp. 186–188.

10. *Using Medical Terminology: A Practical Approach*
    Chapter 16: Reproductive System, pp. 755–832.
    Chapter 17: Pregnancy, Human Development, and Child Health, pp. 833–899.

11. *Pharmacology for Health Professionals*
    Chapter 23: Hormones and Related Drugs, pp. 339–381.
    Chapter 24: Drugs Acting on the Uterus, pp. 382–388.

12. *Understanding Pharmacology for Health Professionals*
    Chapter 23: Obstetric/Gynecologic Drugs, pp. 243–261.

13. *Medical Terminology: The Language of Health Care*
    Chapter 17: Female Reproductive System, pp. 535–584.

SAMPLE REPORTS

The following four reports are examples of reports you might encounter while transcribing obstetrics and gynecology.

OPERATIVE REPORT

SURGEON OF RECORD
John Smith, MD.

RESIDENT SURGEON
Mary Jones, MD.

PREOPERATIVE DIAGNOSIS
Oligohydramnios with breech presentation at 35 weeks estimated gestational age.

POSTOPERATIVE DIAGNOSIS
Oligohydramnios with breech presentation at 35 weeks estimated gestational age.

PROCEDURE
Primary low transverse cesarean section via Pfannenstiel skin incision.

ANESTHESIA
Spinal.

ESTIMATED BLOOD LOSS
Approximately 500 mL.

FINDINGS
A viable male infant in the breech presentation, right sacrum anterior. Normal tubes and ovaries bilaterally. Two small fibroids are noted in the uterus. The infant weighed 5 pounds 12 ounces and Apgar scores were 9 and 9.

PROCEDURE
The patient was taken to the operating room and placed in the dorsal lithotomy position after being given a spinal anesthesia without difficulty. She was then prepped and draped in the usual sterile fashion. A Pfannenstiel skin incision was made with a scalpel and carried through the underlying layer of fascia with the use of electrocautery. The fascial incision was extended laterally, and the superior aspect of the fascial incision was grasped with Kocher clamps, elevated upward, and the rectus muscle was dissected off with the use of cautery. In a similar fashion, this was done at the inferior aspect of the fascial incision.

The muscles were separated. The peritoneum was entered and the incision was extended with the use of a gentle tug. A bladder blade was inserted, and the vesicouterine peritoneum was identified, held with pickups, and entered with Metzenbaum scissors. The incision was extended laterally and a bladder flap was created digitally. The bladder blade was then inserted.

(continued)

The lower uterine segment was incised in transverse fashion, and the incision was extended laterally with the use of bandage scissors. The baby was delivered from a frank breech presentation. The mouth and nose were suctioned and the cord was clamped and cut. Cord blood was sent to pathology, and the infant was then handed off to the awaiting neonatologist.

The placenta was removed manually. The uterus was exteriorized and cleared of all clots and debris. The incision was repaired with #0 Vicryl in running, locked fashion. The uterus was then returned to the pelvis. The gutters were cleared of clots and debris. Hemostasis was assured. The fascia was reapproximated with #0 Vicryl in running fashion. The subcutaneous fat was irrigated, and any bleeders were cauterized and hemostasis was assured. The skin was reapproximated in a subcuticular fashion with the use of 4-0 Vicryl.

The patient tolerated the procedure well. Sponge, instrument, and needle counts were correct x2. The patient was taken to the recovery room in stable condition.

OPERATIVE REPORT

SURGEON
John Smith, MD.

PREOPERATIVE DIAGNOSES
1. Ovarian cyst.
2. Pelvic fluid.

POSTOPERATIVE DIAGNOSES
1. Ovarian cyst.
2. Pelvic fluid.

PROCEDURE
Diagnostic laparoscopy with suction of pelvic fluid for cytology as well as culture and sensitivity.

ANESTHESIA
General endotracheal.

PROCEDURE IN DETAIL
Under satisfactory general anesthesia, the patient was placed in the dorsal lithotomy position, and a tenaculum and cannula were applied to the cervix in the usual manner. The bladder was emptied by simple catheterization. The entire abdomen was then prepped and painted with Betadine soap, cleansed with alcohol solution, and then draped with sterile sheets in the usual manner.

A small, subumbilical, vertical incision was made at the previous scar line. This incision was deepened through the skin. The primary trocar and cannula were inserted into the abdominal cavity and the primary trocar was removed. Through the primary cannula, the laparoscope was introduced, and the pelvic cavity was well visualized. Meanwhile, carbon dioxide gas was insufflated, and we obtained an adequate pneumoperitoneum. A second puncture was made at the McBurney point in the usual manner, and through the second puncture, the retractor was introduced and the abdominal and pelvic cavities were explored.

We found the uterus to be slightly enlarged, with a few leiomyomata noted, which appeared to be more of the intramural type. These were located at the top of the uterine fundus. No other abnormalities were noted. Both tubes revealed evidence of an old tubal ligation. Both ovaries were small and cystic, with no evidence of operation noted. No adhesions were noted. The cul-de-sac was inspected and showed a moderate amount of pelvic fluid which was clear. This fluid was subsequently suctioned in the usual manner and sent for cytology and culture and sensitivity. At this point, the procedure was completed.

The laparoscope and retractors were removed from the abdominal cavity. All carbon dioxide gas was also removed, and both primary and secondary cannulas were removed. The deep fascia of the subumbilical wound was suture ligated with #0 Vicryl using interrupted sutures. The subcutaneous tissue of the wound was suture ligated with 2-0 plain using multiple interrupted simple sutures. The skin was approximated with 3-0 plain using continuous subcuticular stitches. The wound of the second puncture was also approximated with 3-0 plain using single simple sutures. A sterile dressing was placed. The tenaculum and cannulas were removed from the vagina and bleeders were checked.

The patient tolerated the procedure well and was sent to the recovery room in stable condition.

ESTIMATED BLOOD LOSS
Less than 10 mL.

HISTORY & PHYSICAL

CHIEF COMPLAINT
Abdominal pain.

HISTORY OF PRESENT ILLNESS
The patient is a 17-year-old, para 0-0-1-0. Her last menstrual period began 5 days ago. The patient had a sudden onset of sharp, stabbing pain in the right lower quadrant, radiating to her lower back beginning 2 days ago. The patient states she took some Tylenol and ibuprofen for this pain without any relief. On that same evening, she had 3 episodes of vomiting. The patient has also noticed nausea since then, although the patient told me that she ate this morning. The patient states that since the onset of pain, the pain has gotten progressively worse and is now across both lower quadrants, radiating to her lower back. At this time, the patient denies any urinary symptoms. She has had no diarrhea. She notes no unusual vaginal discharge, and she denies having a fever.

PAST MEDICAL HISTORY
The patient denies having any significant medical problems except for treatment of depression and attention deficit hyperactivity disorder. She is on Wellbutrin and Seroquel and has taken those medications since 2000. The patient denies high blood pressure, heart disease, diabetes, thyroid problems, asthma, bronchitis, pneumonia, kidney disease, liver disease, or epilepsy.

MEDICATIONS
She is on Wellbutrin, Seroquel, and Ortho Evra.

PAST SURGICAL HISTORY
The patient has had no previous surgery.

PAST GYNECOLOGIC HISTORY
Menarche at age 13 with cycles every 28 to 30 days lasting for 10 days. The patient has been using Ortho Evra for the past 3 months. On this birth control method, her periods only last 4 days. The patient denies any sexually transmitted diseases. The patient notes no intermenstrual spotting or bleeding.

HABITS
The patient smokes a quarter pack of cigarettes per day. The patient uses ethanol occasionally. She denies any present drug use, although she has used marijuana in the past.

FAMILY HISTORY
Noncontributory.

REVIEW OF SYSTEMS
As noted above.

PHYSICAL EXAMINATION
This is a well-developed, well-nourished female with some abdominal discomfort. Vital signs reveal blood pressure 107/60, pulse 122, respirations 20, and temperature of 99.7. Examination of the head, ears, eyes, nose, and throat reveals no icterus. Her conjunctivae are normal. There are no signs of dehydration. There is no jugular venous distention and no thyromegaly. Her lungs are

(continued)

clear to percussion and auscultation. Heart is regular rhythm. No murmurs or gallops are noted. Breasts reveal no masses. Examination of the abdomen reveals mild upper quadrant tenderness with minimal rebound. She has moderate to severe right and left lower quadrant tenderness, right slightly greater than the left, with positive rebound in both lower quadrants. Her bowel sounds are hypoactive. Examination of the extremities shows no edema and no varicosities. Neurologic exam is grossly normal. Pelvic examination reveals normal external genitalia. Vagina is pink with rugae and a watery discharge. The cervix is pink with a nulliparous os. Cervix measures 2 cm in length. Uterus is markedly tender to motion. Examination of the uterus reveals it to be normal size, anteverted, and extremely tender. Examination of the adnexa reveals severe bilateral adnexal tenderness. I could not palpate any masses in the adnexa.

LABORATORY DATA

CBC reveals white count of 40,000 with a left shift, hemoglobin of 10, hematocrit 31.5, and platelets of 324,000. Pregnancy test is negative. Chemistries show a decreased sodium of 133 and a slightly decreased potassium of 3.4. Urinalysis shows a specific gravity of 1.021. Her leukocyte esterase and nitrite are negative. Albumin is 25 and acetone is 5. Microscopic exam is negative.

STUDIES

The patient had an ultrasound of the pelvis. Preliminary report reveals the uterus and adnexa are normal. There is a small amount of fluid on the right. The appendix is not identified, and no inflammatory masses are noted.

IMPRESSION

1. Probable acute pelvic inflammatory disease.
2. Rule out appendicitis.

PLAN

The patient will be admitted. She will be started on intravenous antibiotic therapy for pelvic inflammatory disease. Surgical consultation has been obtained in the emergency room. Surgery service will follow this patient. A CT scan will also be obtained.

OPERATIVE REPORT

PREOPERATIVE DIAGNOSIS
Fetal malposition, double footling breech.

POSTOPERATIVE DIAGNOSES
1. Fetal malposition, double footling breech.
2. Spigelian hernia.

SURGERY PERFORMED
1. Primary cesarean section, low segment transverse.
2. Spigelian hernia repair.

SURGEON OF RECORD
John Smith, MD.

PROCEDURE IN DETAIL
The patient was taken to the operating theater and given anesthesia without difficulty. She was then sterilely prepped and draped in the usual fashion. A Pfannenstiel skin incision was made transversely, and this was taken down through the anatomical layers. The abdomen was opened atraumatically. A low segment, transverse uterine incision was initiated with the scalpel and bluntly separated with the surgeon's fingers. A breech baby (male) was found in a double footling presentation. Apgar scores were 9 and 9, and the baby weighed 8 pounds 8 ounces. The placenta was delivered spontaneously.

The uterine incision was repaired using #1 Monocryl in a single, running fashion. The peritoneum was well irrigated, and no evidence of active bleeding was noted. The uterus, tubes, and ovaries were found to be within normal limits. The peritoneum was then closed with 2-0 Monocryl in a single, running fashion. The rectus sheath, posterior leaf, was reapproximated at the midline with interrupted #1 sutures of Monocryl for correction of the spigelian hernia. The aponeurosis of the externus and internus were reapproximated using #0 Monocryl in single, running fashion.

The patient tolerated the procedure well without any complications, and she was transferred to the recovery room in stable condition. Skin staples had been applied to the incision site, and these are to be removed 3 days post surgery.

REVIEW QUESTIONS

The goal of these questions is to test your knowledge in the areas of obstetrics and gynecology.

Directions: Select the correct answer for each of the multiple-choice questions provided below. *Answers are provided at the end of this chapter.*

1. What is the term given to the dark pigmented area around the breast nipple?
   A. amnion
   B. areola
   C. chorion
   D. hymen

2. Which of the following combining forms refers to the uterus?
   A. *colp/o*
   B. *hyster/o*
   C. *salpingo/o*
   D. *men/o*

3. Which of the following refers to painful childbirth?
   A. dystocia
   B. dysmenorrhea
   C. placenta previa
   D. abruptio placenta

4. Which of the following is the term given to the region between the vaginal orifice and the anus?
   A. perianal
   B. perineum
   C. peritoneum
   D. peroneal

5. The rounded upper portion of the uterus is called the
   A. corpus.
   B. endometrium.
   C. fundus.
   D. myometrium.

6. The presence of this hormone in the blood and/or urine indicates pregnancy.
   A. estrogen
   B. follicle stimulating hormone
   C. human chorionic gonadotropin
   D. luteinizing hormone

7. The combining form *galact/o* means
   A. discharge.
   B. fluid.
   C. milk.
   D. pus.

8. The combining form *salping/o* refers to
   A. adnexa.
   B. cervix.
   C. tubes.
   D. ovary.

9. A benign tumor which may arise in the uterus or the breast is called a
   A. cervical dysplasia.
   B. cervical neoplasia.
   C. fibroid.
   D. carcinoma in situ.

10. Implantation of the fertilized egg outside the uterine cavity is called
    A. abruptio placentae.
    B. ectopic pregnancy.
    C. placenta previa.
    D. preeclampsia.

11. The use of cold temperatures to destroy tissue is known as
    A. cryosurgery.
    B. conization.
    C. culdocentesis.
    D. exenteration.

12. Cutting or blocking the fallopian tubes in order to prevent fertilization is called
    A. amniocentesis.
    B. dilation and curettage.
    C. protective block.
    D. tubal ligation.

13. What is the correct way to transcribe a patient's obstetric history if she has had three pregnancies and two viable offspring?
    A. gravida 3, para 2
    B. para 3, gravida 2
    C. gravida III, para II
    D. para III, gravida II

14. On examination of a pregnant woman, the distance from the symphysis pubis to the dome (top) of the uterus is referred to as the
    A. abdominal circumference.
    B. fetal station.
    C. fundal height.
    D. myometrial thickness.

15. A fertility drug that is used to stimulate ovulation is
    A. Cialis.
    B. Clomid.
    C. clopidogrel.
    D. Pitocin.

16. Absence of menstruation is
    A. amenorrhea.
    B. menometrorrhagia.
    C. hypermenorrhea.
    D. oligomenorrhea.

17. The thin projections that form a fringe around the ovarian end of the fallopian tube are called
    A. fibrinoids.
    B. fimbriae.
    C. follicles.
    D. oocytes.

18. What is another word for toxemia?
    A. endometriosis
    B. cervicitis
    C. placenta previa
    D. preeclampsia

19. Which of the following is an abbreviation for a procedure to remove the abdominal reproductive organs?
    A. TAH-BSO
    B. LEEP
    C. CVS
    D. ASCUS

20. What is the most common method of assessing a newborn infant?
    A. Allen-Doisy test
    B. Apgar score
    C. Barlow and Ortolani
    D. biophysical profile

21. The ovaries, fallopian tubes, and uterine ligaments collectively are called the
    A. adnexa.
    B. corpus luteum.
    C. fundus.
    D. myometrium.

22. Which of the following would be prescribed for a postmenopausal woman?
    A. HCTZ
    B. BCP
    C. hGH
    D. HRT

23. What is mittelschmerz?
    A. infertility
    B. pain between regular menstrual cycles
    C. premenstrual syndrome
    D. premenopause

24. What is menarche?
    A. an abnormal menstrual cycle
    B. the first menstrual cycle
    C. menstrual pain
    D. postmenopausal bleeding

25. Which of the following provides nutrients to the fetus?
    A. the amniotic fluid
    B. the placenta
    C. the chorionic fluid
    D. the myometrium

26. Which of the following incisions is used for a cesarean section?
    A. clamshell
    B. flank
    C. Pfannenstiel
    D. transmeatal

27. Which of the following is a normal vaginal discharge following childbirth?
    A. lochia
    B. meconium
    C. colostrum
    D. galactorrhea

28. Painless, irregular uterine contractions during pregnancy are called
    A. automatic.
    B. Braxton Hicks.
    C. idiomuscular.
    D. paradoxical.

29. Which monitor would be used to record the force of uterine contractions?
    A. Holter
    B. electronic fetal monitor
    C. tocodynamometer
    D. manometer

30. Which of the following would be given to stop preterm labor?
    A. terbutaline
    B. Mircette
    C. Ortho Tri-Cyclen
    D. testosterone

 Please see the accompanying CD for additional review materials for this section.

ANSWER KEY

REVIEW QUESTIONS ANSWER KEY

1. B	6. C	11. A	16. A	21. A	26. C
2. B	7. C	12. D	17. B	22. D	27. A
3. A	8. C	13. A	18. D	23. B	28. B
4. B	9. C	14. C	19. A	24. B	29. C
5. C	10. B	15. B	20. B	25. B	30. A

15

Ophthalmology

OBJECTIVES CHECKLIST

A prepared exam candidate will know:

- ❏ Combining forms, prefixes, and suffixes related to the body system.
- ❏ Anatomy and physiology of the eye, both internal and external.
- ❏ Visual pathway of light from the cornea to the cerebral cortex.
- ❏ Errors of refraction related to visual acuity.
- ❏ Common pathologic conditions of the eye.
- ❏ Clinical and diagnostic procedures used in the identification of diseases and disorders of the eye.
- ❏ Medications commonly prescribed for symptoms, disorders, and diseases of the eye.

RESOURCES FOR STUDY

1. *Bates' Guide to Physical Examination and History Taking*
   Chapter 6: The Head and Neck, pp. 153–239.

2. *The Language of Medicine*
   Chapter 17: Sense Organs: The Eye and the Ear, pp. 669–689.

3. *Memmler's Structure and Function of the Human Body*
   Chapter 10: The Sensory System, pp. 177–194.

4. *Memmler's The Human Body in Health and Disease*
   Chapter 11: The Sensory System, pp. 222–243; Study Guide, pp. 174–191.

5. *H&P: A Nonphysician's Guide to the Medical History and Physical Examination*
   Chapter 7: Review of Systems: Head, Eyes, Ears, Nose, Throat, Mouth, Teeth, pp. 59–70.

6. *Human Diseases*
   Chapter 18: Diseases of the Eye, pp. 291–314.

7. *Laboratory Tests & Diagnostic Procedures in Medicine*
   Chapter 3: Measurement of Vision and Hearing, pp. 29–38.
   Chapter 7: Endoscopy: Visual Examination of the Eyes, Ears, Nose, and Respiratory Tract, pp. 95–106.

8. *A Manual of Laboratory and Diagnostic Tests*
   Chapter 7: Microbiologic Studies, pp. 456–529.
   Chapter 10: X-Ray Studies, pp. 705–759.
   Chapter 13: Ultrasound Studies, pp. 862–899.
   Chapter 16: Special Systems, Organ Functions, and Postmortem Studies, pp. 1012–1093.

9. *Using Medical Terminology: A Practical Approach*
   Chapter 8: Nervous Systems and Special Senses, pp. 313–377.

10. *Pharmacology for Health Professionals*
    Unit 31: Otic and Ophthalmic Preparations, pp. 526–541.

11. *Understanding Pharmacology for Health Professionals*
    Chapter 20: Ophthalmic Drugs, pp. 217–227.

12. *Medical Terminology: The Language of Health Care*
    Chapter 12: Eye, pp. 386–414.

SAMPLE REPORTS

The following five reports are examples of reports you might encounter while transcribing ophthalmology.

OPERATIVE NOTE

PREOPERATIVE DIAGNOSIS
Medically uncontrolled glaucoma, right eye.

POSTOPERATIVE DIAGNOSIS
Medically uncontrolled glaucoma, right eye.

OPERATION
Trabeculectomy, right eye.

SURGEON
John Smith, MD.

ANESTHESIA
Local with standby.

PROCEDURE
Peribulbar anesthesia of the right eyelids and globe was obtained by injecting 2% Xylocaine into the right eye, and the right eye was sterilely prepped and draped. A lid speculum was inserted, and a 4-0 black silk superior rectus traction suture was placed and additional anesthesia obtained with 2% Xylocaine subconjunctivally. A large, limbal-based, conjunctival flap was fashioned with scissors. The Tenon capsule was excised. Bleeding areas were meticulously cauterized, and a 4 x 4 half-thickness scleral flap was created with a #69 blade.

Mitomycin 0.5 mg/mL was applied to the underside of the flap in the bare sclera for 2 minutes and then copiously irrigated off the eye. The anterior chamber was entered with a #75 blade. A trabeculectomy punch was used to double punch a hole in the trabecular meshwork, and a peripheral iridectomy was performed. The scleral flap was positioned posteriorly with two 10-0 nylon sutures. Irrigation through a side port showed easy flow underneath the flap. The conjunctiva was then closed with running, locked 8-0 Vicryl suture, giving a watertight closure.

At the close of the procedure the chamber was deep and the eye was soft. Ancef and Celestone were injected subconjunctivally. Maxitrol was instilled in the eye. The eye was patched, and the patient tolerated the procedure well.

OPERATIVE NOTE

PREOPERATIVE DIAGNOSIS
Esotropia, both eyes.

POSTOPERATIVE DIAGNOSIS
Esotropia, both eyes.

OPERATION
A 3.5-mm bimedial recession.

SURGEON
John Smith, MD.

ANESTHESIA
General.

PROCEDURE
After successful induction of general anesthesia, both eyes were sterilely prepped and draped in the usual manner for strabismus surgery. Attention was first turned to the right eye.

A lid speculum was inserted, a 5-0 Mersilene limbal traction suture placed, and the eye placed in an abducted position. A limbal peritomy was performed with scissors. The medial rectus was isolated on a muscle hook and attachments to the Tenon capsule cut. At this point, 6-0 Vicryl was threaded through the insertion. The muscle was disinserted and reinserted 3.5 mm from the original point of insertion. The conjunctiva was then closed with a 6-0 plain suture. Maxitrol was instilled into the eye, and the eye was not patched.

Attention was then turned to the left eye where a similar operation was performed by isolating the medial rectus on a muscle hook, recessing it 3.5 mm and closing the conjunctiva with 6-0 plain. Maxitrol was instilled into the eye and the eye was again not patched.

The patient tolerated both procedures well and was taken to the recovery room and then discharged home in excellent condition.

OPERATIVE NOTE

PREOPERATIVE DIAGNOSIS
Pseudophakic bullous keratopathy, right eye.

POSTOPERATIVE DIAGNOSIS
Pseudophakic bullous keratopathy, right eye.

OPERATION
An 8-mm penetrating keratoplasty, right eye.

SURGEON
John Smith, MD.

ANESTHESIA
Local with standby.

PROCEDURE
Peribulbar anesthesia of the right eyelids and globe was obtained by injection of 2% Xylocaine. The right eye was sterilely prepped and draped. A lid speculum was inserted and attention was turned to the donor eye.

The donor was a 47-year-old intracerebral bleed patient who died on 1/05, and the cornea was preserved on the same day and used today. It was removed from the transport medium and placed on the Teflon chopping block epithelial side up. An 8.25-mm button was punched through from the posterior surface. This was flooded with transport media and brought to the operative field.

Attention was returned to the patient, where an 8-mm trephine was placed on the cornea and used to trephine into the anterior chamber. The cornea was cut through with right and left corneal scissors. Healon was used to deepen the fornices in the anterior chamber. The donor button was placed into the recipient bed and sutured in place with four 10-0 nylon cardinal sutures, an additional four 10-0 nylon interrupted sutures and, finally, a 16-bite 10-0 nylon, pulled up once and tied in the wound. The wound was felt to be watertight.

Celestone and Garamycin were injected subconjunctivally, TobraDex instilled in the eye, and the eye patched and shielded. The patient tolerated the procedure well.

DISCHARGE SUMMARY

FINAL DIAGNOSIS
Cataract, right eye.

OPERATION PERFORMED
Kelman phacoemulsification, right eye, with insertion of an AcrySof 19-diopter posterior chamber intraocular lens under local and general anesthesia with microscopic control.

SUMMARY
This is the second outpatient admission for this 65-year-old female who has had decreased vision in both eyes for the last several years. The patient had cataract surgery in the left eye with good visual results. She is now admitted for cataract surgery of the right eye. Her best-corrected vision is 20/80 in the right and 20/40 in the left. Pressures are normal and slit-lamp examination is normal except for corneal scarring. The lens revealed 3+ nuclear sclerosis, and the fundus examination was normal.

DIAGNOSIS
Cataract, right eye.

DISPOSITION
The patient was advised of the above and desired to have cataract surgery. She was seen by a medical doctor and cleared for surgery. She underwent an uncomplicated cataract extraction, right eye, with implant. She tolerated the procedure well and was discharged postoperatively.

She was discharged on Pred Forte drops, Maxitrol drops, patch and shield. She was given postoperative care instructions, and she is to see us for followup in the office in the morning.

OPERATIVE REPORT

PREOPERATIVE DIAGNOSIS
Chronic blepharitis and severe ectropion, left lower lid.

POSTOPERATIVE DIAGNOSIS
Chronic blepharitis and severe ectropion, left lower lid.

OPERATION
Repair of ectropion, left lower lid with excisional biopsy, left lower lid.

SURGEON
John Smith, MD.

ANESTHESIA
Local with standby.

PROCEDURE
Anesthesia of the left lower lid was obtained by injection of 2% Xylocaine in the distribution of the infraorbital nerve and subcutaneously. The left eye was sterilely prepped and draped in the usual manner for major eyelid surgery. An incision was made along the inferior lash line to the lateral canthus, angled out at 15 degrees. A skin and muscle flap was created with Westcott scissors. A 10-mm section of the left lower lid was excised temporally and sent to pathology for permanent section.

The lid was then closed with a 4-0 silk to the grey line, 6-0 silk to the anterior and posterior lid margins, 5-0 chromic to the deep muscle tissues and 6-0 silk to the skin, leaving a good closure. The lid sutures were left long and taped to the face. Maxitrol was applied to the wound and the eye was patched. The patient tolerated the procedure well.

REVIEW QUESTIONS

The goal of these questions is to test your knowledge in the area of ophthalmology.

Directions: Select the correct answer for each of the multiple-choice questions provided below. *Answers are provided at the end of this chapter.*

1. The dark center of the eyes through which light rays enter is called the
   A. ciliary body.
   B. iris.
   C. orbit.
   D. pupil.

2. The opaque white of the eye is called the
   A. cornea.
   B. lens.
   C. retina.
   D. sclera.

3. Which of the following describes the normal adjustment of the eye for seeing objects at various distances?
   A. accommodation
   B. hemianopsia
   C. optic chiasm
   D. refraction

4. Which of the following is the translation for the combining form *blephar/o*?
   A. cornea
   B. eyelid
   C. iris
   D. tears

5. Which of the following is the translation for the combining form *vitre/o*?
   A. glassy
   B. yellow
   C. white
   D. gel-like

6. Defective curvature of the cornea or lens of the eye is called
   A. astigmatism.
   B. hyperopia.
   C. myopia.
   D. presbyopia.

7. Which of the following progressive diseases causes loss of central vision with preservation of peripheral vision?
   A. macular degeneration
   B. retinal detachment
   C. strabismus
   D. stye

8. Double vision, or seeing two overlapping two-dimensional images instead of one three-dimensional image, is called
   A. diplopia.
   B. ectropion.
   C. nystagmus.
   D. papilledema.

9. Which of the following uses a low-power microscope with built-in illumination to examine the conjunctiva, sclera, cornea and anterior chamber?
   A. Snellen test
   B. retinal arteriography
   C. slit-lamp examination
   D. ophthalmoscopy

10. Inflammation of the cornea is called
    A. dacryoadenitis.
    B. conjunctivitis.
    C. keratitis.
    D. uveitis.

11. Swelling of the optic disk, usually due to increased intracranial pressure, is
    A. papilledema.
    B. papilloma.
    C. proptosis.
    D. pupilloplegia.

12. The optic nerve is also known as cranial nerve
    A. I.
    B. II.
    C. VI.
    D. XII.

13. Which of the following moves the eye from side to side and up and down?
    A. extraocular muscles
    B. iridocorneal angle
    C. optic strut
    D. pupillary sphincter

14. Which of the following refers to the protrusion of the eyeball from the socket?
    A. ectropion
    B. exophthalmos
    C. pterygium
    D. xerosis

15. The medical term for nearsightedness is
    A. hyperopia.
    B. keratoconus.
    C. myopia.
    D. presbyopia.

16. Which of these medications would be given for glaucoma?
    A. Fluoracaine
    B. Kenalog
    C. Timoptic
    D. tramadol

17. Tears are secreted through the
    A. corneal tube.
    B. lacrimal duct.
    C. optic disk.
    D. orbicularis oris.

18. Which of the following measures intraocular pressure?
    A. visual field test
    B. pupillometry
    C. sphygmoscopy
    D. tonometry

19. Which of the following is an antibiotic drop used after eye surgery?
    A. Ciloxan
    B. cimetidine
    C. cisplatin
    D. Citracal

20. What is the medical term for pinkeye?
    A. conjunctivitis
    B. anisocoria
    C. presbyopia
    D. retinopathy

21. Which of the following is a medication for itchy eyes?
    A. Parnate
    B. paroxetine
    C. Patanol
    D. Polytrim

22. The abbreviation OD stands for
    A. left eye.
    B. one drop.
    C. right eye.
    D. both eyes.

23. Which of the following is used to treat an eye infection?
    A. Maxitrol
    B. Maxzide
    C. meclizine
    D. Murocel

24. The medical term for crossed eyes is
    A. strabismus.
    B. Strachan-Scott syndrome.
    C. nyctalopia.
    D. hemianopia.

25. Which of the following is an ophthalmic anesthetic?
    A. Cetacaine
    B. Fluoracaine
    C. Polocaine
    D. Solu-Medrol

26. Increased serum bilirubin levels may cause
    A. scleradenitis.
    B. scleral hemorrhage.
    C. scleral icterus.
    D. scleral pallor.

27. Retinopathy is a common complication of
    A. diabetes.
    B. hepatitis.
    C. parkinsonism.
    D. reactive airway disease.

28. Which of the these specialists is concerned with the eye and diseases of the eye?
    A. acupuncturist
    B. optometrist
    C. ophthalmologist
    D. otorhinolaryngologist

29. A scleral buckle is used to repair
    A. presbyopia.
    B. astigmatism.
    C. retinal detachment.
    D. ptosis.

30. The involuntary movement of the eyeball is referred to as
    A. amaurosis.
    B. Bell phenomenon.
    C. nystagmus.
    D. strabismus.

 Please see the accompanying CD for additional review materials for this section.

ANSWER KEY

REVIEW QUESTIONS ANSWER KEY

1. D	6. A	11. A	16. C	21. C	26. C
2. D	7. A	12. B	17. B	22. C	27. A
3. A	8. A	13. A	18. D	23. A	28. C
4. B	9. C	14. B	19. A	24. A	29. C
5. A	10. C	15. C	20. A	25. B	30. C

16

Orthopedics

OBJECTIVES CHECKLIST

A prepared exam candidate will know:

☐ Combining forms, prefixes, and suffixes related to the body system.

☐ Anatomy of the muscles and bones of the musculoskeletal system.

☐ Process of bone formation and the role of cartilage in the development of the bones of the skeleton.

☐ Anatomy and physiology of the supportive structures of the musculoskeletal system (tendons, ligaments, cartilage, etc.).

☐ Anatomy and physiology of the joints as well as the different types of joints.

☐ Physiology of the musculoskeletal system as it coordinates with the nervous system in mobility and ambulation.

☐ Terms used to describe position and direction.

☐ Imaging studies used in the identification and diagnosis of skeletal abnormalities, injuries, diseases, and malformations (congenital and traumatic).

☐ Laboratory studies used in the diagnosis and treatment of musculoskeletal disorders and diseases.

☐ Medications commonly prescribed for musculoskeletal symptoms, disorders, and diseases.

☐ Transcription standards pertaining to the specialty of orthopedics.

RESOURCES FOR STUDY

1. *Bates' Guide to Physical Examination and History Taking*
   Chapter 15: The Musculoskeletal System, pp. 497–571.

2. *The Language of Medicine*
   Chapter 15: Musculoskeletal System, pp. 559–628.

3. *Memmler's Structure and Function of the Human Body*
   Chapter 1: Organization of the Human Body, pp. 3–16.
   Chapter 6: The Skeleton: Bones and Joints, pp. 85–109.
   Chapter 7: The Muscular System, pp. 111–133.

4. *Memmler's The Human Body in Health and Disease*
   Chapter 7: The Skeleton: Bones and Joints, pp. 119–149; Study Guide, pp. 96–121.
   Chapter 8: The Muscular System, pp. 151–175; Study Guide, pp. 122–138.

5. *H&P: A Nonphysician's Guide to the Medical History and Physical Examination*
   Chapter 12: Review of Systems: Neuromuscular, pp. 107–116.
   Chapter 26: Examination of the Back and Extremities, pp. 249–260.

6. *Human Diseases*
   Chapter 17: Musculoskeletal Disorders, pp. 259–274.

7. *Laboratory Tests & Diagnostic Procedures in Medicine*
   Section IV: Medical Imaging (Chapter 10: Plain Radiography, Chapter 11: Contrast Radiography, Chapter 12: Computed Tomography, Chapter 14: Magnetic Resonance Imaging, and Chapter 15: Nuclear Imaging), pp. 127–209.

8. *A Manual of Laboratory and Diagnostic Tests*
   Chapter 9: Nuclear Medicine Studies, pp. 652–704.
   Chapter 10: X-Ray Studies, pp. 705–759.
   Chapter 12: Endoscopic Studies, pp. 819–861.

9. *The AAMT Book of Style for Medical Transcription*
   Orthopedics, pp. 294–299.

10. *Using Medical Terminology: A Practical Approach*
    Chapter 5: Skeletal System, pp. 189–241.
    Chapter 6: Articulations, pp. 243–277.
    Chapter 7: Muscular System, pp. 279–312.

11. *Pharmacology for Health Professionals*
    Chapter 29: Drugs That Affect the Musculoskeletal System, pp. 495–509.

12. *Understanding Pharmacology for Health Professionals*
    Chapter 14: Musculoskeletal Drugs, pp. 137–149.
    Chapter 26: Analgesic Drugs, pp. 296–310.

13. *Medical Terminology: The Language of Health Care*
    Chapter 6: Musculoskeletal System, pp. 144–191.

SAMPLE REPORTS

The following five reports are examples of reports you might encounter while transcribing orthopedics.

CONSULTATION

HISTORY OF PRESENT ILLNESS
The patient is a 56-year-old right-hand-dominant male, status post MVA. He sustained a left open supracondylar humerus fracture that was treated with irrigation and debridement and open reduction and internal fixation with synthetic bone grafting. He also had a splenic injury and a left acetabular fracture. He was initially treated for his left humerus fracture. His postoperative course was complicated by a draining wound. Followup x-rays of his humerus revealed that he had a nonunion/malunion with hardware failure and was referred here for further management. In the interim, he denies any fevers or chills. He denies any sweats or weight loss.

ALLERGIES
He has no known drug allergies.

PAST SURGICAL HISTORY
His past surgical history is significant for left acetabular fracture with ORIF.

MEDICATIONS
None.

SOCIAL HISTORY
He is an engineer. He does not use tobacco. He does not drink alcohol. He likes fishing, swimming, and golf.

PHYSICAL EXAMINATION
On physical examination of his left elbow, there is a well-healed posterior incision. It is warm to touch compared to the right side. There is obvious deformity with swelling. He has intact sensation of the ulnar nerve distribution distally, although he does have a positive Tinel in the ulnar nerve which radiates down into his small finger. He has full digital range of motion. The motion of his elbow is 70 to 90 degrees with 10 degrees of pronation and 40 degrees of supination. His abductor digiti minimi and finger abductors are -4/5.

STUDIES
X-rays reviewed from an outside hospital show a malunion/nonunion of his left supracondylar humerus fracture with fracture collapse and hardware failure.

ASSESSMENT
Left supracondylar humerus fracture, nonunion/malunion with questionable infection.

(continued)

PLAN

We discussed in detail the management of this problem and the difficulty, as we feel that this fracture is possibly infected. The patient will get his medical records, including his operative note and previous injury x-rays. We will send him for an erythrocyte sedimentation rate, C-reactive protein, and complete blood count with differential today. We did an aspiration which was technically difficult due to the distorted anatomy. Therefore, we performed saline washings and sent aspirated washings off for culture and Gram stain. We will follow up with him in 1 week with repeat x-rays of his left elbow, anteroposterior, lateral, and obliques, out of plaster. If cultures return negative, we will again aspirate it under fluoroscopic guidance. We will consider an indium-labeled white cell scan in that instance.

OPERATIVE REPORT

PREOPERATIVE DIAGNOSIS
Hypertrophic bone of 3rd and 4th digits.

POSTOPERATIVE DIAGNOSIS
Hypertrophic bone of 3rd and 4th digits.

PROCEDURE
Ostectomy of proximal phalanx, 3rd and 4th digits.

ANESTHESIA
Monitored anesthesia care.

DESCRIPTION OF PROCEDURE
The patient was transferred to the operating room in apparent good preoperative condition, and no contraindications to the proposed procedure were noted.

Attention was turned to the level of the patient's 3rd digit where an ostectomy was performed at the head of the proximal phalanx and the lateral aspect of the middle phalanx. Also, an incision was made at the dorsal level of the 4th digit where the ostectomies were made at the medial head of the proximal phalanx and the medial aspect of the middle phalanx on the 4th digit. All of these surgical areas where ostectomies were performed were rasped to smoothness and flushed with copious amounts of sterile saline. The soft tissue areas were then apposed and closed with 3-0 Vicryl material, as were the skin edges.

The patient appeared to have tolerated the procedure well and was removed from the operating room in apparent good postoperative condition.

OPERATIVE REPORT

PREOPERATIVE DIAGNOSIS
Right knee degenerative joint disease with degenerative meniscal tear.

POSTOPERATIVE DIAGNOSIS
Degenerative meniscal tear bilaterally, anterior cruciate ligament tear, and severe degenerative joint disease.

SURGEON
John Smith, MD.

ASSISTANT
Jane Smith, ARNP.

PROCEDURE
Diagnostic arthroscopy, bilateral partial meniscectomies, and chondroplasty of the medial femoral condyle, medial tibial plateau, lateral tibial plateau, and undersurface of the kneecap. Notchplasty was performed and craterization and saucerization of the bone to expose the anterior cruciate ligament, which was partially torn and gently débrided and tightened.

ANESTHESIA
General.

ESTIMATED BLOOD LOSS
Minimal.

COMPLICATIONS
None.

SPECIMENS
None.

DRAINS
None.

CULTURES
None.

IV FLUID
IV Ancef preoperatively.

DISPOSITION
To recovery room in stable condition.

HISTORY
The patient is a very pleasant 49-year-old white male well known to me, who in 1992 underwent a horrific car accident with open tib-fib fracture on the left side. He has had multiple surgeries and most recently, about 2 months ago, had a knee scope on the left side. MRIs showed that he had changes on the right side as well, and he has requested arthroscopy. All the complications and indications for the procedure were explained to the patient, and he voiced understanding. Informed consent was obtained.

(continued)

DETAILS OF PROCEDURE

The patient was brought to the operating room and placed on the table in supine fashion. After general anesthesia was induced, he was prepped and draped sterilely. Examination revealed a grossly stable knee. There was no pivot-shift, but he did have 1+ to 2+ positive Lachman. The knee was minimally swollen with palpable crepitus. At this point, standard 3-portal arthroscopy was performed, which revealed a rather large tear of the posterior horn of the medial meniscus and grade 3 changes on the medial femoral condyle, medial tibial plateau, and the undersurface of the patella. There were some grade 2 changes on the lateral tibial plateau and a small tear of the posterior horn of the lateral meniscus. At this point, bilateral partial meniscectomies were undertaken using the shaver, the upbiting rongeur, and the Oratec device. Notchplasty was performed using the shaver and a burr and the Oratec device to widen the arthritic notch to prevent impingement on the ACL. The ACL was gently débrided and tightened. Notchplasty consisted of craterization and saucerization of the bone of the lateral femoral condyle. This also helped to expose the tear of the posterior horn of the lateral meniscus. Chondroplasties were performed as stated previously. The gutters were clear. The knee was copiously irrigated. The portals were closed with interrupted nylon sutures. Then, 0.5% Marcaine with epinephrine and 10 mg of morphine were injected into the knee for postoperative pain control. He was placed in a bulky sterile dressing. He tolerated the procedure well and was sent to the recovery room in stable condition where he will be discharged to home when he is cleared by anesthesia. Followup will be in my office in 2 weeks. We have given him prescriptions for Darvocet, Keflex, and Ativan.

FOLLOWUP NOTE

HISTORY

Postoperative left wrist. The patient returns to the office today with limited complaints on the dorsoradial aspect of her hand. Her swelling is minimal. She was experiencing drainage from her second of 2 proximal pin sites, but this has dried up. She is off the antibiotics, and she only takes an occasional Lortab for pain. She is out of her splint and sling, but she needs to wear the Ace wrap. Her ulnar-sided wrist pain is almost gone, only noting occasional shooting pain.

PHYSICAL EXAM

The patient is neurovascularly intact distally in her left upper extremity. Her pin sites are clean without drainage or erythema. She has full range of motion of her elbow. She pronates to 70 degrees and supinates to 45–50 degrees passively. She can flex her digits and has no soft-tissue swelling or destructive changes. She can nearly make a full fist and has good grip strength. She is nontender. Her ulnar styloid has no soft-tissue swelling.

IMAGING

Three views of the left wrist were obtained. Her hardware is in place without evidence of failure. There is minimal progression of callus formation. There is no loss of alignment. She has evidence of healing of her minimally displaced ulnar styloid fracture with calluses. Her fracture line is less apparent.

DIAGNOSES

1. Approximately 5-1/2 weeks status post ORIF of the left distal radius with additional fixator application of the left wrist.
2. Minimally displaced left ulnar styloid fracture.

TREATMENT RECOMMENDATIONS

1. I explained to the patient my impression and her treatment options. The plan is to remove her external fixator in 2 days. Based on the lack of her ulnar-sided symptoms at this point, and the fact that she is nontender over her styloid, I will hold off on delayed percutaneous pinning of her styloid fracture.
2. Will schedule her for Friday. She will be in a splint briefly postoperatively followed by fabrication of an Orthoplast orthosis.

OPERATIVE NOTE

PREOPERATIVE DIAGNOSIS
Chronic low back pain status post prior laminectomy with postlaminectomy pain syndrome.

POSTOPERATIVE DIAGNOSIS
Chronic low back pain status post prior laminectomy with postlaminectomy pain syndrome.

PROCEDURES
1. Lumbar Racz catheter attempted neuroplasty at L4-5 and L5-S1.
2. Biplanar fluoroscopy.
3. Epidurograms.
4. Lysis of adhesions using Racz catheter and injection of Wydase to soften the scar tissue and to increase the lysis of adhesions.
5. Injection of local anesthetic, narcotic, steroid mixture.

SURGEON
John Smith, MD.

ASSISTANT
Mary Jones, ARNP.

JUSTIFICATION FOR PROCEDURE
This is a 60-year-old African American male with chronic back pain and lumbar radiculopathy down the backs of his legs with a history of laminectomies. MRI findings showed status post L3-4 laminectomy for disk herniation with cephalad migration of disk material. There is also some evidence of canal stenosis, mainly congenital in etiology, noted at the same levels.

As a result of all this, we have decided to do a series of 3 lumbar Racz catheter neuroplasties with lysis of adhesions with the injection of Wydase to widen the spread of the narcotic/steroid mixture as well as to soften any scar tissue. It is hoped that we will be able to relieve any adhesions that might be compressing the respective nerve roots leading to his radiculopathy.

ANESTHESIA
Intravenous sedation due to the patient's apprehension.

PROCEDURE IN DETAIL
The patient was met in the preoperative area where informed consent was obtained in writing. An IV was started in the dorsum of the hand, and the patient was taken to the procedure area where he was placed prone on the radiographic table with pillows below the abdomen. Other pressure points were padded, and monitors were placed to include EKG, Dinamap, and pulse oximetry. Nasal oxygen was given and intravenous sedation with propofol and Versed was started.

Once the desired level of sedation was achieved, the sacral and lower lumbar areas were prepped with Betadine solution and draped in a sterile fashion. Using biplanar fluoroscopy, the sacral cornu was identified and infiltrated with 2% Xylocaine plain.

(continued)

Next, a 16-gauge RK needle was inserted through the anesthetized area, and using biplanar fluoroscopic guidance, the needle was guided into the sacral foramen. Aspiration was carried out and was negative for any blood or cerebrospinal fluid. Next, a Brevi-XL 19-gauge 25-cm catheter was passed through the needle and up into the lower lumbosacral segment. The needle was advanced and at the L5-S1 interspace level was met with some obstruction. By gradual probing with the needle, we were able to advance it to the midbody of L5. At this point, an epidurogram was carried out by injecting Isovue-300 contrast material. The dye was noted to be pooled at the L5-S1 level, and it was then noted to spread in a caudal direction toward the coccyx area. There was no spread in a cephalad direction.

Again, gentle probing with the catheter tip was carried out and 300 units of Wydase was injected. After 2 to 3 minutes, again probing with the tip of the Racz catheter, we were able to advance the catheter up to the L4-5 interspace. Again, an epidurogram was carried out. This again showed dye pooling centrally in a loculated fashion, again suggestive of some adhesions, probably postsurgical, preventing the spread and possibly obliterating the epidural space. Film labeled #8 shows the initial epidurogram and film labeled #9 shows the second injection.

At this point, the Wydase was injected and, again, the spring-loaded tip of the Racz catheter was used to break up the adhesive processes. With this, the dye was noted to spread in a more cephalad direction, crossing the L4-5 level, getting up to the midbody of L4 and now spreading towards the lateral recesses. Again, the tip of the catheter was met with obstruction. Not wanting to puncture the dura, gentle probing was again carried out.

Having made progress from L5-S1 up to the midbody of L4, the decision was made not to carry out any further probing at this time. Therefore, 100 mcg of fentanyl was injected. This was then followed by 80 mg of triamcinolone and 2 mL of 0.25% Chirocaine plain. The total volume was 6 mL plus the 2 mL for the Wydase, for a total of 8 mL. Film labeled #10 shows the final spread of the epidurogram, showing the area of adhesions lysed. This is available in hard copy on the chart. The lateral view confirmed confinement of the dye to the epidural space.

The needles and catheters were then removed, and the back was then cleansed of excess Betadine solution, and antibiotic ointment and dressings were applied. There were no complications noted and the patient tolerated the procedure well. He will be discharged when discharge criteria have been met, and he will be seen in followup in 3 weeks to assess his level of improvement and to perform the second procedure in this series.

REVIEW QUESTIONS

The goal of these questions is to test your knowledge in the area of orthopedics.

Directions: Select the correct answer for each of the multiple-choice questions provided below. *Answers are provided at the end of this chapter.*

1. The bones that are found in the thigh, shins, upper and lower arms are called
   A. flat bones.
   B. long bones.
   C. sesamoid bones.
   D. short bones.

2. Which of the following is another name for the shaft or the middle region of a long bone?
   A. apophysis
   B. diaphysis
   C. epiphysis
   D. metaphysis

3. What is the term for the large process on the femur for attachment of muscles?
   A. condyle
   B. trochanter
   C. tubercle
   D. tuberosity

4. A narrow and deep slit-like opening in a bone is called a
   A. fissure.
   B. foramen.
   C. fossa.
   D. sinus.

5. Which of the following is transcribed correctly?
   A. Imaging studies show nerve-root sleeves fill well.
   B. Imaging studies show nerve-route sleeves fill well.
   C. Imaging studies show nerve-root sleeves feel well.
   D. Imaging studies show nerve-route sleeves feel well.

6. Which of the following is transcribed correctly?
   A. The patient is approximately 6 weeks status post ORIS of the left distal radius.
   B. The patient is approximately 6 weeks status post ORIF of the left ischial radius.
   C. The patient is approximately 6 weeks status post ORIS of the left ischial radius.
   D. The patient is approximately 6 weeks status post ORIF of the left distal radius.

7. The term osteopenia means
   A. fragile bones.
   B. bone deformity.
   C. inadequate bone marrow.
   D. reduced bone mass.

8. The first seven bones of the vertebral column are the
   A. thoracic vertebrae.
   B. cervical vertebrae.
   C. sacral vertebrae.
   D. umbar vertebrae.

9. The flat bone that extends down the midline of the chest is called the
   A. clavicle.
   B. scapula.
   C. sternum.
   D. xiphoid process.

10. The crackling sound produced when ends of bones rub against each other is called
    A. crepitus.
    B. friction.
    C. grind.
    D. rub.

11. Which of the following terms refers to a decrease in bone density with pathologic weakening and fractures?
    A. osteomalacia
    B. osteomyelitis
    C. osteopenia
    D. osteoporosis

12. The sac of fluid located near a joint is called the
    A. bursa.
    B. capsule.
    C. tubercle.
    D. foramen.

13. Movement away from the midline of the body is called
    A. abduction.
    B. adduction.
    C. dorsiflexion.
    D. hyperflexion.

14. Which of the following bones is found in the leg?
    A. fibula
    B. manubrium
    C. lunate
    D. humerus

15. Which of the following bones is found in the wrist?
    A. hamate
    B. ilium
    C. navicular
    D. talus

16. Which of the following is transcribed correctly?
    A. Her fracture line is less apparent, and there is definite callus formation in the distal radius with maintenance of the molar tilt.
    B. Her fracture line is less apparent, and there is definite callous formation in the distal radius with maintenance of the volar tilt.
    C. Her fracture line is less apparent, and there is definite callus formation in the distal radius with maintenance of the volar tilt.
    D. Her fracture line is less apparent, and there is definite callous formation in the distal radius with maintenance of the molar tilt.

17. An injury which involves multiple breaks or splintering of a bone is called a
    A. greenstick fracture.
    B. compound fracture.
    C. comminuted fracture.
    D. Colles fracture.

18. Tests for carpal tunnel syndrome include
    A. Adson and Apley.
    B. fabere and Hawkins.
    C. Phalen and Tinel.
    D. Homans and Spurling.

19. The hallux is more commonly known as the
    A. big toe.
    B. heel.
    C. middle finger.
    D. wrist.

20. Which of the following is an antiinflammatory medication?
    A. Celebrex
    B. Celexa
    C. Coreg
    D. Cialis

21. Abnormal curvature of the spine is called
    A. osteochondritis.
    B. osteoclasis.
    C. rickets.
    D. scoliosis.

22. Anterior and posterior can also be referred to as
    A. cephalad and caudad.
    B. medial and lateral.
    C. proximal and distal.
    D. ventral and dorsal.

23. Replacement of a joint is called
    A. arthroplasty.
    B. chondroplasty.
    C. osteoplasty.
    D. osteotomy.

24. A bimalleolar fracture would be located in the
    A. ankle.
    B. elbow.
    C. jaw.
    D. wrist.

25. The acromioclavicular joint is located in the
    A. hip.
    B. knee.
    C. pelvis.
    D. shoulder.

26. The surgeon smoothed the rough edges of the meniscus and repaired the anterior cruciate ligament. These procedures were performed on the
    A. finger.
    B. hip.
    C. knee.
    D. wrist.

27. Anterior drawer test assesses the stability of the
    A. elbow.
    B. knee.
    C. jaw.
    D. wrist.

28. The incomplete dislocation of the elbow in young children is also known as
    A. little league elbow.
    B. miner's elbow.
    C. nursemaid's elbow.
    D. tennis elbow.

29. Degeneration of the articulating part of the vertebra is called
    A. enterolysis.
    B. homolysis.
    C. litholysis.
    D. spondylolysis.

30. Treatment for osteoporosis may include
    A. Baclofen.
    B. bisacodyl.
    C. Topamax.
    D. Fosamax.

 Please see the accompanying CD for additional review materials for this section.

ANSWER KEY

REVIEW QUESTIONS ANSWER KEY

1. B	6. D	11. D	16. C	21. D	26. C
2. B	7. D	12. A	17. C	22. D	27. B
3. B	8. B	13. A	18. C	23. A	28. C
4. A	9. C	14. A	19. A	24. A	29. D
5. A	10. A	15. A	20. A	25. D	30. D

17

Endocrinology

OBJECTIVES CHECKLIST

A prepared exam candidate will know:

- [ ] All combining forms, prefixes, and suffixes related to endocrinology.

- [ ] Endocrine glands of the human body along with their location and primary function(s) in maintaining homeostasis.

- [ ] Hormones secreted by each gland as well as the hormones secreted by the pituitary gland that stimulate glandular function within the endocrine system.

- [ ] Primary diseases and conditions related to excessive and deficient secretions of the endocrine glands, along with the most common treatment modalities.

- [ ] Common laboratory tests ordered for endocrinologic conditions.

- [ ] Medications commonly prescribed for endocrinologic disorders, symptoms, and diseases.

RESOURCES FOR STUDY

1. *The Language of Medicine*
   Chapter 18: Endocrine System, pp. 719–768.

2. *Memmler's Structure and Function of the Human Body*
   Chapter 11: The Endocrine System: Glands and Hormones, pp. 197–210.

3. *Memmler's The Human Body in Health and Disease*
   Chapter 12: The Endocrine System: Glands and Hormones, pp. 244–260; Study Guide, pp.192–203.

4. *Human Diseases*
   Chapter 15: Disorders of Metabolism, Nutrition, and Endocrine Function, pp. 223–240.
   Chapter 17: Musculoskeletal Disorders (Disorders of Joints), pp. 265–267.

5. *Laboratory Tests & Diagnostic Procedures in Medicine*
   Chapter 20: Chemical Examination of the Blood (Hormones and Blood Sugar), pp. 365–373, 377-378.
   Chapter 24: Laboratory Examination of Urine, Stool, and Other Fluids and Materials, pp. 441–442.

6. *A Manual of Laboratory and Diagnostic Tests*
   Chapter 6: Chemistry Studies, pp. 316–455.
   Chapter 9: Nuclear Medicine Studies, pp. 652–704.

7. *The AAMT Book of Style for Medical Transcription*
   Diabetes Mellitus, pp. 129–132.

8. *Using Medical Terminology: A Practical Approach*
   Chapter 6: Endocrine System, pp. 379–416.

9. *Pharmacology for Health Professionals*
   Chapter 22: Antidiabetic Drugs, pp. 323–338.
   Chapter 23: Hormones and Related Drugs, pp. 339–381.

10. *Understanding Pharmacology for Health Professionals*
    Chapter 21: Endocrine Drugs, pp. 228–235.
    Chapter 22: Antidiabetic Drugs, pp. 236–242.

11. *Medical Terminology: The Language of Health Care*
    Chapter 11: Endocrine System, pp. 358–385.

SAMPLE REPORTS

The following three reports are examples of reports you might encounter while transcribing endocrinology.

THYROID SONOGRAM

PROCEDURE/STUDY
Thyroid sonogram.

CLINICAL INDICATIONS
Enlarged thyroid gland.

TECHNIQUE
Ultrasound examination of the thyroid gland in the longitudinal and transverse planes using a high-resolution linear-array transducer was performed.

REFERENCED EXAM
None.

FINDINGS
There is irregularity of the contour and heterogeneous signal characteristic in both lobes of the thyroid gland consistent with a multinodular goiter. No prominent cystic components are identified. However, there are several small (4-mm and 6-mm) cystic components in the left lobe of the thyroid gland. Therefore, the appearance of the abnormality is most consistent with a multinodular goiter. The thyroid isthmus is prominent in size but within normal limits. No other acute abnormalities are identified.

IMPRESSION
Multiple bilateral nodules in the thyroid gland. The thyroid gland itself is minimally enlarged. There are several small areas of diminished signal intensity consistent with a cystic component. This most likely represents a multinodular goiter. Nonetheless, if there is no history of thyroid disease, then a radionuclide scan may be useful to confirm the presence of a multinodular goiter.

OFFICE VISIT

REASON FOR VISIT
Followup for thyroid cancer.

The patient is a pleasant 69-year-old woman who returns for followup. She had a thyroid biopsy done locally. This was suspicious for papillary or thyroid cancer. She underwent thyroidectomy on 12/17/2003. Multiple small nodules were noted in the thyroid; one was listed as 0.7 cm with a papillary appearance located within the isthmus closest to the right lobe. She had multiple colloid nodules and chronic thyroiditis, but it is unclear from her report whether there was more than one nodule that had papillary thyroid cancer. She reports she underwent a nuclear scan and then received 80 mCi of ^{131}I on 1/14/2004. She then started Synthroid 137 mcg daily on 1/20/2004. She notes she did have typical hypothyroid symptoms and decreased energy, which are only now starting to improve. She was also taking calcium.

MEDICATIONS CURRENTLY
1. Synthroid 137 mcg daily.
2. Nexium.
3. Toprol.
4. Evoxac.
5. Folic acid.
6. Prednisone 30 mg a day.
7. Ambien.
8. Methotrexate.
9. Calcium.

PHYSICAL EXAM
An alert woman in no acute distress. Her blood pressure was 100/70. Her weight was 155. Thyroid exam showed no thyroid tissue palpable. No cervical lymphadenopathy. There was a well-healed neck scar. Cardiac exam showed a regular rhythm. Extremities showed no edema. Neurologic exam showed reflexes were normal. She had cushingoid changes.

IMPRESSION
Papillary thyroid cancer.

PLAN
I reviewed with the patient and her husband that she had appropriate treatment for her papillary thyroid cancer, including thyroidectomy and then subsequently 80 mCi of ^{131}I therapy on 1/14/2004. I told her it was unclear to me by reading her report whether she only had a 0.7-cm nodule that was papillary thyroid cancer or whether there was more than one. I recommended she forward her pathology slides for pathology review. If she really only has one nodule that is under 1 cm, then I think thyroid hormone replacement with target TSH in the lower half of normal would be reasonable. On the other hand, if she had large nodules or multiple nodules, then lowering her TSH below normal would be considered. She has only been on Synthroid about 1 month.

(continued)

I suggested in 6 to 8 weeks after she initiated the Synthroid that she have her TSH, free T_4, and thyroglobulin measured. If she plans on having surgery for her kidneys, she should have her TSH and free T_4 measured before her surgery and ideally have normal thyroid tests before considering another surgery. She will try to get her outside pathology slides and nuclear medicine report forwarded to me. I told her I would be happy to review those, and I could give her a call once we have that information.

OFFICE VISIT

REASON FOR CONSULTATION
Hypercalcemia.

HISTORY
This is a 68-year-old female with a long-standing history of debilitating rheumatoid arthritis. She has had rheumatoid arthritis since age 22 and has been on chronic steroid treatment for the last 40+ years. She has had a history of kidney stones, which has required stent placement over the past several years. She was recently admitted with kidney stones and had urosepsis at the end of January 2005. At that time, apparently her calcium was in the normal range. On 01/31/2005, she was re-admitted with a history of confusion, decreased fluid intake, nausea, and vomiting. At the time of her admission, she was noted to have a creatinine greater than 4 and a calcium of 16. The patient has been on Fosamax and calcium in the past. She has had no previous history of hyperparathyroidism or malignancy. She has had a colostomy for several years. She was given IV fluids, Lasix, and was treated with pamidronate at the time of her admission on 01/31/2005. She had prompt resolution of her hypercalcemia, which went from a high of 16.1 down to the 9 range. Her calcium has since fallen into the range of 5 to 7, with a low albumin. She had one PTH level which was measured on 02/03/2005 at 94. At that time, her calcium was measured at 8.9. A 24-hour urine was obtained. Her serum protein electrophoresis was measured and was essentially unremarkable. The patient is now in the ICU receiving IV fluids and tube feedings. She has recently undergone a swallowing study which was negative.

PAST MEDICAL HISTORY
Her past medical history is significant for her rheumatoid arthritis, causing her to be wheelchair-bound. She has significant ankle deformities and hand deformities as a result. She has had multiple kidney stones and hepatitis C. She has had a colostomy, hysterectomy, and appendectomy.

MEDICATIONS
Fosamax, prednisone, Premarin, Advair, Singulair.

SOCIAL HISTORY
She does not smoke. She occasionally drinks alcohol. She is married.

FAMILY HISTORY
Her mother and father are both deceased.

REVIEW OF SYSTEMS
As per medical review.

PHYSICAL EXAMINATION
Today, her blood pressure is 110/73. HEENT: Pupils are equal, round, reactive to light and accommodation. Extraocular movements are intact. The neck shows no thyromegaly. Chest is clear to auscultation. Cardiovascular: S1 and S2. Neurologic exam is grossly intact. Her extremities show multiple rheumatoid nodules on both hands. She has rheumatoid abnormalities of both her hands and her feet.

(continued)

LABORATORY DATA

Creatinine today is 1.3, calcium 7.3, albumin 1.9, phosphorus 1.2, magnesium 1.8. Her Dilantin level is 15.

IMPRESSION

Hypercalcemia in a patient admitted with renal failure. The etiology of her renal failure is not clear, although it most likely is volume depletion in a patient on calcium and other medications. The patient currently has a low calcium and has received her pamidronate and intravenous fluids initially and now seems to be stabilized as far as this is concerned. It is possible that the kidney stones were a result of her hyperparathyroidism, although I am not convinced that it is the underlying cause of either her kidney stones or her hypercalcemia. Patients who have colostomy, particularly, can have problems with kidney stones also.

PLAN

1. I will discuss these issues with the patient's internist and nephrologist.
2. Consider repeating a complete workup once the patient is out of the ICU and an outpatient, as this would give us a better understanding of her overall calcium balance to see if her levels of PTH are elevated at a time when her calcium is also elevated.
3. Finally, because of all these other complicating variables, I think it is important to have her stable medically before we embark upon any sort of workup or consideration of treatment options. At the present time I do not think that there is any need for any other agents to lower her calcium, as her calcium is in the normal range now. In addition, her kidney function is now normal, and we would expect that to maintain her calcium within the normal range. The plan will be to obtain the workup as an outpatient.

REVIEW QUESTIONS

The goal of these questions is to test your knowledge in the area of endocrinology.

Directions: Select the correct answer for each of the multiple-choice questions provided below. *Answers are provided at the end of this chapter.*

1. Which type of gland secretes hormones directly into the bloodstream rather than into ducts leading to the exterior of the body?
   A. endocrine gland
   B. exocrine gland
   C. serous gland
   D. target gland

2. What is the name of the gland that is composed of a right and left lobe on either side of the trachea?
   A. adrenal gland
   B. parathyroid gland
   C. pituitary gland
   D. thyroid gland

3. Which of the following secrete estrogen and progesterone?
   A. adrenal glands
   B. pineal glands
   C. ovaries
   D. testes

4. Which of the following is secreted by the posterior lobe of the pituitary gland and stimulates contraction of the uterus during labor?
   A. estrogen
   B. oxytocin
   C. progesterone
   D. prolactin

5. Potassium, sodium, and chloride are
   A. catecholamines.
   B. electrolytes.
   C. enzymes.
   D. steroids.

6. The combining form *gonad/o* means
   A. adrenal glands.
   B. pancreas.
   C. sex organs.
   D. thyroid gland.

7. Measurement of T_3, T_4, and TSH is collectively known as
   A. TFTs.
   B. BMP.
   C. LFTs.
   D. CMP.

8. Overactivity of the thyroid gland is called
   A. Addison disease.
   B. Cushing syndrome.
   C. hyperthyroidism.
   D. hypothyroidism.

9. Which of the following is a measure of blood sugar after 4 or more hours of no food?
   A. fasting glucose
   B. glucose tolerance test
   C. microalbumin test
   D. thyroid function test

10. Enlargement of the thyroid gland is called
    A. bruit.
    B. goiter.
    C. moon facies.
    D. thyroiditis.

11. Insulin is produced in the
    A. gallbladder.
    B. kidney.
    C. liver.
    D. pancreas.

12. Which test is used to evaluate blood glucose levels over the previous 2 months?
    A. methemoglobin
    B. C-reactive protein
    C. hemoglobin A_{1c}
    D. prolactin

13. Which of the following would be an appropriate medication for someone with hypothyroidism?
    A. Cymbalta
    B. Levoxyl
    C. Zelnorm
    D. Zithromax

14. Which of the following is a hypoglycemic medication?
    A. Avandia
    B. Ceftin
    C. Lipitor
    D. Prevacid

15. Enlargement of the bones of the hands, feet, and face due to overproduction of growth hormone is called
    A. acromegaly.
    B. Cushing syndrome.
    C. polydactyly.
    D. Addison disease.

16. The "master gland" of the endocrine system, located at the base of the brain, is the
    A. apical gland.
    B. Bartholin gland.
    C. pituitary gland.
    D. thyroid gland.

17. Which gland secretes DHEA and cortisol?
    A. pituitary
    B. adrenal
    C. parathyroid
    D. pineal

18. An excessive or abnormal hair growth, particularly male pattern hair growth on a woman, is called:
    A. Addison disease.
    B. cretinism.
    C. hirsutism.
    D. testotoxicosis.

19. What is a possible diagnosis for a middle-age woman with thinning hair, fatigue, irritability, and weight gain?
    A. hyperthyroidism
    B. hypochondria
    C. hypoparathyroidism
    D. hypothyroidism

20. Which of the following is used to treat diabetes mellitus?
    A. Humalog
    B. Lotrel
    C. Lotensin
    D. Neurontin

21. Severe hypothyroidism characterized by dry, puffy skin, somnolence, slow mentation, and hoarseness is known as
    A. hypoparathyroidism.
    B. myxedema.
    C. pheochromocytoma.
    D. rickets.

22. Graves disease is also known as
    A. hypothyroidism.
    B. parathymia.
    C. hyperinsulinism.
    D. toxic goiter.

23. Which of the following hormones stimulates egg production in the ovaries?
    A. FSH
    B. PSA
    C. TSH
    D. prolactin

24. Which hormone is secreted in the urine of pregnant women?
    A. beta hCG
    B. oxytocin
    C. growth hormone
    D. somatotropin

25. Insulin shock is characterized by
    A. severe hypoglycemia caused by an overdose of insulin.
    B. severe hyperglycemia.
    C. too little insulin in the bloodstream.
    D. an allergic reaction to insulin.

26. Chronic excretion of large amounts of urine of low specific gravity is indicative of
    A. diabetes innocens.
    B. diabetes insipidus.
    C. diabetes intermittens.
    D. diabetes mellitus.

27. Which of the following is a complication of diabetes mellitus?
    A. gastroparesis
    B. exophthalmos
    C. hirsutism
    D. moon facies

28. Elevated glucose levels, especially in obese persons, may be due to
    A. diabetic acidosis.
    B. glucose intolerance.
    C. insulin resistance.
    D. insulin shock.

29. The class of drugs referred to as glitazones are used to treat
    A. diabetes insipidus.
    B. non-insulin-dependent diabetes mellitus.
    C. infertility.
    D. hypothyroidism.

30. Which of the following is transcribed correctly?
    A. The patient was diagnosed with type 1 diabetes at 4 years of age.
    B. The patient was diagnosed with type I diabetes at 4 years of age.
    C. The patient was diagnosed with type I diabetes at 4-years of age.
    D. The patient was diagnosed with type one diabetes at 4 years of age.

 Please see the accompanying CD for additional review materials for this section.

ANSWER KEY

REVIEW QUESTIONS ANSWER KEY

1. A	6. C	11. D	16. C	21. B	26. B
2. D	7. A	12. C	17. B	22. D	27. A
3. C	8. C	13. B	18. C	23. A	28. C
4. B	9. A	14. A	19. D	24. A	29. B
5. B	10. B	15. A	20. A	25. A	30. A

18

Psychiatry/Psychology

OBJECTIVES CHECKLIST

A prepared exam candidate will know the:

❏ Combining forms, prefixes, and suffixes related to psychiatry and psychology.

❏ Role and function of the psychiatrist, psychologist, and other specialists within the discipline of mental health.

❏ Clinical signs, symptoms, and disorders related to psychiatry and mental illness.

❏ Substances associated with abuse and dependence.

❏ Clinical and diagnostic procedures and therapeutic techniques used in the identification and treatment of mental diseases and disorders.

❏ Medications and drug therapies commonly used to treat psychiatric disorders.

❏ Terminology and format related to recording a mental status examination, including testing and classification systems related to mental evaluation and diagnosis.

❏ Role of the *Diagnostic and Statistical Manual of Mental Disorders, Fourth Edition* (DSM-IV) in identifying and classifying psychiatric disorders.

❏ Multi-axial system used in diagnosing psychiatric patients.

RESOURCES FOR STUDY

1. *The Language of Medicine*
   Chapter 22: Psychiatry, pp. 887–924.

2. *H&P: A Nonphysician's Guide to the Medical History and Physical Examination*
   Chapter 13: Review of Systems: Psychiatric, pp. 117–124.
   Chapter 28: The Formal Mental Status Examination, pp. 273–280.

3. *Human Diseases*
   Chapter 20: Mental Disorders, pp. 315–332.

4. *The AAMT Book of Style for Medical Transcription*
   Global assessment of functioning (GAF) scale, p. 75.
   Global assessment of relational functioning (GARF) scale, p. 76.
   Social and occupational functioning assessment scale (SOFAS), p. 79.
   Psychiatric diagnoses, pp. 133–134.

5. *Using Medical Terminology: A Practical Approach*
   Chapter 18: Mental Disorders, pp. 901–955.

6. *Pharmacology for Health Professionals*
   Chapter 5: Psychiatric Drugs, pp. 63–91.

7. *Understanding Pharmacology for Health Professionals*
   Chapter 25: Psychiatric Drugs, pp. 279–295.

8. *Medical Terminology: The Language of Health Care*
   Chapter 10: Nervous System, pp. 310–357.

The following five reports are examples of reports you might encounter while transcribing psychiatry and psychology.

CONSULTATION

IDENTIFICATION DATA
The patient is a 33-year-old African American male with no prior psychiatric contacts. He was admitted to the inpatient mental health service by Dr. Jones secondary to an acute overdose. The patient apparently overdosed on Pamelor and Tylenol (approximately 15 tablets). The patient was intending to hurt himself secondary to his recent divorce.

CHIEF COMPLAINT
"Yeah, I've been depressed."

HISTORY OF PRESENT ILLNESS
The patient is a 33-year-old African American male with no prior psychiatric contact who was admitted to the inpatient mental health service through the courtesy of Dr. Jones secondary to a possible overdose. The patient stated, "I took the pills but then I called my pastor."

The patient relates that he has been depressed over the past few years secondary to his mother dying. Shortly after his mother's death 2 years ago, he relates that he discovered he was adopted and he became even more despondent. Early last month, his wife of 3 years filed for divorce, and that has been worsening his mood. He apparently moved to Indiana after the divorce "to find a job" but moved back to Iowa over the past week and moved into his mother's old home. He states that he has been living in a home with no running water and no utilities and has been increasingly despondent secondary to this. He states that he took the pills "without thinking." The patient also reported drinking about a 24-ounce can of beer prior to taking the overdose, stating, "I just got more depressed after I drank." The patient also has a history of cannabis use but denies recent use.

The patient requests discharge and is enthusiastic about the job that he has waiting for him in Iowa. The patient relates that he went through orientation on the job last Thursday and felt that his life was taking a turn for the better, but he then became acutely depressed on the day prior to admission, drank some alcohol, and took the pills. The patient states, "I did it without thinking, and after I took the pills, I called my pastor right away. Then I called my cousin and they told me to come to the hospital."

PAST PSYCHIATRIC HISTORY
The patient has a history of depression, by his report, over the past 2 years. The patient reports decreased interest in daily activities but has no sleep disturbance, and his appetite has been "fine." He has some guilt about not being able to provide for his biological children in a consistent fashion and occasionally feels helplessness. There are no feelings of hopelessness or worthlessness. The patient is actually hopeful about the future, and there are no psychotic symptoms in evidence and no manic symptoms either. The patient downplays his cannabis use and denies alcohol use on a regular basis.

(continued)

PAST MEDICAL HISTORY

The patient denies any active medical problems, but he is status post overdose with 15 tablets of Pamelor and Tylenol, as above. The patient does have a history of a gunshot wound to the left shoulder, which the patient describes as an "accident" after he got into an argument with someone. He states he has no access to handguns or firearms and states that the mother of his biological children has all of his firearms. He is reluctant to allow disclosure of information regarding why he is in the hospital.

SOCIAL/FAMILY HISTORY

The patient was born in Ohio and raised in this area. He was raised by his adoptive mother. He had no contact with his biological parents. He has a twelfth-grade education. He also went to college and studied pre-law at the local community college. He has worked in the past doing various jobs and plans to start work tomorrow as previously mentioned. His 3 children with his previous girlfriend include a daughter, age 12, and 2 sons, ages 8 and 10.

INVENTORY OF ASSETS

The patient is physically healthy, has gainful employment, a supportive pastor, a supportive cousin, and supportive ex-girlfriend.

MENTAL STATUS EXAMINATION

In general, the patient appears cooperative, pleasant, and interactive. Psychomotor activity is within normal limits. Speech is normal in amount and tone. Mood is "better." Affect is bright. The patient denies suicidal or homicidal ideations, plans, or intents. He also denies auditory or visual hallucinations, and he has concrete plans for the future, including starting his job tomorrow morning in Iowa. He states that he has a "good job" with "good benefits" and states, "Someone like me will not have this opportunity again."

He was alert and oriented x3. The patient is very emotional about the overdose attempt and is also ashamed, stating, "I don't know what I was thinking." The patient was able to recall 3/3 items after 1 minute and 3/3 items after 5 minutes. Serial sevens were intact. Abstractions are concrete.

ADMITTING DIAGNOSES

Axis I   Adjustment disorder with mixed disturbance of emotions and conduct; rule out major depression, not otherwise specified.

Axis II   None.

Axis III   Please refer to the internal medicine notes.

Axis IV   Recent divorce. Recent occupational history, which has actually improved, and death of his mother 2 years ago.

Axis V   Global assessment of functioning = 75–80. Highest in the past year not known.

PLAN

At the present time, the patient will be discharged to the outpatient setting. The patient denied suicidal or homicidal ideation and does not pose a threat to himself or others, and this seems to have been an impulsive gesture after drinking alcohol and possible use of cannabis. In addition, the patient states he has concrete plans for the future, including starting to work tomorrow morning at his new job.

(continued)

The patient will be started on Wellbutrin SR 150 mg p.o. every morning for 3 days and increase to 150 mg b.i.d. thereafter. The patient will receive a 2-week supply of this medication through my office in the form of samples. The risks, benefits, and side effects of the medications were discussed with the patient, and he gave informed consent to treatment.

The patient will follow up with Comprehensive Mental Health or my office within 2 weeks after discharge.

The patient was advised to go to the nearest emergency room if he has any suicidal thoughts, and the patient was strongly recommended to abstain from alcohol and drug use.

CONSULTATION

IDENTIFICATION DATA
Please refer to her detailed mental status assessment and diagnosis.

CHIEF COMPLAINT
Please refer to her detailed mental status assessment and diagnosis.

HISTORY OF PRESENT ILLNESS
Please refer to her detailed mental status assessment and diagnosis.

DIAGNOSES UPON DISCHARGE
Axis I   Major depression with psychotic features, as well as cocaine abuse.
Axis II   Personality disorder; not otherwise specified.
Axis III   History of colostomy secondary to perforated diverticulum, as well as gastroesophageal reflux disease and hypertension.
Axis IV   Chronic mental illness and multiple medical issues.
Axis V   Global assessment of functioning = 20–25; highest in the past year 55–60.

HOSPITAL COURSE
This patient was admitted to the inpatient psychiatric service for evaluation and treatment of suicidal ideation as well as cocaine abuse. The patient was increasingly depressed secondary to news that her colostomy would be irreversible, and she verbalized suicidal thoughts. The patient was placed on routine precautions after being admitted on April 22 and started on Xanax 0.5 mg t.i.d., Remeron 15 mg nightly, and Prozac 20 mg every morning. She was also started on Zyprexa 5 mg at 8 p.m. on April 23. Surgical nursing was consulted for ostomy supplies. Zyprexa was increased to 7.5 mg at 8 p.m. on April 25, and she continued to be monitored for depressive symptoms. A GI consultation was ordered for Dr. Jones to see the patient for abdominal pain on April 26. Social work referred the patient to ARTS, as the patient was reluctant to go to our inpatient treatment program. She was also referred to the partial hospitalization program.

She was discharged to her home on April 30 with her husband and was scheduled to follow up with Dr. Jones within 2 weeks of discharge and to follow up at her regular hospital for colostomy care the day after discharge from this facility.

At the time of discharge, the patient denied suicidal or homicidal ideation. Her psychotic symptoms have cleared, and she is more interactive, pleasant, and no longer tearful.

MEDICATIONS UPON DISCHARGE
Remeron 15 mg nightly, Prevacid 30 mg daily, Norvasc 5 mg daily, Colace 100 mg b.i.d., Metamucil b.i.d., Prozac 20 mg every morning, Zyprexa 7.5 mg nightly, Premarin 0.625 mg daily, and Xanax 0.5 mg t.i.d.

PROGNOSIS AT TIME OF DISCHARGE
Guarded, secondary to the patient's substance abuse issues, minimizing of symptoms, and sporadic compliance. At the time of discharge, the patient was strongly advised to abstain from the use of cocaine secondary to its deleterious effects on her health, and the patient agreed to follow with the inpatient program for relapse prevention.

CONSULTATION

HISTORY OF PRESENT ILLNESS

The patient is a 59-year-old female admitted on an emergency basis because of a confusional state, irritability, walking out of her home, not sleeping, and feeling very anxious. The patient was taken to the emergency room 2 days ago, her blood sugar and other medical problems were checked, and she was sent back home. Then her sister, with whom she had been living, called on April 22, 2004, to report that at odd hours the patient walks out of the house, apparently in a confused state, and she is not eating or sleeping well. She is also not making much sense most of the time.

I recommended admission, but the patient declined to go to the hospital, so her sister brought her to the office this morning. She appeared to be drowsy, lethargic, mumbling to herself, and hearing voices. However, she is under the impression that she has some medical problems and that her diabetes is out of control. Therefore, she wants to go to the medical floor. Her blood sugar has been pretty stable, according to the sister. Finally, the patient agreed to be admitted to the psychiatric floor.

PAST PSYCHIATRIC HISTORY

The patient has a long history of having had psychiatric problems. She has had one admission here in 2002. Prior to that, she was living in Alabama and had multiple admissions there. She has had psychotic symptoms practically all of her adult life. During the past 6 months, she has grown quite resistant to taking her psychotropic medications. These consist of Risperdal 3 mg b.i.d. and Depakote-ER 500 mg 3 nightly. Her Risperdal was reduced at her request because she claimed she was sleeping too much, but the reality was that she sleeps through the day and stays up at night. Her Depakote was decreased about 1 month ago, but this was again because of complaints that she was gaining weight, etc. She did not want to take Depakote any longer. I had warned both the patient and her sister that she might have increased symptoms, and not surprisingly, within 2 weeks, she began deteriorating, getting confused, and hearing voices.

FAMILY HISTORY

Unchanged from previous admissions.

REVIEW OF SYSTEMS

The patient offers no specific complaints, but she thinks her tiredness, confusion, drowsiness, etc., are because of her diabetes.

PHYSICAL EXAMINATION

HEAD: Normocephalic.
NECK: Supple.
CHEST: Symmetrical.
LUNGS: Clear to percussion and auscultation.
HEART: No murmur.
ABDOMEN: Soft and nontender; no organomegaly or masses palpable.
NEUROLOGICAL EXAMINATION: Gait and coordination normal.

(continued)

MENTAL STATUS EXAMINATION

The patient looks older than her stated age. She is glum and wary. She mumbles often and has difficulty expressing her thoughts in a relevant fashion. She is not able to answer questions appropriately. She is reasonably oriented to date, place, and person. Sensorium, in that sense, is fairly clear, but she lacks clarity of thinking. She looks very depressed, somewhat perplexed, and is mildly confused. She always has excessive worry about things. Insight and judgment are poor.

DIAGNOSES

Axis I   Schizoaffective disorder, depressed-type, with acute relapse.

Axis II   None.

Axis III Type 2 diabetes mellitus, hypertension, coronary artery disease, obesity, hypothyroidism, history of chronic obstructive pulmonary disease, and history of congestive cardiac failure.

Axis IV   Psychosocial stressors: None.

Axis V   Global assessment of functioning at the time of admission: 55.

CONSULTATION

SUMMARY OF INFORMATION

The patient is a 42-year-old male who was admitted to this facility with a variety of complaints, not the least of which was a low mood, agitation, and getting into violent fights. He said he had to come and get checked out to see for himself. He wanted to know if he handled things responsibly. These were his words, which are a bit unusual for this man. Of course, he has had several years of college training, and we have worked rather hard with him trying to get a stable place for him to live, because none of his family seems to take any interest in him.

FAMILY HISTORY

His father has diabetes and his mother is hypertensive. He has a brother with HIV and a sister who is supposedly bipolar, just as he is.

He had been doing fairly well with his once-a-month office visits and his occasional need for long-acting medicines, but recently he has become quite irritable, easily agitated, takes umbrage at the slightest thing, mopes around a great deal, and is noncompliant in general.

He has had no injuries or operations since the last time we saw him. Medications have been given, and his caretaker has seen to it that he at least gets his medicine. Whether he actually swallows it or not is a different story, and she cannot be sure of this one way or the other.

PHYSICAL EXAMINATION

GENERAL: He is very well developed and well nourished, with good muscle structure, good station and gait.

VITAL SIGNS: He is 180 pounds now. He had been about 160 before we got him stabilized. He is 5 feet 10 inches. He has a blood pressure of 124/64. Temperature, pulse, and respiratory rate are normal.

HEENT: No masses of the head, neck, chest, or abdomen. Extraocular movements are normal. He is quite expressive when he wants to be. Sometimes he becomes a bit grandiloquent and is hard to follow. He has the notion that he and his family are better off than they really are, and yet he cannot explain the fact that no one comes to visit him and no one will take him in.

CHEST: Lungs are clear.

HEART: No murmurs are appreciated.

ABDOMEN: Normal and very muscular.

EXTREMITIES: His extremities are also muscular.

MENTAL STATUS EXAMINATION

Aside from having some hostile display, irritability, and attitudes of being withdrawn, he has not had gross hallucinations, though there seems to be a paranoid delusional system simmering in him at this point. He is rather flippant in his affect except when he is trying to explain himself. He thinks he has business to take care of and does not think that this hospital stay should be very long. Indeed, it probably will not be.

PLAN

The patient will be admitted, and we will make sure that he gets restarted on his medications. We will contact his boarding home caretaker to make sure there is medicine at the house upon discharge.

(continued)

READMISSION DIAGNOSES

Axis I   Schizoaffective disorder.

Axis II   Paranoid personality.

Axis III No pathology.

Axis IV   Questionable compliance with treatment protocols.

Axis V   Current global assessment of functioning is 50.

CONSULTATION

CHIEF COMPLAINT/HISTORY OF PRESENT ILLNESS
The patient is a 20-year-old female with ingestion of an overdose of aspirin because she wanted to kill herself after an argument with her mother about 15 minutes prior to presentation in our emergency room.

CURRENT MEDICATIONS
Unknown at this time.

ALLERGIES
Unknown.

PHYSICAL EXAMINATION
VITAL SIGNS: Temperature 96.3, pulse 120, respirations 24, blood pressure 146/68. She is morbidly obese.
GENERAL: The patient appears to be in some distress.
HEENT: Normocephalic. Eyes normal. ENT normal.
NECK: Supple.
CHEST: Clear.
HEART: Tachycardia.
ABDOMEN: Soft and nontender.
GENITALS: Deferred.
RECTAL: Deferred.
EXTREMITIES: Limbs are normal.
NERVOUS SYSTEM: No sign of focal deficit. No sign of meningismus.

DIAGNOSTIC STUDIES
Her salicylate level was 6 mg/dL. Tylenol level was less than 10.

EMERGENCY DEPARTMENT COURSE
The patient was given 50 g of charcoal mixed with sorbitol, and a normal saline IV was started to run at 125 mL/hr. She also received Zantac 300 mg and Maalox 1 ounce. Dr. Jones was consulted, and the patient will be admitted for an aspirin overdose in a suicide attempt. The psychiatrist will evaluate her with regard to her suicide attempt.

FINAL DIAGNOSES
Aspirin overdose.
Suicide attempt.
Morbid obesity.

REVIEW QUESTIONS

The goal of these questions is to test your knowledge in the areas of psychiatry and psychology.

Directions: Select the correct answer for each of the multiple-choice questions provided below. *Answers are provided at the end of this chapter.*

1. In psychiatry, the abnormality described by the absence of emotions and lack of interest or emotional involvement is called
   A. amnesia.
   B. anxiety.
   C. apathy.
   D. autism.

2. An exaggerated feeling of well-being, also known as a "high," is called
   A. delusion.
   B. dysphoria.
   C. euphoria.
   D. conversion.

3. In psychiatry, this disorder is characterized by recurrent thoughts and repetitive acts that dominate the patient's behavior.
   A. agoraphobia
   B. claustrophobia
   C. obsessive-compulsive disorder
   D. posttraumatic stress disorder

4. Which of the following is used to describe the symptoms caused by withdrawal from chronic, excessive alcohol intake?
   A. delirium tremens
   B. delusions
   C. dementia
   D. dissociation

5. Which of the following terms describes depression which recurs at the same time of the year?
   A. bipolar disorder
   B. dysphoric disorder
   C. dysthymic disorder
   D. seasonal affective disorder

6. A person with a grandiose sense of self-importance or uniqueness and preoccupation with fantasies of success and power is said to be
   A. borderline.
   B. narcissistic.
   C. paranoid.
   D. schizoid.

7. The disorder characterized by withdrawal from reality into an inner world of disorganized thinking and conflict is called
   A. hypochondriasis.
   B. voyeurism.
   C. paranoia.
   D. schizophrenia.

8. A patient presenting with no facial expressions is said to have
   A. dysaphia.
   B. disorganized thinking.
   C. a flat affect.
   D. impaired interpersonal functioning.

9. Developed by Sigmund Freud, this long-term form of therapy seeks to influence behavior and resolve internal conflict by allowing patients to bring their unconscious emotions to the surface.
   A. cognitive behavior therapy
   B. group therapy
   C. hypnosis
   D. psychoanalysis

10. Which of the following is transcribed correctly?
    A. His judgment is intact, and he is experiencing no hallucinations or paranoid illusions.
    B. His judgment is intact, and he is experiencing no illuminations or paranoid delusions.
    C. His judgment is intact, and he is experiencing no hallucinations or paranoid delusions.
    D. His judgment is intact, and he is experiencing no illuminations or paranoid illusions.

11. A physician with medical training in the diagnosis, prevention, and treatment of mental disorders is called a
    A. physiologist.
    B. psychiatrist.
    C. psychologist.
    D. psychoanalyst.

12. The name of the defense mechanism by which unacceptable thoughts, feelings, and impulses are automatically pushed into the unconscious is called
    A. amnesia.
    B. delusion.
    C. depression.
    D. repression.

13. Which of the following is the translation for the combining form *hypn*/o?
    A. mind
    B. nerve
    C. sleep
    D. treatment

14. Which of the following is the translation for the combining form *somat*/o?
    A. body
    B. depressed
    C. distressed
    D. split

15. In a psychiatric diagnosis, the abbreviation NOS stands for
    A. new onset of symptoms.
    B. no other symptoms.

    C. no outstanding symptoms.
    D. not otherwise specified.

16. Which of the following medications is an antidepressant?
    A. Levaquin
    B. Levoxyl
    C. Lexapro
    D. lisinopril

17. Which of the following medications is used to treat anxiety?
    A. Adderall
    B. albuterol
    C. Ativan
    D. Avelox

18. A medication that is similar to morphine and is used for treatment of heroin addiction is
    A. metformin.
    B. methadone.
    C. Neurontin.
    D. Nexium.

19. A disorder characterized by refusal to maintain minimally normal body weight and intense fear of gaining weight is
    A. anorexia nervosa.
    B. compulsive neurosis.
    C. dysphagia globosa.
    D. hypothymic personality disorder.

20. The medical term for mild, chronic depression is
    A. anaphoria.
    B. dysthymia.
    C. hedonophobia.
    D. cyclothymia.

21. In an emergency room, a "banana bag" would be given to treat a patient with
    A. acetaminophen overdose.
    B. alcohol intoxication or withdrawal.
    C. obsessive-compulsive disorder.
    D. vascular dementia.

22. Electroconvulsive therapy is used to treat
    A. severe depression.
    B. dementia.

C. psychosis.

D. schizophrenia.

23. Which of the following describes a person who has been appointed by a judge to protect the interests of a person who is deemed incompetent?

A. conservator

B. lawyer

C. malefactor

D. power of attorney

24. The global assessment of function is transcribed under which of the following headings?

A. Axis V

B. criteria

C. differential

D. DSM-IV

25. A loss of memory is

A. amnesia.

B. aphasia.

C. apraxia.

D. aphagia.

26. Which of the following is transcribed correctly?

A. He states he is having significant martial problems and has been placed on probation at his job. He has a significant body odor, and his hair and clothes are unkept.

B. He states he is having significant marital problems and has been placed on probation at his job. He has a significant body odor, and his hair and clothes are unkept.

C. He states he is having significant martial problems and has been placed on probation at his job. He has a significant body odor, and his hair and clothes are unkempt.

D. He states he is having significant marital problems and has been placed on probation at his job. He has a significant body odor, and his hair and clothes are unkempt.

27. In psychology, the treatment of anxiety, phobias, and other disorders by changing behavior patterns and responses is known as

A. cognitive behavior therapy.

B. hypnosis.

C. play therapy.

D. psychoanalysis.

28. Anxiolytic drugs are used to help treat

A. anxiety.

B. dementia.

C. depression.

D. obsessive-compulsive disorder.

29. The psychoactive component of marijuana is

A. cannabis.

B. cocaine.

C. heroin.

D. morphine.

30. Which of the following is an antipsychotic drug used in treatment of schizophrenia?

A. Geodon

B. Klonopin

C. trazodone

D. Xanax

 Please see the accompanying CD for additional review materials for this section.

ANSWER KEYS

REVIEW QUESTIONS ANSWER KEY

1. C	6. B	11. B	16. C	21. B	26. D
2. C	7. D	12. D	17. C	22. A	27. A
3. C	8. C	13. C	18. B	23. A	28. A
4. A	9. D	14. A	19. A	24. A	29. A
5. D	10. C	15. D	20. B	25. A	30. A

19

Pulmonology

OBJECTIVES CHECKLIST

A prepared exam candidate will know:

❑ Combining forms, prefixes, and suffixes related to the body system.

❑ Anatomical structures of the respiratory system.

❑ Physiologic process of respiration and the pathway of air from the nose to the lung capillaries.

❑ Difference between external (pulmonary) respiration and internal (cellular) respiration.

❑ Terminology and definitions related to auscultated breath sounds.

❑ Signs, symptoms, and diseases related to the respiratory system.

❑ Diagnostic studies used in the diagnosis and treatment of respiratory symptoms, disorders, and diseases.

❑ Respiratory therapies.

❑ Imaging studies used in the identification and diagnosis of respiratory diseases.

❑ Laboratory studies used in the diagnosis and treatment of respiratory symptoms, disorders, and diseases.

❑ Common medications prescribed for respiratory symptoms, disorders, and diseases.

❑ Transcription standards related to pulmonary and respiratory terms.

RESOURCES FOR STUDY

1. *Bates' Guide to Physical Examination and History Taking*
   Chapter 7: The Thorax and Lungs, pp. 241–277.

2. *The Language of Medicine*
   Chapter 12: Respiratory System, pp. 441–486.

3. *Memmler's Structure and Function of the Human Body*
   Chapter 16: Respiration, pp. 289–303.

4. *Memmler's The Human Body in Health and Disease*
   Chapter 18: Respiration, pp. 362–383; Study Guide, pp. 278–291.

5. *H&P: A Nonphysician's Guide to the Medical History and Physical Examination*
   Chapter 9: Review of Systems: Respiratory, pp. 83–88.
   Chapter 24: Examination of the Lungs, pp. 227–234.

6. *Human Diseases*
   Chapter 10: Diseases of the Respiratory System, pp. 141–152.

7. *Laboratory Tests & Diagnostic Procedures in Medicine*
   Chapter 4: Measurement of Temperature, Rates, Pressures and Volumes (Respiratory Measurements), pp. 48–50.
   Chapter 7: Visual Examination of the Eyes, Ears, Nose and Respiratory Tract, pp. 95–106.
   Chapter 10: Plain Radiography (Chest X-ray), pp. 137–138.
   Chapter 20: Chemical Examination of the Blood (Acid-Base Balance, pp. 357–360, and Arterial Blood Gases, p. 362).

8. *A Manual of Laboratory and Diagnostic Tests*
   Chapter 7: Microbiologic Studies, pp. 456–529.
   Chapter 9: Nuclear Medicine Studies, pp. 652–704.
   Chapter 10: X-ray Studies, pp. 705–759.
   Chapter 11: Cytologic, Histologic, and Genetic Studies, pp. 760–818.
   Chapter 12: Endoscopic Studies, pp. 819–861.
   Chapter 14: Pulmonary Function, Arterial Blood Gases (ABGs), and Electrolyte Studies, pp. 900–972.

9. *The AAMT Book of Style for Medical Transcription*
   Pulmonary and Respiratory Terms, pp. 338–340.

10. *Using Medical Terminology: A Practical Approach*
    Chapter 13: Respiratory System, pp. 571–631.

11. *Pharmacology for Health Professionals*
    Unit III: Drugs That Affect the Respiratory System (Chapters 11–13), pp. 169–197.

12. *Understanding Pharmacology for Health Professionals*
    Chapter 18: Pulmonary Drugs, pp. 192–204.

13. *Medical Terminology: The Language of Health Care*
    Chapter 9: Respiratory System, pp. 269–309.

SAMPLE REPORTS

The following four reports are examples of reports you might encounter while transcribing pulmonology.

FOLLOWUP REPORT

HISTORY OF PRESENT ILLNESS
The patient is a 56-year-old white female with rheumatoid arthritis and bronchiectasis. She had a right upper lobe cavity develop on CT scan. When I saw her in January, she had had an upper respiratory tract infection. She felt better with antibiotics, and then as she came off the antibiotics her symptoms worsened. By phone, I prescribed Avelox for 21 days. She is 1 week into her therapy and feels significantly better. On a scale of 1–10 (with 10 being normal), she is about a 7 or 8 now, in her opinion, and previously had been as low as a 4, by her description, when she first became ill. She has not had any hemoptysis. She had chills but they resolved. No sweats. No fevers. No chest pain. Appetite is acceptable but not quite normal. She has also had Mycobacterium avium (MAI) in her sputum. She has never had cyclic antibiotics, because she has had minimal symptoms and normal PFTs. Her most recent set of PFTs in January 2004, despite fairly extensive radiographic studies, was unremarkable.

PHYSICAL EXAMINATION
Physical exam today is unremarkable.

DIAGNOSTIC STUDIES
A CT scan of the thorax today, compared with January, shows that the cavitary lesion in the right upper lobe has not significantly changed other than more opacity within the cavity suggesting retained secretions. She has diffuse bronchiectatic changes throughout including all areas of confluence.

ASSESSMENT
I had a very long discussion with her today regarding bronchiectasis and its interaction with MAI and the difficulties in treating MAI, including 18 months of therapy with triple-drug combinations. Because she is clinically feeling well, her PFTs are normal, and her exercise tolerance has always been good, our current plan is to continue with the Avelox until it is completed at 21 days. We will check sputum for MAI between now and then, and I will see her back in 1 month with CT and PFTs at that time.

I have given her a web site to look for information regarding nontuberculous mycobacterium and have discussed the disease in great detail with her. I highlighted the controversies with regard to management and the appropriate timing of beginning antimycobacterial therapy. I also discussed our lack of good knowledge regarding temporal changes in PFTs over time.

I will see the patient in 1 month. I have invited her to call me if she develops any interim problems. She appears to be agreeable to this plan and is anxious to proceed as outlined.

CONSULTATION

HISTORY OF PRESENT ILLNESS

The patient is a 73-year-old white female originally from Europe. She is seeking evaluation here at the clinic for left upper abdominal pain. She is seen in the pulmonary clinic today for evaluation of chronic lung disease. She is a previous smoker, having smoked until 2 years ago. She also has a history of childhood "bronchitis" and also previous pneumonia. She has cough and dyspnea but not much in the way of phlegm production. It sounds as if she may have also had a positive tuberculin skin test, but never had active TB as far as she is aware. The remainder of her history and physical examination is as documented by her primary care physician. I highlight that she is on nocturnal oxygen, but she is not wearing it during the day. She is only on inhalers with beta agonists and ipratropium. She is not on any inhaled steroid. She has had deleterious side effects with systemic steroids.

PHYSICAL EXAMINATION

Physical exam today is limited by her discomfort. Lung exam is most notable for very diminished breath sounds and a few wheezes with poor air exchange throughout.

DIAGNOSTIC STUDIES

Chest x-ray shows changes of hyperinflation with increased retrosternal air space and a flattened hemidiaphragm. PFTs show severe obstructive lung disease with relatively preserved diffusion capacity and some reversibility. The ratio is 37.7. FEV_1 is 0.87, which is 37% of predicted, and it increases to 1.08 or 24% after bronchodilators. Lung volumes show increased TLC and increased RV/TLC. Diffusion capacity is 61% and resting saturation is 88%.

ASSESSMENT AND PLAN

Chronic obstructive lung disease with some reversibility and mildly reduced diffusion capacity. I do not suspect her pain has anything to do with her lung disease. I am uncertain if her underlying lung disease is a fixed asthma, bronchiectasis, or changes of chronic bronchitis, although her clinical history does not suggest that. I would like to perform a CT scan to better characterize her lung disease. If it appears that this is predominantly bronchiectasis, there will not be strong indications for inhaled corticosteroids. However, if this is asthma that still maintains reversibility, then proceeding with inhaled steroids in addition to other therapies would be of benefit. Next, I am not certain that her Singulair is offering her much benefit, and discontinuation of this would be appropriate.

BRONCHOSCOPY

PROCEDURE PERFORMED
Bronchoscopy.

PREOPERATIVE DIAGNOSIS
Nodular density in the right lower lobe, etiology uncertain.

POSTOPERATIVE DIAGNOSIS
Nodular density in the right lower lobe, etiology uncertain.

FINDINGS
No endobronchial lesions seen.

INDICATIONS FOR PROCEDURE
This is a patient with what appears to be neurofibromatosis and was found to have a density in the right midlung field, felt by the radiologist to be in the lower lobe. Bronchoscopy is being done for further evaluation. He has a past smoking history. He came in with left-sided pleurisy.

PREOPERATIVE MEDICATIONS
Demerol 30 mg IM plus atropine 0.6 mg IM.

DESCRIPTION OF PROCEDURE
The patient was brought to Endoscopy, where topical anesthesia was administered. The bronchoscope was introduced through the right transnasal approach. The nasopharynx appeared normal. The vocal cords were normal. The trachea, main carina, right mainstem, right upper lobe, right middle lobe, and right lower lobe segments appeared normal. No lesions were seen. The left mainstem and left upper lobe segments appeared normal. There was some mild extrinsic compression of the left lower lobe orifice. There was no evidence of any endobronchial lesions seen. The bronchoscope was then reintroduced into the right upper lobe where the areas were reexamined, and no lesions were seen. The bronchoscope was then reintroduced into the right lower lobe where multiple washings were taken from the right basilar segments and the superior segment of the right lower lobe. Brushings were taken from the superior segment of the right lower lobe and sent for cytology also.

COMPLICATIONS
None so far. A postprocedure chest x-ray is pending.

SPECIMENS
1. Bronchial washings from the right lower lobe are being sent for routine culture and sensitivity, fungal culture, acid-fast bacillus smear, acid-fast bacillus culture, and routine viral cultures, since the patient did have some left chest pain on admission.
2. Bronchial brushings from the superior segment of the right lower lobe were sent for cytology.

CONDITION TO RECOVERY
Stable.

EXAMINATION PRE-PROCEDURE
Lungs were clear to auscultation and percussion. Heart had a regular rhythm with no murmurs, rubs, or gallops.

(continued)

EXAMINATION POST PROCEDURE
Lungs were clear to auscultation and percussion. Heart had a regular rhythm with no murmurs, rubs, or gallops.

TELEMETRY
Sinus rhythm throughout without any arrhythmias. Oxygen saturation was well above 90% throughout the procedure on 50% oxygen via mask. Post procedure on room air, the oxygen saturation was 96%. The blood pressure did increase during the procedure, but the patient indicated that he felt fine.

DISPOSITION
The patient will have a post-procedure chest x-ray done and will be monitored over the next few hours.

PULMONARY FUNCTION STUDIES

PROCEDURE
Pulmonary function testing.

LUNG VOLUMES
There is a moderate decrease in FVC. There is a marked reduction in TLC, RV, and FRC.

LUNG FLOWS
Moderate decrease in FVC, marked reduction in FEV_1, mild reduction in FEV_1/FVC. Marked decrease in $FEF_{25-75\%}$.

RESPONSE TO BRONCHODILATORS
There is a significant improvement in the FEV_1 and $FEF_{25-75\%}$ post-bronchodilator administration.

MVV AND PEF
None.

FLOW VOLUME LOOP
No evidence of upper airway obstruction.

DIFFUSING CAPACITY
Marked reduction in lung diffusion. The corrected DLCO [DL/VA] is moderately reduced.

ARTERIAL BLOOD GASES
None.

IMPRESSION
1. This study is suggestive of severe restrictive lung disease.
2. No evidence of upper airway obstruction.
3. Significant response to bronchodilators was seen.
4. Moderate reduction in the corrected DLCO [DL/VA].
5. The patient's obesity is probably related to the decrease in lung diffusion, at least in part.
6. At least a mild degree of coexisting airway obstruction is suspected. Clinical correlation is indicated.
7. The marked reduction in FRC and other lung volumes may be erroneous. Clinical correlation is indicated.

REVIEW QUESTIONS

The goal of these questions is to test your knowledge in the area of pulmonology.

Directions: Select the correct answer for each of the multiple-choice questions provided below. *Answers are provided at the end of this chapter.*

1. The nasal cavity is lined with a mucous membrane and fine hairs called
   A. alveoli.
   B. cilia.
   C. papillae.
   D. sacs.

2. The flap of cartilage attached to the root of the tongue that prevents choking or aspiration of food is called the
   A. epiglottis.
   B. larynx.
   C. oropharynx.
   D. pharynx.

3. The smallest of the bronchial branches are known as
   A. alveoli.
   B. bronchi.
   C. bronchioles.
   D. capillaries.

4. A pulmonary embolism is often secondary to a
   A. history of smoking.
   B. viral infection.
   C. bacterial infection.
   D. blood clot in the leg.

5. Which of the following gasses is produced as the end-product of metabolism and exhaled through the lungs?
   A. carbon dioxide
   B. carbon monoxide
   C. nitrogen
   D. oxygen

6. Which of the following is the muscle that separates the chest and the abdomen?
   A. latissimus dorsi
   B. diaphragm
   C. piriformis
   D. pectoralis major

7. The combining form *cyan/o* means
   A. air sac.
   B. blue.
   C. epiglottis.
   D. lobe.

8. The combining form *phon/o* means
   A. air.
   B. diaphragm.
   C. pleura.
   D. voice.

9. Listening to sounds within the body for diagnostic purposes is called
   A. auscultation.
   B. palpation.
   C. percussion.
   D. succussion.

10. Which of the following is the term for an abnormal crackling sound heard during inspiration when there is fluid, blood, or pus in the alveoli?
    A. pleural rub
    B. rales
    C. stridor
    D. wheezes

11. The acute viral infection most common in infants and children in which there is an obstruction of the larynx, barking cough, and stridor is called
    A. croup.
    B. diphtheria.
    C. asthma.
    D. pertussis.

12. Persistent blockage of air flow through the bronchial tubes and lungs is
    A. asbestosis.
    B. mesothelioma.
    C. chronic obstructive pulmonary disease.
    D. pulmonary fibrosis.

13. The procedure in which a rigid endoscope is inserted into the bronchial tubes for diagnosis, biopsy, or collection of specimens is called
    A. bronchoscopy.
    B. endotracheal intubation.
    C. laryngoscopy.
    D. mediastinoscopy.

14. The surgical procedure to remove fluid from the pleural space is called
    A. thoracentesis.
    B. thoracoscopy.
    C. tracheostomy.
    D. thoracotomy.

15. The medical term for snoring is
    A. Cheyne-Stokes respiration.
    B. Kussmaul respiration.
    C. stertor.
    D. stridor.

16. Which of the following drugs would be used to treat Mycobacterium tuberculosis (TB)?
    A. NicoDerm
    B. Serevent Diskus
    C. isoniazid
    D. Proventil

17. Which of the following has been transcribed correctly?
    A. He has a previous history of constructive sleep apnea treated with CPAT.
    B. He has a previous history of obstructive sleep apnea treated with CPAT.
    C. He has a previous history of obstructive sleep apnea treated with CPAP.
    D. He has a previous history of constructive sleep apnea treated with CPAP.

18. A respiratory therapist uses clapping and vibration on the patient's chest wall during
    A. auscultation and percussion.
    B. bronchial lavage.
    C. chest physiotherapy.
    D. inhalation therapy.

19. Which of the following medications is used to treat asthma?
    A. albuterol
    B. atenolol
    C. Lotrel
    D. Pravachol

20. Which of the following is transcribed correctly?
    A. PA and lateral x-rays show early pneumonia. Examination reveals diminished breath sounds throughout.
    B. BA and lateral x-rays show early pneumonia. Examination reveals diminished breath sounds throughout.
    C. PA and lateral x-rays show early pneumonia. Examination reveals diminished breathe sounds throughout.
    D. TA and lateral x-rays show early pneumonia. Examination reveals diminished breathe sounds throughout.

21. Which of the following is used in the treatment of obstructive sleep apnea?
    A. continuous positive airway pressure
    B. nasal cannula
    C. sequential compression device
    D. spirometer

22. When treating breathing disorders, inhaled medication is delivered via a (an)
    - A. PE tube.
    - B. nasal cannula.
    - C. inspirometer.
    - D. nebulizer.

23. Which of the following connect the trachea with the lungs?
    - A. alveoli
    - B. bronchi
    - C. lobes
    - D. ventricles

24. The uppermost portion of the lung is the
    - A. apex.
    - B. diaphragm.
    - C. hilum.
    - D. mediastinum.

25. The combining form *phren/o* means
    - A. air sac.
    - B. chest.
    - C. diaphragm.
    - D. lung.

26. Decreased oxygen in the blood is known as
    - A. anemia.
    - B. hypokalemia.
    - C. hypercapnia.
    - D. hypoxemia.

27. Which of the following means difficulty breathing?
    - A. dyspnea
    - B. apnea
    - C. hyperpnea
    - D. tachypnea

28. Incomplete expansion of the alveoli is called
    - A. atelectasis.
    - B. pneumothorax.
    - C. rales.
    - D. stridor.

29. The expectoration of blood from the larynx, trachea, bronchi, or lungs is known as
    - A. hematemesis.
    - B. hemoptysis.
    - C. hemorrhage.
    - D. hemothorax.

30. Tachypnea is
    - A. slow breathing.
    - B. labored breathing.
    - C. rapid breathing.
    - D. shallow breathing.

Please see the accompanying CD for additional review materials for this section.

ANSWER KEY

REVIEW QUESTIONS ANSWER KEY

1. B	6. B	11. A	16. C	21. A	26. D
2. A	7. B	12. C	17. C	22. D	27. A
3. C	8. D	13. A	18. C	23. B	28. A
4. D	9. A	14. A	19. A	24. A	29. B
5. A	10. B	15. C	20. A	25. C	30. C

20

Urology

OBJECTIVES CHECKLIST

A prepared exam candidate will know:

❏ Combining forms, prefixes, and suffixes related to the urological system.

❏ Anatomical structures of the urinary system.

❏ Anatomical structures of the male reproductive system.

❏ Physiology of waste removal and urine production.

❏ Physiology of sperm production and the sequence of structures through which sperm passes, from the seminiferous tubules to exiting the body.

❏ Sequence of structures through which urine is produced and eliminated from the body, from glomerular filtration to micturition.

❏ Role of the kidneys as endocrine organs and the purpose and function of the substances secreted.

❏ Signs, symptoms, and diseases related to the urinary system.

❏ Signs, symptoms, and diseases related to the male reproductive system, including sexually transmitted diseases.

❏ Imaging studies used in the identification and diagnosis of urinary and male reproductive diseases and disorders.

❏ Laboratory studies used in the diagnosis and treatment of urinary disorders and male reproductive symptoms, disorders, and diseases.

❏ Common medications prescribed for urinary and male reproductive symptoms, disorders, and diseases.

❏ Transcription standards related to urology.

RESOURCES FOR STUDY

1. *Bates' Guide to Physical Examination and History Taking*
   Chapter 11: Male Genitalia and Hernias, pp. 411–427.

2. *The Language of Medicine*
   Chapter 7: Urinary System, pp. 213–252.
   Chapter 9: Male Reproductive System, pp. 305–332.

3. *Memmler's Structure and Function of the Human Body*
   Chapter 19: The Urinary System and Body Fluids, pp. 337–353.
   Chapter 20: The Male and Female Reproductive Systems, pp. 357–372.

4. *Memmler's The Human Body in Health and Disease*
   Chapter 22: The Urinary System, pp. 432–451; Study Guide, pp. 332–348.

5. *H&P: A Nonphysician's Guide to the Medical History and Physical Examination*
   Chapter 11: Review of Systems: Genitourinary, pp. 97–106.
   Chapter 25: Examination of the Abdomen, Groins, Rectum, Anus, and Genitalia, pp. 235–248.

6. *Human Diseases*
   Chapter 12: The Excretory System, the Male Reproductive System, and Sexually Transmitted Diseases, pp. 173–188.

7. *Laboratory Tests & Diagnostic Procedures in Medicine*
   Chapter 8: Endoscopy, Examination of the Digestive Tract and Genitourinary System, pp. 107–118.
   Chapter 20: Blood Chemistry (Osmolality, Electrolytes and Acid-Base Balance, Minerals, and Waste Products), pp. 371–400.
   Chapter 24: Examination of Urine, Stool, and Other Fluids and Materials, pp. 437–454.

8. *A Manual of Laboratory and Diagnostic Tests*
   Chapter 3: Urine Studies, pp. 163–263.
   Chapter 9: Nuclear Medicine Studies, pp. 652–704.
   Chapter 10: X-ray Studies, pp. 705–759.
   Chapter 11: Cytologic, Histologic, and Genetic Studies, pp. 760–818.
   Chapter 12: Endoscopic Studies, pp. 819–861.
   Chapter 13: Ultrasound Studies, pp. 862–899.

9. *The AAMT Book of Style for Medical Transcription*
   Gleason tumor grade, p. 53.
   Jewett classification of bladder carcinoma, p. 54.
   Specific gravity, p. 233.
   Urinalysis, p. 407.

10. *Using Medical Terminology: A Practical Approach*
    Chapter 15: Urinary System, pp. 707–753.
    Chapter 16: Reproductive Systems, pp. 755–832.

11. *Pharmacology for Health Professionals*
    Chapter 19: Diuretics, pp. 275–288.
    Chapter 20: Urinary Anti-Infectives and Miscellaneous Urinary Drugs, pp. 289–298.

12. *Understanding Pharmacology for Health Professionals*
    Chapter 12: Urinary Tract Drugs, pp. 102–714.
    (Review anti-infectives for the treatment of STDs).

13. *Medical Terminology: The Language of Health Care*
    Chapter 15: Urinary System, pp. 482–508.
    Chapter 16: Male Reproductive System, pp. 509–534.

SAMPLE REPORTS

The following five reports are examples of reports you might encounter while transcribing urology.

OPERATIVE REPORT

PREOPERATIVE DIAGNOSES
1. Urethral stricture.
2. Hypospadias.
3. Urethrocutaneous fistula.

POSTOPERATIVE DIAGNOSES
1. Urethral stricture.
2. Hypospadias.
3. Urethrocutaneous fistula.

PROCEDURE
1. Retrograde urethrogram.
2. Cystoscopy.
3. Placement of suprapubic catheter.
4. Placement of scrotal drains.

ANESTHETIC
General.

HISTORY
The patient is a 59-year-old gentleman with a history of a previous urethroplasty of the pendulous urethra who was seen in the office with urinary retention, urinary tract infection, and dysuria with a slow urinary stream. Attempts at dilation in the office were frustrated by patient discomfort and a very tight, pendulous urethra. The patient is scheduled now for cystoscopy, urethral dilation, and urethrogram.

The patient was aware of the potential for bleeding, infection, pain, and numbness, as well as bladder, bowel, or other organ injury.

PROCEDURE IN DETAIL
General anesthesia was given by the anesthesia staff. The patient was placed in a left lateral oblique position by rotating the table. A 14-French Foley catheter was placed in the fossa navicularis, actually more proximally due to a coronal hypospadias. There was also evidence of a urethrocutaneous fistula at the penoscrotal junction. Contrast material was injected in a retrograde fashion under fluoroscopy. There appeared to be some extravasation of the contrast at the distal urethra; otherwise, this was a fairly normal appearing urethra.

The catheter was removed and the patient was placed in the dorsal lithotomy position. A 17-French panendoscope was introduced into the urethra with difficulty due to poor visualization of the actual urethra. There was a false passage, which appeared at about the level of the penoscrotal junction, but I was able to feed a filiform stylet into the appropriate channel. This was followed alongside by the 17-French panendoscope.

(continued)

The prostatic urethra appeared to have a markedly elongated median lobe. The bladder neck was slightly elevated, and the interior of the bladder revealed median lobe intrusion into the lumen. The trigone was difficult to see due to floating debris and bladder wall trabeculation. There did not appear to be any neoplasia. There appeared to be some acellular debris floating in the bladder. The scope was removed along with the filiform stylet.

My feeling was that the 17-French scope did pass, and I felt it would be fairly reasonable to expect a 16-French coude tip Foley catheter to follow the same tract; however, this was not the case. The tissue in the penoscrotal junction was quite friable and allowed for passage of the coude tip Foley in different directions except for the proper channel. Attempts at trying to relocate the proper channel by the cystoscope and passage of the filiform stylet again were unsuccessful, with a progressively enlarging scrotum from accumulation of irrigant solution.

At this point, I elected to discontinue irrigating and looking for the urethra with the cystoscope, as tissue plane dissection was continuing. I did locate the bladder suprapubically with a spinal needle and instilled it through a 30-mL syringe until it presented a large enough target so that I could safely place a Rush-type suprapubic catheter blindly into this distended bladder. This was accomplished and the balloon was inflated to 10 mL. There was prompt return of the irrigant solution. The catheter was placed for gravity drainage.

Following this, I did make stab wounds in the scrotum to allow for placement of Penrose drains for dependent drainage of the accumulated irrigation solution. This has been dressed with 4 x 4's, ABDs and the mesh shorts.

At this point, the procedure was ended, anesthesia was ended, and the patient was returned to the recovery room in satisfactory condition.

It should be noted that previous urine cultures were growing gram-positive organisms. The patient received 2 g of Ancef IV piggyback during the course of the procedure.

OPERATIVE REPORT

PREOPERATIVE DIAGNOSIS
Right kidney stone.

POSTOPERATIVE DIAGNOSIS
Right kidney stone.

OPERATION
1. Right stent placement.
2. Right extracorporeal shock-wave lithotripsy.

ANESTHESIA
General.

COMPLICATIONS
None.

DRAINS
6-French, 26-cm stent.

INDICATIONS FOR THE PROCEDURE
The patient is a 35-year-old male who presented with a right kidney stone, and after discussing all options, risks, and complications, including hemorrhage, sepsis, perforation, need for nephrostomy tube, hypertension, etc., he decided to undergo ESWL with stent placement.

FINDINGS
On cystoscopy, the urethra appeared normal. The prostate appeared bilobar. The ureteral orifice was quickly localized and the stent glided all the way up the ureter without difficulty. Following this, the patient was taken to the ESWL suite.

PROCEDURE IN DETAIL
The patient was taken to the operating suite, and under satisfactory general anesthesia, he was prepped and draped in the usual sterile fashion using Betadine soap.

The 21-French cystoscope was introduced into the bladder. The right ureteral orifice was quickly localized, and a Glidewire was threaded all the way up under fluoroscopic control. This was followed by insertion of a 6-French, 26-cm stent that curled up nicely in the renal pelvis and in the bladder after removing the Glidewire.

The bladder was then emptied, and the patient was taken to the lithotripsy suite, where the treatment was carried out with 2400 shock waves to the right kidney. Fragmentation appeared to be excellent. The patient tolerated the procedure well and was transferred to the recovery room in good condition.

OPERATIVE REPORT

PREOPERATIVE DIAGNOSIS
Right renal mass.

POSTOPERATIVE DIAGNOSIS
Right renal mass.

PROCEDURE
Right radical nephrectomy.

ANESTHESIA
General endotracheal anesthesia.

DESCRIPTION OF THE PROCEDURE
After being properly identified and consented, the patient was taken to the operating room and placed under general endotracheal anesthesia. Under sterile conditions, a 16-French Foley catheter was placed.

The patient was positioned in the right flank position with the table flexed, and the right flank was prepped and draped. A skin incision overlying the 12th rib was made. The incision was taken down through the subcutaneous fat, and the muscles overlying the flank were incised. The incision was taken down onto the rib. The intercostal muscles were separated from the upper portion of the 12th rib using Bovie electrocautery, and the tip of the rib was dissected away from its attachments.

Once all the muscles of the flank were divided and the tip of the rib was mobilized, we entered the Gerota space right where it meets the tip of the 12th rib. We then used the periosteal elevator to remove the diaphragmatic pleural attachments to the posterior aspect of the 12th rib. Using Bovie electrocautery to remove the intercostal muscles from the superior portion of the 12th rib, and using the periosteal elevator as described, the rib was completely mobilized away from the muscles, pleura and diaphragm, all the way to the posterior aspect of this rib, and the intercostal ligament was identified and incised with Metzenbaum scissors.

At this point, the pleura was identified as well as the peritoneum. The peritoneum was swept away medially from the Gerota fascia, and the diaphragmatic and pleural attachments to the Gerota fascia were dissected away as well. The Burford retractor was placed in between the 11th and 12th ribs and the Gerota space exposed appropriately.

Once proper exposure of the right kidney and Gerota fascia was accomplished, we incised the Gerota fat and entered into the perinephric fat. The perinephric fat was then dissected away from the kidney using Bovie electrocautery, and the kidney was mobilized posteriorly, superiorly, and inferiorly, away from the fat, using right-angle dissection and Bovie electrocautery. We then mobilized the anterior aspect of the kidney.

The ureter was identified inferior to the kidney and it was isolated, with a vessel loop placed around it. Once the kidney was completely mobilized up to the hilum, we identified the right renal artery, and from a posterior dissection, we were able to completely dissect it out and place a vessel loop around it. From an anterior approach, we then dissected out the right renal vein, and we were able to put a vessel loop around that as well.

(continued)

At this point, 12.5 g of mannitol was given IV. The right renal artery and renal vein were clamped using Fogarty clamps, a bowel bag was placed around the kidney, and slush ice was placed around the kidney. The kidney was cooled for 10 minutes, and then we approached the renal mass.

Bovie electrocautery was used to circumscribe the renal mass, and then the Bovie cautery was used to continue the dissection around the renal mass deep into the renal substance. We cut into several segmental veins as well as the collecting system and realized that this tumor was just too deep to resect with a partial nephrectomy, and we decided that we would perform a radical nephrectomy as a curative cancer procedure.

The bowel bag was removed and the ice was removed. A right-angle clamp was placed on the right renal artery, and #0 silk ties were placed, two on the patient's side and one on the specimen side, and the artery was divided. We then placed #0 silk sutures around the right renal vein, two ties on the patient's side and one on the specimen side, and the renal vein was divided. Then #0 chromic sutures were placed around the ureter, and the ureter was divided.

At this point, a right-angle clamp was placed around any remaining tissue attaching the kidney to the retroperitoneum. The tissue was divided and the specimen removed. Following this, #0 silk sutures were placed underneath the right-angle clamp.

There was barely any bleeding and hemostasis was perfect. Estimated blood loss at this point was about 50 mL. We then closed the flank muscles in 2 layers, using interrupted #0 Vicryl sutures. The skin was then reapproximated using skin staples. The wound was cleaned. Sterile drapes were removed, and the patient was extubated and taken to the recovery room in good condition.

OFFICE NOTE

PROBLEM LIST
Recurrent urinary tract infections.
Vesical dyskinesia.
Urethral syndrome.
History of urethral stricture.
Recent proteus infection.

HISTORY OF PRESENT ILLNESS
The patient returns today for further workup and evaluation because of her recurrent infections. Infections have been resistant to a large number of antibiotics. Because of her history of proteus infection, I believe it will be prudent for us to obtain x-rays of her kidneys to make sure she does not have a stone or some other anatomical abnormality.

PHYSICAL EXAMINATION
GENERAL: Well-nourished white female, not acutely ill.
ABDOMEN: Soft, nontender, no masses. No CVA tenderness. The liver and spleen are not palpable. No hernia.
PELVIC: External genitalia: Normal general appearance without evidence of discharge or lesions, normal hair distribution. Vagina: Normal. Urethra: Without evidence of masses, tenderness, or scarring. There was no hypermobility noted. Cervix: Normal appearance and no lesions, cervical motion tenderness, or discharge. Bladder: Tender to palpation. No fullness or palpable mass. Anus and perineum: Normal in appearance.

DATA REVIEWED
Urinalysis: pH 6.5, specific gravity 1.005. Microscopically and chemically negative on a catheterized specimen.

ASSESSMENT
1. Recurrent urinary tract infections.
2. Vesical dyskinesia.
3. Urethral syndrome.
4. History of urethral stricture.
5. Recent proteus infection.

PLAN
1. Send her for an IVP.
2. Put her on tetracycline as a suppressive.
3. Return in 3 weeks for repeat exam and to go over the results of her IVP.

OFFICE NOTE

PROBLEM LIST
Benign prostatic hypertrophy.
Bladder neck obstruction.
Hypertension.
Hypothyroidism.
Elevated PSA.
Probable prostatitis.

CHIEF COMPLAINT
Benign prostatic hypertrophy and prostatitis.

HISTORY OF PRESENT ILLNESS
The patient returns today with signs and symptoms consistent with prostatitis. He also has been found to have an elevated PSA in the past, which has been thought to perhaps be due to infection. He now comes for further workup and evaluation.

PHYSICAL EXAMINATION
GENERAL: Well-nourished white male, not acutely ill.
PSYCHIATRIC: The patient is oriented in time, place, and person.
ABDOMEN: Soft, nontender, no masses. No CVA tenderness. The liver and spleen are not palpable. No hernia.
RECTAL/GENITAL: Scrotum: Without lesions, cysts, or rashes. Testes: Equal in size and symmetry and descended bilaterally, without tenderness, masses, spermatoceles, or hydroceles. Epididymides: Examination of the epididymides revealed equal size and symmetry with no masses or tenderness. Urethra: Normal urethral location and size with no lesions or discharge. Penis: Normal circumcised penis without plaques, lesions, or masses. Prostate: Symmetrical, 1+ hypertrophy with no evidence of nodularity or induration. Tender to palpation. Seminal vesicles: Symmetrical and nonpalpable with no evidence of masses. Rectal/anus: Anus and perineum are normal in appearance; normal rectal tone; no hemorrhoids or masses.

DATA REVIEWED
Catheterized urine specimen: pH 6.0, specific gravity 1.005. Microscopically shows 4-5 RBC/hpf and 4-5 WBC/hpf, but no bacteria. PSA 4.2.

ASSESSMENT
1. Benign prostatic hypertrophy.
2. Bladder neck obstruction.
3. Hypertension.
4. Hypothyroidism.
5. Elevated PSA.
6. Probable prostatitis.

PLAN
1. Give the patient Cipro 400 mg b.i.d., #56.
2. Refill Flomax.
3. Return in 6 weeks for repeat exam and be prepared to repeat his PSA at that time.

REVIEW QUESTIONS

The goal of these questions is to test your knowledge in the area of urology.

Directions: Select the correct answer for each of the multiple-choice questions provided below. *Answers are provided at the end of this chapter.*

1. The outer region of the kidney is called the
   A. cortex.
   B. hilum.
   C. medulla.
   D. ureter.

2. The small cup-like regions of the renal pelvis are called
   A. calices.
   B. nephrons.
   C. renal tubules.
   D. ureters.

3. An opening of a canal or tubular structure is called a
   A. cortex.
   B. meatus.
   C. medulla.
   D. trigone.

4. Which of the following is the term for the act of voiding or urination?
   A. filtration
   B. hydronephrosis
   C. micturition
   D. reabsorption

5. Which of the following is a nitrogenous waste excreted by the kidneys?
   A. erythropoietin
   B. potassium
   C. sodium
   D. creatinine

6. The combining form *nephr/o* means
   A. calyx.
   B. kidney.
   C. meatus.
   D. urinary bladder.

7. The combining form *dips/o* means
   A. sugar.
   B. water.
   C. nitrogen.
   D. thirst.

8. The examination of the urine to determine the presence of abnormal elements is called a (an)
   A. VCUG.
   B. BUN.
   C. IVP.
   D. UA.

9. Elevated levels of glucose in the urine may be indicative of
   A. diabetes mellitus.
   B. gout.
   C. pregnancy.
   D. urinary tract infection.

10. A diagnostic imaging procedure using x-rays and contrast material which is placed in the ureters and kidney by way of the bladder is called a (an)
    A. CT scan.
    B. KUB.
    C. retrograde pyelogram.
    D. sonogram.

11. The process of removing waste materials from the bloodstream when the kidneys no longer function is called
    A. cystoscopy.
    B. dialysis.
    C. extracorporal shock wave lithotripsy.
    D. renal angioplasty.

12. A term that means no urine production is
    A. anuria.
    B. hematuria.
    C. hypouresis.
    D. nocturia.

13. A term that means surrounding the urinary bladder is
    A. pericecal.
    B. perinephric.
    C. perirenal.
    D. perivesical.

14. Which of the following is a plain x-ray of the urinary tract?
    A. KUB
    B. BUN
    C. IVP
    D. renography

15. A dilation, or out-pouching, of the ureter is called a
    A. ureterocele.
    B. ureteroileostomy.
    C. urethrocele.
    D. urethrocystitis.

16. Which of the following measures the amount of urea in the blood?
    A. BUN
    B. IVP
    C. KUB
    D. PSA

17. Which of the following is a gland located below the bladder and surrounding the male urethra?
    A. Bartholin
    B. epididymis
    C. prostate
    D. seminal vesicle

18. Failure of one or both testicles to descend into the scrotum is called
    A. anorchism.
    B. cryptorchism.
    C. epispadias.
    D. phimosis.

19. Benign prostatic hyperplasia is characterized by
    A. dilation of the ureter.
    B. shrinkage of glandular tissue.
    C. absence of glandular tissue.
    D. enlargement of glandular tissue.

20. Benign prostatic hypertrophy can be treated with
    A. CABG.
    B. ESWL.
    C. meatotomy.
    D. TURP.

21. Which of the following is a lab test used to screen for cancer of the prostate?
    A. CEA
    B. DHEA
    C. PSA
    D. AFP

22. What portion of the penis is removed by circumcision?
    A. prepuce
    B. shaft
    C. glans penis
    D. vas deferens

23. The Gleason score indicates the prognosis of
    A. bladder cancer.
    B. kidney cancer.
    C. prostate cancer.
    D. testicular cancer.

24. Surgical removal of a testicle is called
    A. cystectomy.
    B. vasectomy.
    C. nephrectomy.
    D. orchiectomy.

25. Obstruction of the normal flow of urine from the kidneys causes
    A. glomerulonephritis.
    B. hydronephrosis.
    C. nephrocalcinosis.
    D. perinephritis.

26. The term for scanty or diminished urine production is
    A. azoturia.
    B. glucosuria.
    C. hyperketonuria.
    D. oliguria.

27. Which of the following is transcribed correctly?
    A. Cystoscopy showed normal reflux from the ureters.
    B. Cystoscopy showed normal reflex from the ureters.
    C. Cystoscopy showed normal efflux from the ureters.
    D. Cystoscopy showed normal afflux from the ureters.

28. Which of the following is transcribed correctly?
    A. Testis are equal in size and symmetry and descended bilaterally.
    B. Testes are equal in size and symmetry and distended bilaterally.
    C. Testes are equal in size and symmetry and descended bilaterally.
    D. Testis are equal in size and symmetry and distended bilaterally.

29. Which of the following would be prescribed for a urinary tract infection?
    A. Accupril
    B. Keflex
    C. Neurontin
    D. Zantac

30. A bacterial infection involving the renal parenchyma, calices, and renal pelvis is called
    A. hydronephrosis.
    B. pelvic inflammatory disease.
    C. pyelonephritis.
    D. cystitis.

 Please see the accompanying CD for additional review materials for this section.

ANSWER KEY

REVIEW QUESTIONS ANSWER KEY

1. A	6. B	11. B	16. A	21. C	26. D
2. A	7. D	12. A	17. C	22. A	27. C
3. B	8. D	13. D	18. B	23. C	28. C
4. C	9. A	14. A	19. D	24. D	29. B
5. D	10. C	15. A	20. D	25. B	30. C

Radiology/Nuclear Medicine

OBJECTIVES CHECKLIST

A prepared exam candidate will know:

☐ Terminology related to radiology, nuclear medicine, and radiation therapy.

☐ Fundamentals of x-rays and CT scans and common diagnostic techniques employed in the x-ray process, including terminology related to x-ray positioning.

☐ Radiographic studies that require the use of contrast media and the various types of contrast media used for this purpose.

☐ Fundamentals of ultrasonography, including common ultrasound studies.

☐ Fundamentals of MRI and MRA, including common diagnostic studies.

☐ Fundamentals of nuclear medicine, including terminology related to radionuclides and common diagnostic studies.

☐ Common radiopharmaceuticals administered to obtain scans of specific organs of the body.

☐ Difference between *in vitro* and *in vivo* procedures in nuclear medicine.

☐ Terminology and application of radiation therapy, including external-beam radiation and brachytherapy.

RESOURCES FOR STUDY

SAMPLE REPORTS

The following five reports are examples of reports you might encounter while transcribing radiology and nuclear medicine.

PET SCAN

HISTORY
This is a 69-year-old female with a history of lung carcinoma.

TECHNIQUE
A dose of 15 mCi of fluorine-19 FDG was infused. Images were obtained from the base of the skull through the midthighs utilizing a fixed, full-ring PET scanner. Tomographic and volumetric images are reviewed.

This study is compared to a previous PET scan dated August 21, 2004, and a previous CT scan of the chest dated November 10, 2004.

FINDINGS
Again demonstrated is a stable, linear, moderate, increased metabolic activity extending from the left hilum to the left lateral chest wall. This region of increased metabolic activity measured 1.7 standard uptake value on the previous study and measures 1.8 standard uptake value on the current study. This region of abnormal linear increased metabolic activity corresponds to lung parenchyma fibrosis and scarring extending from the hilum to the lateral chest wall, demonstrated on CT scan. The remainder of the lungs demonstrates no abnormal increased metabolic activity.

The remainder of the body scan demonstrates no abnormal increased metabolic activity.

IMPRESSION
1. The stable, linear, increased metabolic activity corresponding to parenchymal scarring on CT scan in the left lung is compatible with expected uptake from parenchymal granulation and scarring.
2. There is a low probability for residual, recurrent, or metastatic lung carcinoma.
3. A 6-month interval followup PET scan is recommended to ensure continued stability.

MRI

HISTORY
The patient is a 48-year-old female with previous MRI from August 25, 2004.

TECHNIQUE
MRI of the left knee was performed at 0.7 Tesla field strength, utilizing an open-configuration magnet. Coronal T1 and fast IR, axial fat-suppressed proton-density, sagittal fat-suppressed proton-density, and fast T2 images were obtained.

FINDINGS
The examination again shows a large joint effusion with distension of the joint capsule and suprapatellar pouch. A multiloculated large cyst is seen in the popliteal fossa, more towards the medial side along the medial head of the gastrocnemius muscle. The cyst measures up to 10 cm craniocaudad, centered at the level of the joint line and up to 3.5 cm in AP diameter. Internal septations and nodularity along the wall are seen. There is some fluid intensity around the outer margins of the cystic collection, more diffusely in the soft tissues, more evident inferiorly.

Evaluation of the articular cartilage and the menisci shows no focal defects. The bone marrow signal under the weightbearing area appears normal. The collateral ligaments and cruciate ligaments appear intact. Patellar tendon and quadriceps tendon are within normal limits in dimension and signal intensity.

When compared to the previous examination, a similar appearance is noted in the contour of the popliteal cyst and also in the distribution of joint effusion. The distention of the lateral recesses of the axillary pouch appears similar. On sagittal fat-suppressed images, pericapsular soft tissue edema also appears nearly similar, with mild reduction seen on the medial aspect in the soft tissues.

IMPRESSION
1. The examination shows no significant interval change in the appearance of the left knee, showing a prominent joint effusion and nodularity along the synovial linings suggesting synovitis.
2. A large popliteal cyst with inflammatory reaction around it is seen posteromedially as described above.
3. No new areas of intraarticular abnormalities or in the periarticular soft tissues identified.

MRI

HISTORY
The patient is a 95-year-old female with dizziness and suspected CVA.

TECHNIQUE
MRI of the brain was performed at 0.7 Tesla field strength, utilizing an open-configuration magnet. Sagittal T1, coronal fast IR, axial T1, FLAIR, and fast T2 images were obtained. Also, diffusion-weighted images in the axial plane were obtained.

FINDINGS
The examination shows moderate prominence of the cortical sulci and fissures and basal cisterns. There is moderate proportionate enlargement of the ventricular system. On T2 and FLAIR images, confluent increased high-intensity signal is seen along the body of the lateral ventricles and a few scattered punctate foci are seen deeper in the white matter. No dominant focal lesions are seen at the level of the basal ganglia or thalami. A few CSF-intensity lesions are seen in the subinsular region bilaterally with tubular configuration. Also, striated T2 high-intensity areas are seen along the convexity bilaterally, consistent with dilated perivascular spaces.

No signal changes suggestive of hemorrhage are seen. There is no mass effect. No abnormal localizing extraaxial collections are seen.

The flow-related signal void in intracranial arteries and venous sinuses appears normal. Signal in the calvaria is normal. Paranasal sinuses and mastoid cells appear aerated, with some mucosal thickening seen in the ethmoid cells along the left side. No fluid levels are seen.

IMPRESSION
1. The examination shows moderate involutional changes with mild a pattern of ischemic leukomalacia.
2. No signs of mass lesion, hydrocephalus, or evidence of hemorrhage are seen.
3. Incidentally on sagittal images, advanced degenerative changes at the craniocervical juncture are seen, with erosive changes of the odontoid. Correlation with lateral plain radiographs of the cervical spine are suggested for additional assessment of bony detail.

ULTRASOUND-GUIDED BIOPSY

PROCEDURE ORDERED
Ultrasound-guided biopsy of a nodule in the left lobe of the thyroid.

CLINICAL HISTORY
This is a 70-year-old male with a history of a cold nodule in the left lobe of the thyroid.

REPORT
After the benefits (to try to obtain samples of tissue to submit to the laboratory for analysis), risks (bleeding, infection, nerve damage, and the need for emergency surgery), and alternatives (possible surgery or doing nothing) of the procedure were explained to the patient and the opportunity to ask questions given, written consent was obtained and witnessed.

The patient is anticoagulated due to a left ventricular thrombus and atrial fibrillation. The increased risk of bleeding due to the anticoagulation was also discussed with the patient. The patient was awake and alert and wished to proceed.

Using real-time sonographic imaging, the nodule in the left lobe of the thyroid was localized. The nodule is located in the mid and lower pole of the left lobe and extends inferiorly off the supraclavicular fossa and left clavicle. The nodule measured approximately 4 cm in greatest diameter. A spot was then marked with ink on the overlying skin of the neck. The patient's neck was then prepped and draped in the usual sterile fashion. Local anesthesia was administered with 1% lidocaine. Using sterile ultrasound gel, a sterile ultrasound probe cover, and sterile technique, a 25-gauge needle was directed into the nodule in the left lobe of the thyroid and a sample of tissue obtained and submitted to the cytotechnologist who was in attendance. This was repeated two times for a total of three passes that were made and three samples of tissue that were obtained.

At the end of the procedure, there was approximately a 1-cm hematoma in the subcutaneous tissues at the biopsy site. The patient's skin was cleansed with sterile saline and antibiotic ointment applied. A sterile overlying dressing was then applied. The patient tolerated the procedure well and left the angiography suite in good, stable condition.

IMPRESSION
Successful ultrasound-guided biopsy. Small post-procedural hematoma noted, as described above.

CT SCAN

PROCEDURE ORDERED
CT scan of the abdomen and pelvis.

TECHNIQUE
Helical imaging of the abdomen and pelvis was performed from the lung bases to the symphysis pubis with 7-mm collimation after the administration of oral and the intravenous injection of 125 mL of Visipaque. No prior cross-sectional imaging studies of the abdomen or pelvis are available at this time.

The AP scout film of the abdomen and pelvis demonstrates gas density within the wall of the urinary bladder and surgical clips projecting over the right upper quadrant of an obese patient. There are no nodules in the imaged portions of the lung bases. There is no pericardial or pleural effusion in the imaged portions of the lower thorax.

There is gas in the wall of the urinary bladder. No Foley catheter is present within the urinary bladder. There is no evidence of free intraperitoneal air or fluid. The uterus is atrophic. The abdominal aorta is nonaneurysmal, and there are no pathologically enlarged retroperitoneal lymph nodes.

Surgical clips are located in the gallbladder fossa; the gallbladder is absent. The attenuation of the liver is slightly less than that of the spleen. The hepatic and portal veins enhance with contrast, and there is no intrahepatic biliary dilatation. The spleen and adrenal glands are within normal limits. The pancreas is atrophic. The cortex of each kidney is thin. Both kidneys enhance with contrast, and there is no hydronephrosis. There is degenerative change of the lumbar spine.

IMPRESSION
1. Emphysematous cystitis.
2. Status post prior cholecystectomy.
3. Mild fatty infiltration of the liver.
4. Bilateral renal atrophy.
5. Lumbar spondylosis.

REVIEW QUESTIONS

The goal of these questions is to test your knowledge in the areas of radiology and nuclear medicine.

Directions: Select the correct answer for each of the multiple-choice questions provided below. *Answers are provided at the end of this chapter.*

1. Which of the following diagnostic procedures uses x-rays and contrast media to evaluate the bile ducts?
   A. arthrography
   B. cholangiography
   C. myelography
   D. pyelography

2. The x-ray procedure that uses a fluorescent screen instead of a photographic plate to create a visual image is called
   A. pyelography.
   B. CT scan.
   C. fluoroscopy.
   D. MRI.

3. Which of the following is transcribed correctly?
   A. T1, flair, and fast T2 images were obtained.
   B. T1, FLARE, and fast T2 images were obtained.
   C. T1, flare, and fast T2 images were obtained.
   D. T1, FLAIR, and fast T2 images were obtained.

4. The most common chest x-ray in which x-rays travel from the patient's back toward the front is a (an)
   A. posteroanterior (PA) view.
   B. anteroposterior (AP) view.
   C. lateral view.
   D. oblique view.

5. The body is separated left to right by the
   A. sagittal plane.
   B. transverse plane.
   C. dorsal plane.
   D. axial plane.

6. Which of the following is an imaging position which has the patient lying on their side with the x-ray beam projecting horizontally?
   A. lateral decubitus
   B. prone
   C. recumbent
   D. supine

7. Which of the following means turning outward?
   A. anteversion
   B. extension
   C. flexion
   D. eversion

8. Doppler imaging technology uses
   A. magnets.
   B. x-rays.
   C. radionuclides.
   D. sound waves.

9. The time required for a radioactive substance to lose half its radioactivity by disintegration is called
   A. half-life.
   B. ionization.
   C. tagging.
   D. uptake.

10. Which of the following is transcribed correctly?
    A. MRI of the brain shows no midline shift or evidence of intracranial mass.
    B. MRI of the brain shows no midline lift or evidence of intracranial mass.
    C. MRI of the brain shows no midline shift or evidence of inner cranial mass.
    D. MRI of the brain shows no midline shift or evidence of intracranial mast.

11. The combining form *is/o* means
    A. luminous.
    B. sound.
    C. the same.
    D. the opposite.

12. A ventilation/perfusion lung scan is performed to rule out
    A. pulmonary embolus.
    B. cardiopulmonary edema.
    C. pleural effusion.
    D. peribronchial cuffing.

13. An instrument used to measure exposure to radiation is a
    A. Vernier gauge.
    B. roentgenograph.
    C. spectrogram.
    D. dosimeter.

14. A radioactive iodine uptake test is used to assess the
    A. bone marrow.
    B. thyroid.
    C. kidney.
    D. lung.

15. Which of the following is transcribed correctly?
    A. The AP scalp film of the abdomen and pelvis shows surgical clips in the right upper quadrant.
    B. The AP scout film of the abdomen and pelvis shows surgical blips in the right upper quadrant.
    C. The AP spout film of the abdomen and pelvis shows surgical clips in the right upper quadrant.
    D. The AP scout film of the abdomen and pelvis shows surgical clips in the right upper quadrant.

16. On x-ray film, a radiopaque image appears
    A. black.
    B. clear.
    C. white.
    D. absent.

17. Palliative radiation therapy
    A. alleviates pain.
    B. is curative.
    C. aids in a diagnosis.
    D. is performed intraoperatively.

18. A form of radiation therapy in which implants are positioned within the body in or near the tissue to be treated is
    A. interventional radiation.
    B. brachytherapy.
    C. scintigraphy.
    D. pyretotherapy.

19. Which of the following tests would be ordered to rule out a cerebrovascular accident?
    A. CT scan
    B. MUGA scan
    C. KUB
    D. V/Q scan

20. A Cardiolite stress test is performed to evaluate the function of the
    A. heart.
    B. lungs.
    C. muscles.
    D. brain.

21. A handheld device which sends and receives sound waves is a
    A. tracer.
    B. gamma camera.
    C. transducer.
    D. plate.

22. Echocardiography is useful for detecting
    A. coronary artery stenosis.
    B. carotid artery stenosis.
    C. pulmonary embolism.
    D. heart valve defects.

23. Which of the following is a contrast media used in gastrointestinal studies, angiography, and urography?
    A. Hyzaar
    B. Hypaque
    C. Hyoscine
    D. Hytrin

24. During this noninvasive study, a radionuclide is administered and a two-dimensional image is obtained of the radioactive tissues with a special camera.
    A. scintigraphy
    B. echocardiography
    C. tomography
    D. stereoradiography

25. Which of the following is transcribed correctly?
    A. There is a 3.5-cm soft tissue mass in the colon which is worrisome for malignancy. A barium enema is recommended for further evaluation.
    B. There is a 3.5-cm soft tissue mass in the colon which is worrisome for malignancy. A bare minima is recommended for further evaluation
    C. A 3.5 cm soft tissue mass in the colon which is worrisome for malignancy. A flair enema is recommended for further evaluation.
    D. A 3.5 cm soft tissue mass in the colon which is worrisome for malignancy. A barium enema is recommended for further evaluation

26. Which anatomical plane divides the body into superior and inferior sections?
    A. sagittal
    B. median
    C. transverse
    D. frontal

27. Which anatomical plane runs through the midline, transecting the nose, naval, and spine?
    A. frontal
    B. transverse
    C. median
    D. coronal

28. Cephalic indicates a direction toward the
    A. head.
    B. tail.
    C. front.
    D. back.

29. Oblique means
    A. up and down.
    B. side to side.
    C. slanted.
    D. parallel.

30. An in vitro test is performed
    A. inside the body.
    B. outside the body.
    C. after a diagnosis.
    D. at the point of origin.

 Please see the accompanying CD for additional review materials for this section.

ANSWER KEY

REVIEW QUESTIONS ANSWER KEY

1. B	6. A	11. C	16. C	21. C	26. C
2. C	7. D	12. A	17. A	22. D	27. C
3. D	8. D	13. D	18. B	23. B	28. A
4. A	9. A	14. B	19. A	24. A	29. C
5. A	10. A	15. D	20. A	25. A	30. B

English Language

Grammar

OBJECTIVES CHECKLIST

A prepared exam candidate will know the:

- ❏ Identification and function of all eight (8) parts of speech utilized in the English language.

- ❏ Component parts of a sentence, including compound constructions.

- ❏ Identification and function of the five (5) types of phrases utilized in sentence construction.

- ❏ Identification and function of both independent and dependent clauses.

- ❏ Six types of dependent, or subordinate, clauses.

- ❏ Classification of sentences by structure.

- ❏ Classification of sentences by purpose.

RESOURCES FOR STUDY

1. *The AAMT Book of Style for Medical Transcription*
   Adjectives, pp. 12–13.
   Adverbs, pp. 14–15.
   Appositives, pp. 29–30.
   Articles, pp. 31–32.
   Clause, pp. 79–82.
   Elliptical construction, p. 160.
   Grammar, p. 196.
   Nouns, pp. 274–275.
   Phrases, pp. 314–316.
   Pronouns, pp. 334–336.
   Sentences, pp. 357–360.
   Verbs, pp. 409–413.

2. *The Gregg Reference Manual: A Manual of Style, Grammar, Usage, and Formatting*

3. *American Medical Association Manual of Style*

PART 1: PARTS OF SPEECH

There are eight (8) classes into which words are grouped according to their uses in a sentence:

1. **Noun:** the name of a person, place, object, idea, quality, or activity.

   a. **abstract noun:** the name of a quality or general idea.

   Examples: *faith, hope, love*

   b. **collective noun:** a noun that represents a group of people, animals, or things.

   Examples: *team, herd, audience*

   c. **common noun:** the name of a class of people, places, or things.

   Examples: *parent, student, teacher, dog*

   d. **predicate noun:** a word or phrase that follows a linking verb, completes the sense of the verb, and explains the subject.
   A predicate noun is also identical to the subject.

   Examples:
   Sally is our <u>president</u>.
   Mr. Jones was <u>principal</u> of my high school.

   e. **proper noun:** the official name of a particular person, place, or thing.

   Examples: *George Washington, Florida, Great Dane, White House.*

2. **Verb:** a word or phrase used to express action or a state of being.

   a. **helping verb:** a verb that helps in the formation of another verb.
   The primary helping verbs are *be, can, could, do, have, may, might, must, ought, shall, should, will,* and *would*. They precede other verbs to form the predicate.

   Examples:
   He <u>might</u> go to the meeting.
   I <u>will</u> walk the dog later.

   b. **transitive verb**: a verb that requires an object to complete its meaning.

   Example:
   He has cancelled the meeting. (the verb *has cancelled* requires the object *meeting*)

   c. **intransitive verb:** a verb that does *not* require an object to complete its meaning.

   Examples:
   Member participation has increased.
   The wind blows.

   d. **linking verb**: a verb that connects a subject with the predicate adjective, noun, or pronoun.
   The most common linking verbs are the various forms of the verb "to be."

   Examples:
   He will be team captain. (the verb *will be* links *He* and *captain*)
   The company is happy with its growth. (the verb *is* links *company* and *happy*)

3. **Adjective:** a single word, phrase, or clause that answers the question *what kind, how many,* or *which one* and modifies the meaning of a noun or pronoun.
The articles *(a, an,* and *the)* are also considered adjectives.

Examples:

excellent prognosis	*eight* grandchildren
the latest results	*green* sputum
a man *of great integrity*	*silly* me
open incision	*lovely* girl

4. **Adverb:** a single word, phrase, or clause that answers the question *when, where, why, in what manner,* or *to what extent* and modifies the meaning of a verb, adjective, or another adverb.
Hint: Adverbs often end in "ly."

Examples:
She spoke <u>clearly</u> when giving her instructions.
The physician seemed <u>sincerely</u> concerned about his patients.
The patient was <u>well</u> developed and <u>well</u> nourished.

5. **Pronoun:** a word used in place of a noun.
Exception: Possessive pronouns function as adjectives in the sentence because they precede and modify a noun rather than replace it.

a. **personal:** *I, you, he, she, it, we, they*

b. **possessive:** *my/mine, his, her/hers, its, our/ours, their/theirs,* and *your/yours*

c. **demonstrative:** *this, that, these, those*

d. **indefinite:** *each, either, any, anyone, someone, few, all,* etc.

e. **intensive:** *myself, yourself, himself, herself,* etc.

f. **interrogative:** *who, which, what,* etc.

g. **relative:** *who, whose, whom, which, that,* and compounds like *whoever, whomever,* etc.

6. **Preposition:** a word used to show the relation of a noun or pronoun to some other word in the sentence.
A preposition always appears in a phrase (called the *prepositional phrase)*, with the preposition usually at the beginning and the noun/pronoun at the end of the phrase as the *object*. Together, the preposition and noun (along with any modifiers) form a phrase that describes another word in the sentence.

Example:

The beautiful painting <u>on the wall</u> is a DaVinci. (on is the preposition, wall is the object, and the prepositional phrase on the wall describes the noun painting)

<u>Commonly Used Prepositions</u>

about	at	but (meaning "except")
above	before	by
across	behind	concerning
after	below	down
against	beneath	during
along	beside	except
amid	besides	for
among	between	from
around	beyond	in

Note: Prepositions are often directional, and the old schoolhouse hint was that prepositions were "anything an airplane could do to a cloud," meaning that the preposition describes the directional relationship between the airplane and a cloud.

7. **Conjunction:** a word or phrase that connects words, phrases, or clauses.

   a. **coordinating conjunction:** connects words, phrases or clauses of equal rank. The coordinating conjunctions are *and, but, or, nor,* and *for.*

   b. **correlative conjunction:** conjunction consisting of two elements used in pairs.

   Examples: *both. . .and, not only. . .but (also), either. . .or,* and *neither. . .nor*

   c. **subordinating conjunction:** used to join subordinate, or dependent, clauses to independent clauses; however, it does not need to link the dependent clause to the independent clause. It often can occur at the *beginning* of a sentence to introduce the subordinate clause.

   Examples:
   We stayed indoors <u>until</u> the storm abated.
   <u>When</u> I take a test, I get very nervous. (simply a recasting of the sentence, *I get very nervous <u>when</u> I take a test.*)

8. **Interjection:** a word that shows emotion, usually without grammatical connection to other parts of a sentence.

   Examples:
   Oh!   My goodness!   Hurry!   Ah!   Ouch!   Wow!

REVIEW EXERCISE: PARTS OF SPEECH

The following paragraph contains numbered, italicized words. For each, indicate the part of speech (noun, verb, adjective, adverb, pronoun, preposition, conjunction, or interjection). For the nouns, verbs, pronouns, and conjunctions, indicate the type.

The (1) *patient* presented to the office (2) *with* a complaint of (3) *shortness* of breath (4) *and* productive cough (5) *although* it (6) *has* been of (7) *short* duration. On (8) *my* evaluation (9) *today*, she appeared (10) *tired* and ill. (11) *Her* skin was (12) *slightly* dry, indicating (13) *some* dehydration. There was some (14) *redness* of the throat, and her nose showed moist (15) *but* congested (16) *mucous* membranes. (17) *When* I auscultated (18) *the* lungs, they were clear (19) *bilaterally*, and breath sounds were equal on (20) *both* sides.

PART 2: PARTS OF A SENTENCE

1. **Subject and Predicate**

   A sentence consists of two parts: the *subject* and the *predicate*. The *subject* of the sentence is that part about which something is being said. The *predicate* is that part which says something about the subject.

   Examples:

Subject	Predicate
Faculty and students	*planned a new class schedule.*
The beautiful woman	*kissed the handsome man.*

   a. **simple subjects and verbs**

   The whole subject is called the *complete subject*, but the *simple subject* is the principal word or group of words in the subject.

   Example:
   The old book on the table was a favorite of her grandmother's.
   Subject: *The old book on the table*
   Simple subject: *book*

   The whole predicate is called the complete predicate, but the principal word or group of words in the predicate is called the simple predicate, or the verb.

   Example:
   The teachers planned a dynamic new course curriculum.
   Predicate: *planned a dynamic new course curriculum.*
   Simple predicate, or verb: *planned*

   b. **compound subjects and verbs**

   A *compound subject* consists of two or more subjects that are joined by a conjunction and have the same verb. The usual connecting words are *and* and *or*.

   Example:
   The White House and the Pentagon called an emergency press conference.
   Compound subject: *White House and Pentagon*

   A *compound verb* consists of two or more verbs that are joined by a conjunction and have the same subject.

   Example:
   The team improved its defensive strategy and performed much better in their next few games.
   Compound verb: *improved* and *performed*

2. **Complements**

   Some sentences express a complete thought by means of a subject and verb only.

   Examples:

Subject	Verb
The girl	*cried.*
Everybody	*left.*

However, most sentences have one or more words in the predicate that complete the meaning of the subject and verb. These completing words are called *complements.*

Examples:

Subject	Verb	Complement
John and Ed	*caught*	*five wide-mouthed <u>bass</u>.*
She	*handed*	<u>*me*</u> *a stack of books.*
Your brother	*seems*	*very <u>happy</u>.*

Complements fall into two categories: *objects and subject complements.*

a. **objects**

Complements that receive or are affected by the action of the verb are called *objects.* The *direct object* of the verb receives the action of the verb or shows the result of the action. It answers the question *What?* or *Whom?* after an action verb.

Examples:
I took my <u>lunch</u> with me. (I took what?)
The patient told <u>me</u> she was in pain. (The patient told whom?)
He tried <u>to reason with her</u>. (He tried what?)

The *indirect object* of the verb precedes the direct object and usually tells *to whom* or *for whom* the action of the verb is done.

Examples:
Fed-Ex delivered the package <u>to me</u>. (package—direct object; to me—indirect object)
The salesman showed <u>me</u> the latest arrivals. (arrivals—direct object; me—indirect object)

b. **subject complements**

Complements that refer to (describe, explain, or identify) the subject are *subject complements.* A *predicate nominative* is a noun or pronoun complement that refers to the same person or thing as the subject of the verb. *It follows a <u>linking verb</u>.*

Examples:
Aunt Clara is my oldest <u>relative</u>. (relative refers to Aunt Clara)
He will be <u>president</u> next year. (president refers to He)

A *predicate adjective* is an adjective complement that modifies the subject of the verb. It also follows a linking verb.

Example:
The stray dog was very <u>thin</u>. (thin refers to dog)

c. **compound complements**

Two or more complements joined by a conjunction are called compound complements.

Examples:
Andrew gave David and me two tickets to the concert. (David and me—compound indirect object)
She was tired and hungry. (tired and hungry—compound predicate adjective)

REVIEW EXERCISE: PARTS OF A SENTENCE

For each of the 10 sentences below, identify the subject(s), verb(s), direct objects, indirect objects, predicate nominatives, and predicate adjectives.

1. The laboratory results showed protein in the urine.

2. The daughter and son told me the story.

3. Examination revealed exquisite tenderness and guarding of the abdomen.

4. Dr. Smith is a specialist in reproductive health and excellent with this particular problem.

5. Upon admission, the patient received fluids and oxygen and improved on this regimen.

6. Despite aggressive chemotherapy, the tumor was unaffected and continued its progression.

7. She was given at-home care directions and told to follow up with me.

8. Take the medicine with food and call me tomorrow.

9. Whatever is wrong will be determined by diagnostic testing.

10. The patient never claimed to be disoriented but did seem confused on questioning.

PART 3: PHRASES

1. **Phrase:** a group of words not containing a verb and its subject.
   Phrases are used as a single part of speech.

   a. **prepositional phrase:** a group of words beginning with a preposition and usually ending with a noun or pronoun that functions as the *object* of the preposition.
   Prepositional phrases are usually used as *adjective phrases* (modifying a noun) or as *adverb phrases* (modifying a verb). Adverb phrases answer the question *how, when, where, to what extent,* or *why.* Occasionally, prepositional phrases are used as nouns.

   Examples:
   The book <u>on the table</u> is mine. (on the table is an *adjective phrase* modifying the noun *book)*
   The falcon can fly <u>at great speeds</u> <u>for long distances.</u> (at great speeds and *for long distances* are *adverb phrases* modifying the verb *can fly)*
   <u>After dinner</u> will be too late. (after dinner is the subject and is used as a noun*)*

   b. **participles and participial phrases**
   A *participle* is a verb form (often identified by its present tense *-ing* ending or by its past tense *-ed, -d, -t, -en,* or *-n* endings) that is used as an adjective.

   Examples:
   The <u>developing</u> storm threatened to ruin the picnic.
   A <u>watched</u> pot never boils.
   I found him <u>sleeping</u> in the hammock.

   A *participial phrase* is a phrase containing a participle and any complements or modifiers it may have. The participle usually introduces the phrase, and the entire phrase acts as an adjective to modify a noun or pronoun.

   Examples:
   Michael Jordan, <u>playing with skill</u>, led the Bulls to victory. (phrase modifies the noun *Michael Jordan)*
   <u>Getting up at 5 a.m.</u>, we got an early start. (phrase modifies the noun *we)*
   The firefighters arrived on the scene to find the church <u>destroyed by fire</u>. (phrase modifies the noun *church)*

   c. **gerunds and gerund phrases**
   A gerund is a verb form ending in *-ing* that is used as a noun.

   Examples:
   <u>Swimming</u> is good exercise.
   Good <u>writing</u> comes from much practice.
   It takes a lot of <u>studying</u> to pass that examination.

   A *gerund phrase* is a phrase consisting of a gerund and any complements or modifiers it may have. Like the gerund alone, the gerund phrase may be used in any place that a noun would be used.

   Examples:
   <u>Wearing a flag pin</u> is a great way to express patriotism. (phrase functions as the subject)
   Her idea of <u>selling tickets to raise money</u> is a good one. (phrase functions as the object of the preposition *of)*
   The school advises <u>paying your registration fees</u> by tomorrow. (phrase functions as the direct object of the verb *advises)*

d. **infinitives and infinitive phrases**

An *infinitive* is a verb form, usually preceded by the word *to*, that is used as a noun or a modifier. Sometimes the word *to* is implied in an infinitive expression.

Examples:
We want <u>to go</u> to the beach on Sunday.
<u>To achieve success</u>, a person must work hard.
To forgive is divine.
He helped me [<u>to</u>] <u>do</u> my homework.

Note: Do not confuse infinitives that begin with the word *to* with prepositional phrases that begin with *to*.

He gave the medicine <u>to me</u>. (prepositional phrase)
He gave the medicine <u>to help me</u>. (infinitive phrase)

An *infinitive phrase* consists of an infinitive and any complements or modifiers it may have. Like infinitives alone, infinitive phrases can be used as nouns or modifiers.

Examples:
*We tried <u>to reason with her</u>. (*phrase as direct object of *tried)*
<u>To save money</u> became her obsession. (phrase as subject)
I am too busy <u>to go to the store with you tonight</u>. (phrase modifies the adjective *busy)*
His plan is <u>to go to graduate school next year</u>. (phrase as predicate nominative)

e. **appositives**

An *appositive* is a noun or pronoun—often with modifiers—set beside another noun or pronoun to explain or identify it.

Examples:
My brother <u>Todd</u> is coming over for dinner.
John's father, <u>a physician</u>, chaired the committee last year.

An *appositive phrase* is a phrase consisting of an appositive and its modifiers. An appositive phrase usually follows the word it explains or identifies, but it may precede it.

Examples:
He donated the car, <u>an old Volkswagen Beetle</u>, to a local charity.
<u>A fascinating thriller</u>, the book is still one of my favorites.

REVIEW EXERCISE: PHRASES

The following paragraph contains numbered, italicized phrases. For each, indicate the type of phrase (prepositional, participial, gerund, infinitive, or appositive); in the case of prepositional phrases, indicate whether the phrase is used as an adjective or an adverb phrase.

As technology advances (1) *by leaps and bounds*, the healthcare industry faces the potential (2) *for great change*. One obvious way (3) *to embrace this evolving science* is (4) *to focus on advanced treatment technologies*. (5) *Looking for treatment solutions* is one way to drive the development (6) *of technology*. (7) *For years*, patients have benefited (8) *from life-saving advances* (9) *in technology*. Refined surgical instrumentation, (10) *a critical area of developing technologies*, has been one outcome of this area of scientific focus. (11) *Using statistical data based on treatment outcomes*, technology experts are able (12) *to develop advanced tools* (13) *for improving patient care*. Such tools, (14) *in the hands* of a skilled practitioner, can generate improved treatment outcomes, (15) *a desirable goal for any healthcare provider*. (16) *For many reasons*, this is good news (17) *for the industry*, (18) *pressured to lower costs and improve patient care*. The quality of patient care (19) *in the future* can only benefit from (20) *developing more advanced technology solutions*.

PART 4: CLAUSES

A *clause* is a group of words containing a subject and predicate and used as a part of a sentence. Clauses are classified according to grammatical completeness. Those that can stand alone when removed from their sentences are called *independent clauses.* Those that do not express a complete thought and cannot stand alone are called *dependent,* or *subordinate,* clauses.

1. **Independent Clauses**

   When removed from its sentence, an *independent clause* makes complete sense. When written with a capital at the beginning and a period at the end, it becomes a *simple sentence.* It is only referred to as an *independent clause* when it exists in a larger sentence with one or more additional clauses, whether independent or dependent.

   Examples:
   The patient was discharged. (simple sentence)
   Once her condition improved, <u>the patient was discharged</u>. (independent clause within the sentence)

2. **Dependent Clauses**

   Dependent clauses, which cannot stand alone as sentences, are used as nouns or modifiers in the same way as single words and phrases. A dependent clause is always combined in some way with an independent clause. A dependent clause, like a sentence, has a verb and a subject and may contain complements and modifiers. It is the *entire* clause that functions as the noun or modifier, and it is important not to confuse these with *independent clauses* merely because they contain a subject and verb.

   Examples:
   <u>Whoever knows the song</u> may join in.
   We ordered spaghetti, <u>which everyone in the family likes</u>.
   <u>As she had guessed</u>, her car was out of gas.

   a. **adjective clauses**

      Like a phrase, an *adjective clause* is a dependent clause that functions as an adjective by modifying a noun or pronoun.

      Examples:
      The house <u>where he was born</u> was still in very good condition. (clause modifies *house*)
      The letter, <u>which I wrote to the editor last month</u>, is going to be published in the next issue. (clause modifies *letter*)

      Note: Adjective clauses often begin with a relative pronoun *(who, whom, which,* or *that)* the relative adjective *whose,* or the relative adverb *where* or *when.* These refer to, or are *related* to, a noun or pronoun that has come before. The noun or pronoun to which these relative terms refer is called the *antecedent.*

      A relative pronoun, adjective or adverb does three things: (1) it refers to a preceding noun or pronoun; (2) it connects its clause with the rest of the sentence; (3) it performs a function within its own clause by serving as the subject, object, etc., of the dependent clause.

      Examples:
      Richard is a friend <u>whom</u> we can trust. (refers to *friend,* links the clause to the sentence and serves as the direct object of the verb *trust* within its clause)
      He is a coach <u>whose</u> record has been amazing. (refers to *coach,* links the clause to the sentence and serves as an adjective modifying *record*)

b. **noun clauses**

A *noun clause* is a dependent clause that is used as a noun.

Examples:
<u>Whoever wins the election</u> will have big shoes to fill. (clause functions as subject)
The details of <u>what she does</u> are not known to me. (clause functions as the object of the preposition *of*)
I know <u>whose car this is</u>. (clause functions as the direct object of the verb *know*)

c. **adverb clauses**

An *adverb clause* is a dependent clause that, like an adverb, modifies a verb, adjective, or adverb. Adverb clauses often begin with a *subordinating conjunction*, a conjunction that joins the clause to the rest of the sentence.

<u>Common Subordinating Conjunctions</u>

after	because	so that	whenever
although	before	than	where
as	if	though	wherever
as if	in order that	unless	whether
as long as	provided that	until	while
as though	since	when	

Examples:
She writes in her diary <u>like she is in a great hurry</u>. (how?)
She writes in her diary <u>before she goes to sleep</u>. (when?)
She writes in her diary <u>wherever the light is strongest</u>. (where?)
She writes in her diary <u>because she enjoys it</u>. (why?)
She writes in her diary <u>as often as she can</u>. (to what extent?)
She writes in her diary <u>if she gets to bed early</u>. (under what conditions?)

d. **elliptical clauses**

Sometimes in our writing and speaking, we do not complete the adverb clauses we use. The omitted part of the clause is implied and is said to be *elliptical*.

Examples:
I am stronger than you (are).
While (I was) *waiting for the doctor, the patient fell asleep.*

REVIEW EXERCISE: CLAUSES

Each of the following sentences contains one or more dependent clauses in italics. Indicate whether it is an adjective, noun, or adverb clause.

1. *When you draw blood from a patient*, you should wear appropriate gloves, *which can protect both you and the patient.*

2. The last chemotherapy trial worked better *than the first one did.*

3. Only children *who are under the age of two* should receive this immunization.

4. He had no explanation for *what he was doing.*

5. *Whatever the patient says* has to be clinically correlated *so that we can accurately document the present illness.*

6. She is confident *that her test results will be negative.*

7. I know *where she lives,* and *driving there* will take awhile.

8. The brace *that I gave her on her last visit* has greatly improved her symptoms, *which were rather severe at that time.*

9. Patients *whose symptoms are unrelieved by steroid injection* will likely not respond well to surgical intervention.

10. He works for the clinic *where you had your previous surgery.*

PART 5: SENTENCE CLASSIFICATION

1. **Sentences Classified by Structure**

   Classified according to their structure, there are four kinds of sentences: *simple, compound, complex,* and *compound-complex.*

   a. **simple sentence**

   A *simple sentence* is a sentence with one independent clause and no dependent clauses.

   Examples:
   Great literature stirs the imagination.
   Great literature stirs the imagination and challenges the intellect. (compound predicate in a simple sentence)

   b. **compound sentence**

   A *compound sentence* is a sentence composed of two or more independent clauses but no dependent clauses.

   Example:
   Great literature stirs the imagination, and it challenges the intellect. (two independent clauses joined by the conjunction *and*)

   c. **complex sentence**

   A *complex sentence* is a sentence that contains one independent clause and at least one dependent clause.

   Example:
   Great literature, which stirs the imagination, also challenges the intellect. (single independent clause with an interruptive dependent clause)

   d. **compound-complex sentence**

   A *compound-complex sentence* is a sentence that contains two or more independent clauses (compound) and at least one dependent clause (complex).

   Example:
   Great literature, which challenges the intellect, is sometimes difficult, but it is also rewarding. (two independent clauses joined by the conjunction *but,* with an interruptive dependent clause in the first independent clause)

2. **Sentences Classified by Purpose**

   Classified according to their purpose, there are four kinds of sentences: *declarative, imperative, interrogative,* and *exclamatory.*

   a. **declarative sentence**

   A *declarative sentence* is a sentence that makes a statement.

   Examples:
   In 1492, Columbus discovered the Americas.
   The dog was sleeping on the back porch.

   b. **imperative sentence**

   An *imperative sentence* is a sentence that gives a command or makes a request.

   Examples:
   Stop talking and finish eating your supper.
   Please give me a chance to explain.
   Don't ride a motorcycle without a helmet.

c. **interrogative sentence**

An *interrogative sentence* is a sentence that asks a question.

Examples:
Which medication did you take?
Are you going to the theater on Friday night?

d. **exclamatory sentence**

An *exclamatory sentence* is one that expresses a strong feeling.

Examples:
How amazing!
It's a miracle!
Freeze!

REVIEW EXERCISE: SENTENCE CLASSIFICATION

For each of the following sentences, indicate the classification by structure and purpose.

1. According to the patient, she has had a long history of urinary tract infections, and she is used to taking antibiotics periodically for these.

2. After you spent all those years in college, why would you decide to become a bartender?

3. We really needed her help in developing a new strategy for membership growth and marketing our benefits.

4. The patient complained of severe restrictive chest pain, but we ruled out an MI with EKG and cardiac enzymes.

5. If you touch me, I will call the police!

6. Let me have your order tomorrow if you can.

7. Despite her mild improvement on this regimen, I am going to try her on a different protocol, and we'll see if we get better results.

8. Watch out!

9. Take this medication, which I'm giving you a prescription for, and be sure to call me if your symptoms don't improve.

10. How much longer do we have to wait for the doctor to arrive?

ANSWER KEYS

REVIEW EXERCISES ANSWER KEY

Part 1: Parts of Speech

1. noun (common)

2. preposition

3. noun (abstract)

4. conjunction (coordinating)

5. conjunction (subordinating)

6. verb (linking)

7. adjective

8. pronoun (possessive) *Note: Adjective is also an acceptable answer.*

9. adverb

10. adjective

11. pronoun (possessive) *Note: Adjective is also an acceptable answer.*

12. adverb

13. adjective

14. noun

15. conjunction (coordinating)

16. adjective

17. conjunction (subordinating)

18. adjective

19. adverb

20. adjective

Part 2: Parts of a Sentence

1. *results* (subject), *showed* (verb), *protein* (direct object)

2. *daughter* and *son* (compound subject), *told* (verb), *me* (indirect object), *story* (direct object)

3. *Examination* (subject), *revealed* (verb), *tenderness* and *guarding* (compound direct object)

4. *Dr. Smith* (subject), *is* (verb), *specialist* (predicate nominative), *excellent* (predicate adjective)

5. *patient* (subject), *received* and *improved* (compound verb), *fluids* and *oxygen* (compound direct object of *received*)

6. *tumor* (subject), *was* and *continued* (compound verb), *progression* (direct object of *continued*), *unaffected* (predicate adjective)

7. *She* (subject), *was given* and *told* (compound verb), *directions* (direct object of *was given*) and *to follow up with me* (direct object of *told*)

8. *You* (implied subject), *take* and *call* (compound verb), *medicine* (direct object of *take*) and *me* (direct object of *call*)

9. *Whatever is wrong* (subject), *will be determined* (verb)

10. *patient* (subject), *claimed* and *seemed* (compound verb), *to be disoriented* (direct object of *claimed*), *confused* (predicate adjective)

Part 3: Phrases

1. prepositional (adverb)

2. prepositional (adjective)

3. infinitive

4. infinitive

5. gerund

6. prepositional (adjective)

7. prepositional (adverb)

8. prepositional (adverb)

9. prepositional (adjective)

10. appositive

11. participial

12. infinitive

13. prepositional (adjective)

14. prepositional (adverb)

15. appositive

16. prepositional (adverb)

17. prepositional (adjective)

18. participial

19. prepositional (adverb)

20. gerund

Part 4: Clauses

1. adverb, adjective

2. adverb

3. adjective

4. noun

5. noun, adverb

6. adverb

7. noun, noun

8. adjective, adjective

9. adjective

10. adjective

Part 5: Sentence Classification

1. compound-complex, declarative

2. complex, interrogative

3. simple, declarative

4. compound, declarative

5. complex, exclamatory

6. complex, imperative

7. compound-complex, declarative

8. simple, exclamatory

9. compound-complex, imperative

10. simple, interrogative

23

Punctuation Rules

OBJECTIVES CHECKLIST

A prepared exam candidate will know the:

- ☐ Identification and function of the three forms of terminal punctuation.
- ☐ Rules and exceptions governing the use and placement of colons.
- ☐ Rules and exceptions governing the use and placement of semicolons.
- ☐ Rules and exceptions governing the use and placement of commas.
- ☐ Difference between commas that separate and commas that set off.

RESOURCES FOR STUDY

1. *The Gregg Reference Manual: A Manual of Style, Grammar, Usage and Formatting*
2. *The AAMT Book of Style for Medical Transcription*
   Colons, pp. 85–87.
   Commas, pp. 87–91.
   Periods, pp. 310–311.
   Punctuation, p. 340.
   Semicolons, pp. 354–356.

OVERVIEW

As with all other areas of usage and style, the goal of punctuation in formal documentation is to promote clarity and consistency throughout the record. Punctuation, particularly commas and semicolons, should be applied with reasonable and prudent consideration for the standards that govern their usage. They should never be applied in random or haphazard fashion, without a sense of purpose or reasonable function. The "rules" that exist in language texts of authority (such as *The Gregg Reference Manual*) and those summarized in *The AAMT Book of Style* outline specific and concrete definitions for either including or omitting a particular form of punctuation. To attempt to delineate them all here would be exhaustive, but a great many of the itemized rules for commas, for example, can be summarized in some general statements about usage that will enable the MT to graduate to a more consistent application of these standards based on knowledge.

TERMINAL PUNCTUATION

Terminal punctuation, or the punctuation that ends a sentence, should always be included throughout the document and should be chosen to express tone and purpose. For most sentences in a medical report, obviously, the terminal punctuation is going to be a *period*. Rarely does a physician request or even dictate in a tone that implies the need for an *exclamation point* or *question mark*. It is important to note here, however, that often dictators will provide direct quotes from the patient or other involved parties, in which a question mark or other punctuation might often be included. Remember, terminal punctuation usually falls within the quotation marks in these instances.

Examples:
The patient was brought to the ER by ambulance.
The patient was repeatedly crying out "Why me?" and complaining of unrelenting pain.
She says the symptoms "have been coming and going."

INTERNAL PUNCTUATION

Internal punctuation exists *within* a sentence and is used primarily to set off or separate one word or phrase from another.

A. Colons

1. Between Independent Clauses

Use a colon between two independent clauses when the second clause explains or illustrates the first clause and there is no coordinating conjunction or transitional expression linking the two clauses.

Example:
I have two goals in this year: lose 50 pounds and remodel my kitchen.

2. Before Lists and Enumerations

a. Place a colon before such expressions as *for example, namely,* and *that is* when they introduce words and phrases.

Example:
Visa provides identity-theft insurance; for example, if someone steals your card, you are protected from the charges incurred by that individual.

b. When a clause contains an anticipatory expression (such as *the following, as follows, thus,* and *these*) and directs attention to a series of explanatory words, phrases, or clauses, use the colon between the clause and the series.

Example:
The following items will be deleted from our website menu: Events, News, and Contacts.

3. In Expressions of Time or Proportions

a. When hours and minutes are expressed in figures, separate them with a colon.

Example: *6:35 p.m.*

b. Use a colon to represent the word *to* in ratio expressions.

Examples: *2:1, epinephrine 1:250,000*

4. In References to Books/Publications

a. Use a colon to separate the title and the subtitle of a book or article.

Example:
Meg Cox wrote *The Heart of the Family: Searching America for New Traditions that Fulfill Us.*

b. Use a colon to separate volume number and page number in footnotes and references.

Example: *8:763–766*

B. Commas

While the incorrect placement of a comma in a medical document is rarely quality-critical, the *correct* placement of them and a thorough understanding of their grammatical implications reflect a skill set that should be the goal of any quality-driven MT. In most instances, these standards rely on a fundamental understanding of and ability to identify both *independent* phrases and clauses and *dependent* phrases and clauses. In those examples below, the independent (or stand-alone) clauses are underlined to differentiate them from the dependent clauses in the sentences.

1. **Commas That Separate**

   a. Two or more adjectives describing the same noun.

   Example:

   It was a long, hot summer.

   b. Two or more items in a simple series.

   Examples:

   Temperature was 98.6, pulse 80, respirations 22, and blood pressure 132/74.

   The area was prepped with Betadine, draped with sterile drapes, and completely anesthetized.

   c. Lines of a full address when listed horizontally and/or within a sentence.

   Example:

   The clinic address is 2152 Park Street, Jacksonville, Florida 99999.

   d. A person's name from his/her credential or title.

   Examples:

   John A. Smith, Jr., MD
   Lea M. Sims, CMT

   e. Two or more independent clauses.

   Examples:

   She was evaluated in triage, and she was found to be hypotensive.
   A bladder flap was created, and upon identification of the fundus, a transverse incision was made and widened with blunt dissection.
   The abdomen was insufflated with CO$_2$ gas, and a trocar inserted into both ports under direct visualization.

2. **Commas That "Set Off"**

   a. Nonessential words or phrases that introduce an independent clause.

   Examples:

   After discussion of her case with the tumor panel, it was felt that she would best benefit from a course of chemotherapy and concomitant radiation treatment.
   About a week ago, the patient suffered a fall from the stairs.
   Without consent from the parent, I felt we could not move forward with surgery.

   b. Nonessential words or phrases that interrupt the flow from subject to verb or from verb to object within an independent clause.

   Examples:

   The problem, if I remember correctly, was related to the patient's diet.
   We made an incision, careful not to damage the underlying structures, with a #11 blade.
   The alternative, as I told the patient, is to let this heal in by secondary intention.

   c. Nonessential words or afterthoughts that occur at the end of an independent clause.

   Example:

   There is very little we can offer her at this point, unfortunately.

d. Appositives or Direct Address

Examples:
I have requested a consult with a pulmonologist, Dr. Jones, for respirator management.
Thank you, John, for allowing me to participate in this patient's care.

e. Nonessential or dependent clauses within an independent clause.

Examples:
The patient, whom I have seen in consultation before, was admitted by Dr. Smith for exacerbation of COPD. (nonessential)
The mass, which was biopsied in September, is unchanged on today's exam. (nonessential)
The mass that was biopsied in September is unchanged on today's exam. (essential)
She was seen by a cardiologist who was on call for the ER. (essential)
She was seen by Dr. Smiley, who was on call for the ER. (nonessential).
The area was thoroughly explored for hemostasis, with no evidence of bleeding or hemorrhage noted. (nonessential)
The area was infiltrated using Marcaine 5% with epinephrine. (essential)

f. Month, day, and year when all three are written.

Example:
On July 1, 1998, she underwent successful CABG.

g. Full-sentence quotations from the rest of the independent clause.

Example:
The patient's husband stated, "I found her on the kitchen floor unresponsive and not breathing."

C. Semicolons

1. To Separate Clauses

Semicolons are often misunderstood and either over-utilized or erroneously applied in documentation. They should serve to occasionally separate two closely related sentences, particularly when the second sentence contains a transitional word or phrase (like *however* or *therefore*). When in doubt about their application, it is always safer to separate the two sentences with a period.

Examples:
She was told not to return to work at this time; we will re-evaluate that on her next visit.
He was given an aggressive course of IV antibiotics; however, his condition did not improve.

2. In a Complex Series

The second instance of utilizing a semicolon is to separate items in a complex series. A *simple series*, whose examples were provided above, is one whose items are separated by commas. A *complex series* is one in which at least one of the items contains an internal comma or commas, thereby making it necessary to separate the items themselves with alternate punctuation, namely a semicolon.

Example:
The patient has older twin sisters, one of whom died of breast cancer in 1998; a brother that died of rectal cancer earlier this year; and a younger sister who is alive and in good health.

REVIEW EXERCISES

Given the information provided in this chapter, can you correctly punctuate the following sentences? These were taken from in-the-trenches, real dictation, but be careful. Not all of them need correction.

1. "I explained to her and her daughter the severity of this injury and that her wrist would never function the same."

2. "She was admitted and monitored and no neurological injury was found."

3. "This is an 81-year-old male with whom I am quite familiar who has an underlying problem of a more serious nature which is diabetes that has caused him to have premature atherosclerotic heart disease."

4. "The red cells appeared normal with a rare fragmented cell seen."

5. "The patient is a pleasant 51-year-old black male who presented to the office of his new primary care physician Dr. Williams on the day of admission complaining of an episode of chest pain and palpitations which occurred about a week earlier."

6. "He complained of palpitations and to rule out cardiac dysrhythmia a consultation with a cardiologist was obtained."

7. "Over the past few months she has had episodic left-sided abdominal pain and pain behind her left breast which became severe and eventually she states she collapsed."

8. "Again in light of the fact that she has been on corticosteroids it would be somewhat unusual to develop pneumonitis and an atypical infection should also be in our differential."

9. "He became combative violent and abusive and security had to be involved in subduing the patient and haloperidol 5 mg and Ativan 2 mg IM was used to help control the patient."

10. "We then made a lateral incision beginning at the greater trochanter and extending distally and carried it down through the deeper subcutaneous tissues."

ANSWER KEY

REVIEW EXERCISES

1. No commas needed.

2. monitored,

3. male,
   familiar,
   nature,
   diabetes,

4. normal,

5. physician,
   Williams,
   (no comma after "palpitations"; phrase that
   follows is essential because it relates to
   onset/duration of symptoms)

6. palpitations,
   dysrhythmia,

7. months, (optional)
   severe,
   eventually,
   states,

8. Again,
   corticosteroids,
   pneumonitis,

9. combative,
   violent, (optional)
   abusive,
   patient,

10. incision,
    distally,

English Usage

OBJECTIVES CHECKLIST

A prepared exam candidate will know the:

❏ Rules and exceptions related to agreement, both for subjects/verbs and pronouns/antecedents.

❏ Rules and exceptions governing the use and placement of interrogative and relative pronouns.

❏ Correct use of modifiers, both adjective and adverb forms, including compound modifiers.

❏ Principles related to diction and the most commonly confused words encountered in English usage.

RESOURCES FOR STUDY

1. *The Gregg Reference Manual: A Manual of Style, Grammar, Usage and Formatting*

2. *The AAMT Book of Style for Medical Transcription*
   Compound modifiers, pp. 91–98.
   Pronouns, pp. 334–336.
   Subject-verb agreement, pp. 376–378.
   Who, whom, p. 422.

3. Appendix 2: Medical Soundalikes (*found at the end of this text*)

PART I: AGREEMENT

A. SUBJECTS AND VERBS

1. **Rule of Agreement.** A verb must agree with its subject in number and person.

   Examples:
   I <u>know</u> that he is my friend.
   She <u>is coming</u> to spend the weekend with me.

   Note: A plural subject is always required after the use of the word *you*, whether *you* is singular or plural.

   Examples:
   You alone <u>have made</u> it possible to complete this project.
   You both <u>have been</u> on my mind all day.

2. **Subjects joined by *and*.**

   If the subject consists of two or more words connected by *and* or by *both . . . and*, the subject is plural and requires a plural verb.

   Examples:
   The teacher and her students <u>have been working</u> hard on the play.
   The sales projections and the estimated costs <u>are</u> reasonable.

   Use a singular verb when two or more subjects connected by *and* refer to the same person or thing.

   Example:
   Our President and committee chair is Lisa Smith.

   Use a singular verb when two or more subjects connected by *and* are preceded by *each, every, many a,* or *many an.*

   Examples:
   Every member <u>has</u> a right to a vote.
   Each puppy <u>needs</u> a good home.

3. **Subjects joined by *or*.**

   If the subject consists of two or more *singular* words connected by *or, either. . . . or, neither. . . . nor,* or *not only. . . . but also,* the subject is singular and requires a singular verb.

   Example:
   Either May or June <u>is</u> a good month for the wedding.

   If the subject consists of two or more *plural* words that are connected by *or, either. . . . or, neither . . . nor,* or *not only. . . . but also,* the subject is plural and requires a plural verb.

   Example:
   Neither dogs nor cats <u>like</u> cold weather.

   If the subject consists of both singular and plural words connected by *or, either. . . . or, neither . . . nor,* or *not only. . . . but also,* the verb agrees with the nearer, or closest, subject.

   Example:
   Neither the board members nor the Executive Director <u>is</u> in favor of spending money on that project.

Note: When establishing agreement between subject and verb, ignore any intervening, and potentially distracting, phrases or clauses.

Examples:
The order for new textbooks <u>is</u> on the table.
The key consideration in this argument, the budgetary feasibility of the project, <u>is not being given</u> sufficient weight in the analysis.

B. PRONOUNS AND ANTECEDENTS

Rule of Agreement. A pronoun agrees with its antecedent in number and gender. The antecedent of a pronoun is the word to which the pronoun refers, either in the same sentence or in a previous one.

Examples:
<u>He</u> should have thought of that <u>himself</u>.
Mary is devoted to <u>her</u> career.

The words *each, neither, either, one, everyone, everybody, no one, nobody, anyone, anybody, someone, somebody* are referred to by a singular pronoun—*he, him, his, she, her, hers, it,* and *its*. Intervening phrases do not change the number of the antecedent.

Example:
<u>Each</u> of the women had removed <u>her</u> shoes.

Two or more singular antecedents joined by *or* or *nor* should be referred to by a singular pronoun.

Example:
<u>Neither</u> Greg <u>nor</u> John had <u>his</u> keys with <u>him</u>.

Two or more antecedents joined by *and* should be referred to by a plural pronoun.

Example:
Greg <u>and</u> John had <u>their</u> keys in <u>their</u> pockets.

REVIEW EXERCISE: AGREEMENT

For each of the following sentences, indicate correct subject/verb or pronoun/antecedent agreement by selecting the word or phrase in parentheses that completes the sentence.

1. One out of every 20 patients (*respond/responds*) to this medication.

2. Each of the women told the reporter what (*she/they*) had seen.

3. Neither of the proposed amendments (*was/were*) accepted in their entirety.

4. Each of the articles featured in *JAAMT* (*was/were*) good.

5. (*Has/Have)* either of the orders been sent?

6. Neither the nursing home nor the paramedics (*has/have*) the patient's DNR papers.

7. Neither Jeremy nor Paul used (*his/their)* tickets to the show.

8. Many an at-home medical transcriptionist (*has/have)* felt isolated.

9. The frequency of fatal traffic accidents (*is/are*) rising.

10. A certain degree of privacy and security (*seem/seems*) appropriate.

PART 2: INTERROGATIVE AND RELATIVE PRONOUNS

A. *WHO* AND *WHOM; WHOEVER* AND *WHOMEVER*

All four of these pronouns are both *interrogative* when they are used in asking questions and are *relative* when they are used to relate to or refer to a noun in the main clause.

Examples:
Who is going to the party?
My sister is the one who is going to the party.
To whom should I send this bill?
Dr. Smith, whom I have never met, runs that program.

These pronouns may be either singular or plural in meaning.

Examples:
Who is speaking?
Who are going?

Who (or *whoever*) is the nominative (or subjective) form. Use *who* whenever *he, she, they, I,* or *we* could be substituted in the *who* clause.

Examples:
Who is arranging the meeting next month?
Who did they say was presenting to the group?
The matter of who to appoint to the task force was not addressed.
Mary is the one who can best do the job.

Whom (or *whomever*) is the objective form. Use *whom* whenever *him, her, them,* or *me* could be substituted as the object of the verb or object of the preposition in the *whom* clause.

Examples:
Whom did you meet yesterday?
To whom did you write your letter?
I will hire whomever I believe will get the job done.
It depends on whom they elect to office.

B. *WHO, WHICH,* AND *THAT*

Who and *that* are used when referring to persons. Select *who* when referring to an individual person or individuality of a group, and select *that* when referring to a class, species, or type.

Examples:
He is the only person in my family who understands how I feel.
She is the kind of boss that employees really respond to.

Which and *that* are used when referring to places, objects, and animals. *Which* is used to introduce nonessential clauses (set off by commas) and *that* is usually used to introduce essential clauses (no commas).

Examples:
Bonnie's report on membership benefits, which I read on the website, should be of some help.
The report that I told you about is now up on the website.

REVIEW EXERCISE: INTERROGATIVE AND RELATIVE PRONOUNS

For each of the following sentences, indicate the pronoun's correct form by selecting the word in parentheses that completes the sentence.

1. In *Romeo and Juliet*, the two characters (*who/whom*) I loved the most were Tybalt and Mercutio.

2. If I had known (*who/whom*) you were referring to, I could have given you that information.

3. Next month's issue will feature (*whoever/whomever*) the editor selects.

4. Since I did not know (*who/whom*) the member wanted to speak to, I took a message.

5. Everybody (*who/whom*) receives *Plexus* will get the poster insert in May.

6. Only the members (*who/whom*) have paid their dues are allowed to vote.

7. She was one of those (*who/whom*) the politicians could not influence.

8. No one has figured out to (*who/whom*) the anonymous letter was referring.

9. The association is looking for someone (*who/whom*) it can appoint to chair this committee.

10. You may tell anyone (*who/whom*) you think is interested that the group is having an informational meeting next Friday.

PART 3: COMPOUND MODIFIERS

A compound modifier consists of two or more words that act as a unit modifying a noun or pronoun. The use of hyphens to join these words varies depending on the type of compound modifier, as indicated below.

Some compound modifiers are so commonly used together, or are so clear, that they are automatically read as a unit and do not need to be joined with hyphens.

Examples:
dark brown lesion
deep tendon reflexes
1st trimester bleeding
jugular venous distention
left lower quadrant
low back pain
ST-T wave abnormality
3rd degree burn

A. ADJECTIVE ENDING IN -LY

Use a hyphen in a compound modifier beginning with an adjective that ends in *-ly*. (This requires distinguishing between adjectives ending in *-ly* and adverbs ending in *-ly*.) Do not use a hyphen with compound modifiers containing an adverb ending in *-ly*.

Example:
scholarly-looking patient
<u>but</u> *quickly paced steps*

B. ADJECTIVE-NOUN COMPOUND

Use a hyphen in an adjective-noun compound that precedes and modifies another noun.

Examples:
second-floor office
<u>but</u>
The office is on the second floor.

C. ADJECTIVE WITH PREPOSITION

Use hyphens in most compound adjectives that contain a preposition.

Example: *finger-to-nose test*

D. ADJECTIVE WITH PARTICIPLE

Use a hyphen to join an adjective to a participle, whether the compound precedes or follows the noun.

Examples:
good-natured, soft-spoken patient
The patient is good-natured and soft-spoken.

E. ADVERB WITH PARTICIPLE OR ADJECTIVE

Use a hyphen to form a compound modifier made up of an adverb coupled with a participle or adjective when they precede the noun they modify but not when they follow it.

Examples:
well-developed and well-nourished woman
<u>but</u>
The patient was well developed and well nourished.
fast-acting medication
<u>but</u>
The medication is fast acting.

F. ADVERB ENDING IN -LY

Do not use a hyphen in a compound modifier to link an adverb ending in *-ly* with a participle or adjective.

Examples:
recently completed workup
moderately acute pain
financially stable investment

G. ADVERB PRECEDING A COMPOUND MODIFIER

Do not use a hyphen in a compound modifier preceded by an adverb.

Example: *somewhat well nourished patient*

H. VERY

Drop the hyphen in a compound modifier with a participle or adjective when it is preceded by the adverb *very*.

Example: *very well developed patient*

I. DISEASE-ENTITY MODIFIERS

Do not use hyphens with most disease-entity modifiers even when they precede the noun. Check appropriate medical references for guidance.

Examples:
cervical disk disease
oat cell carcinoma
pelvic inflammatory disease
sickle cell disease
urinary tract infection
<u>but</u>
insulin-dependent diabetes mellitus and non-insulin-dependent diabetes mellitus

J. EPONYMS

Use a hyphen to join two or more eponymic names used as multiple-word modifiers of diseases, operations, procedures, instruments, etc.

Do not use a hyphen if the multiple-word, eponymic name refers to a single person.

Use appropriate medical references to differentiate.

Examples:
Osgood-Schlatter disease (named for US orthopedic surgeon Robert B. Osgood and Swiss surgeon Carl Schlatter)
Chevalier Jackson forceps (named for Chevalier Jackson, US pioneer in bronchoesophagology)

K. EQUAL, COMPLEMENTARY, OR CONTRASTING ADJECTIVES

Use a hyphen to join two adjectives that are equal, complementary, or contrasting when they precede or follow the noun they modify.

Examples:
anterior-posterior infarction
physician-patient confidentiality issues
His eyes are blue-green.

L. FOREIGN EXPRESSIONS

Do not hyphenate foreign expressions used in compound adjectives, even when they precede the noun they modify (unless they are always hyphenated).

Examples:
in vitro experiments
carcinoma in situ
cul-de-sac (always hyphenated)
ex officio member

M. HIGH- AND LOW-

Use a hyphen in most *high-* and *low-* compound adjectives.

Examples:
high-density mass
low-frequency waves
high-power field

N. NOUN-ADJECTIVE COMPOUND

Use a hyphen to join some noun-adjective compounds (but not all). Check appropriate references (dictionaries and grammar books). When a hyphen is appropriate, use it whether the noun-adjective compound precedes or follows the noun it is modifying.

Examples:
It is a medication-resistant condition.
The condition was medication-resistant.
This is a symptom-free patient.
The patient was symptom-free.
Stool is heme-negative.

O. NOUN WITH PARTICIPLE

Use a hyphen to join a noun and a participle to form a compound modifier whether it comes before or after a noun.

Examples:
bone-biting forceps
She was panic-stricken.
mucus-coated throat (the throat was coated with mucus, not mucous)
callus-forming lesion (the lesion was forming callus, not callous)

P. NUMERALS WITH WORDS

Use a hyphen between a number and a word forming a compound modifier preceding a noun.

Examples:
3-week history
5 x 3 x 2-cm mass
2-year 5-month-old child
8-pound 5-ounce baby girl

Q. PROPER NOUNS AS ADJECTIVE

Do not use hyphens in proper nouns even when they serve as a modifier preceding a noun.

Examples:
John E Kennedy High School
New Mexico residents

Do not use hyphens in combinations of proper noun and common noun serving as a modifier.

Example: *Tylenol capsule administration*

R. SERIES OF HYPHENATED COMPOUND MODIFIERS

Use a suspensive hyphen after each incomplete modifier when there is a series of hyphenated compound modifiers with a common last word that is expressed only after the final modifier in the series.

Examples:
10- to 12-year history
3- to 4-cm lesion
full- and split-thickness grafts

If one or more of the incomplete modifiers is not hyphenated, repeat the base with each, hyphenating or not, as appropriate.

Example: *preoperative and postoperative diagnoses (not pre- and postoperative diagnoses)*

S. TO CLARIFY OR TO AVOID CONFUSION

Use a hyphen to clarify meaning and to avoid confusion, absurdity, or ambiguity in compound modifiers. The hyphen may not be necessary if the meaning is made clear by the surrounding context.

Example: *large-bowel obstruction (obstruction of the large bowel, not a large obstruction of the bowel)*

T. HYPHENATED COMPOUND MODIFIERS

Use a hyphen or en dash to join hyphenated compound modifiers or a hyphenated compound modifier with a one-word modifier.

Example:
non-disease-entity modifier
<u>or</u>
non–disease-entity modifier

Use a hyphen or en dash to join two unhyphenated compound modifiers.

Example:
the North Carolina-South Carolina border
<u>or</u>
the North Carolina–South Carolina border

Use a hyphen or en dash to join an unhyphenated compound modifier with a hyphenated one.

Example:
beta-receptor-mediated response
<u>or</u>
β-receptor–mediated response

Use a hyphen or en dash to join an unhyphenated compound modifier with a one-word modifier.

Example:
vitamin D-deficiency rickets
<u>or</u>
vitamin D–deficiency rickets

REVIEW EXERCISE: COMPOUND MODIFIERS

The following sentences contain potential compound modifiers. Identify the sentences that are correct with a "C" and the sentences that are incorrect with an "I."

1. He smiled at the lovely looking lady in the front row.

2. She responded with an ear-to-ear grin.

3. She noticed that he was well-groomed and well-dressed.

4. The patient had a recently acquired hesitation in his gait.

5. Exam revealed a very well-developed female.

6. She complained of a 2–3 day headache.

7. He indicated that he spent the weekend doing back-breaking activities, like moving furniture for a friend.

8. X-rays revealed an area of small bowel distention.

9. He gave a 3-week history of decreased appetite and fatigue.

10. The patient was pain free after the procedure.

ANSWER KEYS

REVIEW EXERCISES ANSWER KEY

Part 1: Agreement

1. responds
2. she
3. was
4. was
5. Has
6. have
7. his
8. has
9. is
10. seems

Part 2: Interrogative and Relative Pronouns

1. whom
2. whom
3. whomever
4. whom
5. who
6. who
7. whom
8. whom
9. who
10. who

Part 3: Compound Modifiers

1. I
2. C
3. I
4. I
5. I
6. I
7. C
8. I
9. C
10. I

The Healthcare Record

25

Medicolegal Issues

OBJECTIVES CHECKLIST

A prepared exam candidate will know the:

❑ Basic tenets of health information privacy and security, including the roles of HIM professionals within the documentation domain.

❑ Role of risk management in the healthcare setting and the correlation between documentation and risk management.

❑ Role and function of the Joint Commission on Accreditation of Healthcare Organizations (JCAHO) in establishing standards at the acute care provision level.

❑ Fundamental legal terms encountered in healthcare delivery, particularly as they pertain to patient privacy, safety, and security of health information.

❑ Purpose and principles associated with the Health Insurance Portability and Accountability Act (HIPAA).

❑ Seven patient rights as defined by HIPAA.

❑ Fundamentals of HIPAA compliance as they pertain to medical transcription and the patient care documentation process.

❑ Definitions related to covered entities and business associates, as well as the provisions and stipulations related to each.

RESOURCES FOR STUDY

1. *HIPAA for MTs*
2. *Legal Aspects of Health Information Management*
3. *Glencoe Law and Ethics for Medical Careers*

OVERVIEW

Information is one of the healthcare industry's most important resources. Health information management (HIM) professionals serve the healthcare industry and the public by managing, analyzing, and utilizing data that is necessary for patient care, including transcription, statistics, birth data, death statistics, coding (reimbursement), tumor registry, and correspondence. Once transcribed, reports are charted on the patient's medical record. This is done on a daily basis to provide continuity of care. Confidentiality of patient records is an important aspect of HIM. The HIM director is the first line of defense in maintaining the integrity of the patient's protected health information (PHI). With the enactment of HIPAA, the role of the HIM Director, in conjunction with the Information Systems Director, has become more vital to managing confidential patient information. The HIM Department is also an integral member of the team when the hospital undergoes Joint Commission on Accreditation of Healthcare Organizations (JCAHO) review.

The Risk Management Department works closely with the HIM Department. The Department of Risk Management has the responsibility of identifying, analyzing, evaluating, and reducing or eliminating the risk of possible injury to patients, visitors, staff, and the institution itself. The Risk Manager has duties including liability claims management, participating in safety and security programs, and monitoring loss prevention and reduction. This department is also involved in risk management education for its employees.

The JCAHO evaluates and accredits more than 15,000 healthcare organizations and programs in the United States. An independent, not-for-profit organization, the Joint Commission is the nation's predominant standard-setting and accrediting body in healthcare. The review is used internally by health care organ-izations to support performance improvement and externally, to demonstrate accountability to the public. Participation in Joint Commission accreditation is voluntary at for-profit hospitals, but mandatory for all government hospitals. Participation in Joint Commission Accreditation is mandatory for those hospitals receiving reimbursement from Medicare/Medicaid. Accreditation standards are published in the Accreditation Manual for Hospitals (AMH).

Joint Commission standards address the organization's level of performance in key functional areas, such as patient rights, patient treatment, and infection control, and the standards focus not simply on an organization's ability to provide safe, high-quality care, but on its actual performance as well. Standards set forth performance expectations for activities that affect the safety and quality of patient care. If an organization does the right things and does them well, there is a strong likelihood that its patients will experience good outcomes. The Joint Commission develops its standards in consultation with healthcare experts, providers, measurement experts, purchasers, and consumers.

MEDICOLEGAL TERMS

As medical transcriptionists, we are familiar with the terminology that relates specifically to our profession—disease processes, anatomy and physiology, diagnoses, treatments, etc., but how familiar are we with some of the terms and concepts in our medicolegal system?

When looking at the legal and medical professions, probably the first area of law that comes to people's minds is that of medical malpractice. Medical malpractice is a controversial topic and becomes a highly debated political issue, especially at election time. Another area in the legal field that has come into its own in recent years is that of health law. The increasing costs of healthcare, financing this care, care for the uninsured and indigent, privacy, confidentiality, and security of patient care have given rise to many new laws.

GLOSSARY OF TERMS

Abuse (as in Medicare/Medicaid fraud and abuse): incidents or practices that may directly or indirectly cause financial losses to government health programs, beneficiaries, or recipients.

Advance directive: power of attorney that gives someone decision-making powers upon the person's incompetence.

ADA: Americans with Disabilities Act.

Common law: body of law made up of judicial opinions and precedents as opposed to legislatively created laws or statutes.

Damages: money compensation paid through the courts to persons who have suffered an injury or detriment due to the negligence or omission of another.

DNR (Do Not Resuscitate Order): this order specifies what efforts should or should not be taken in order to revive a patient who has experienced cardiac or pulmonary arrest and what level of care should be provided in the case of an arrest.

Electronic signature: electronic method of authenticating or signing a legal document.

ERISA: an abbreviation for Employee Retirement Security Income Act—covers employee benefit plans such as health plans and pensions.

Ethical behavior: behavior that conforms to accepted professional standards of conduct.

Ethics: a set of moral principles or behavior.

Family and Medical Leave Act (FMLA): the Family and Medical Leave Act of 1993 entitles a covered employee to take up to 12 weeks of leave in a 12-month period for the birth or adoption of a child, or the serious health condition of the employee or the employee's child, spouse, or parent.

Fraud: an "intentional" misrepresentation or deception that an individual knows to be false and could result in unauthorized benefit to himself or some other person. A criminal intent to defraud is when the misrepresentation or deception is made willingly. (An example would be Medicare fraud—charges knowingly submitted for treatment not provided.)

Good Samaritan Acts: according to the 7th edition of Black's Law, this is "A statute that exempts from liability a person (such as an off-duty physician) who voluntarily renders aid to another in imminent danger but negligently causes injury while rendering aid." This type of legislation is passed on a state-by-state basis.

Grandfather clause: a provision of law that exempts certain persons or pre-existing conditions from the scope of a regulation or requirement.

Healthcare directive: any statement made by a competent individual about preferences for future medical treatment in the event that the patient is unable to make decisions at the time of treatment.

Indemnification: the act of compensating for loss or damage.

Independent contractor: an individual who is hired to complete a specific project but who is free to do that work as he or she wishes; it is not based on how the person is paid, how often the person is paid, or whether the person works part-time or full-time. An independent contractor is not an employee, thus cannot sue an employer for a wrongful act or injury suffered on the job. The independent contractor will receive a 1099 form for tax reporting purposes.

Informed consent: a person's agreement to allow something to happen after the person has been informed of all the risks involved and the alternatives.

Life-sustaining procedure: a medical procedure that uses mechanical or artificial means to sustain a person's vital functions and basically just serves to postpone a person's death.

Malpractice: negligence or incompetence on behalf of an individual, usually applied to professionals such as attorneys or physicians.

Medicaid: a program that helps pay for medically necessary medical services for needy and low-income persons. It uses state and federal government money. It is covered under Social Security Act Title XIX.

Medicare: a federal insurance program for people age 65 and older and certain disabled people. The Centers for Medicare & Medicaid Services (CMS) operates Medicare. The Medicare program consists of two parts, Medicare Part A (hospital insurance) and Medicare Part B (supplemental medical insurance). It is covered under Social Security Act Title XVIII.

Negligence: the most common cause of action in medical malpractice cases. It will arise where injury results from a failure of the wrongdoer to exercise due care.

Occupational Safety and Health Act (OSHA): the federal occupational safety and health agency. It enforces the Occupational Safety and Health Act (the OSH Act), which provides the legal framework for the work of OSHA. OSHA has established federal health and safety rights for all workers in the U.S. whether or not they are United States citizens.

Pain and suffering: includes the loss of physical abilities, such as the use of your hand or foot, and physical discomfort, such as chronic backache or stiffness in your neck. The term also includes any emotional pain you might suffer, such as worry, anxiety, embarrassment, and the loss of the pleasures and enjoyment of life.

Risk management: in healthcare, this is preventive medicine. This calls for identifying problems and forestalling incidents that could lead to claims. Accurate and proper documentation of healthcare provided is vital in risk management. Often what is omitted from the medical record can be more harmful to the healthcare provider than what is included.

Sexual harassment definition: Title VII of the Civil Rights Act of 1964 makes it unlawful for an employer to discriminate against any individual with respect to compensation, terms, conditions, or privileges of employment, because of such individual's sex.

Standard of care: the standard of care used in malpractice cases has been stated as "A physician is bound to bestow such reasonable and ordinary care, skill, and diligence as physicians and surgeons in good standing in the same neighborhood, in the same general line of practice, ordinarily have and exercise in like cases."[1]

Statutory employee: workers deemed to be employees by statute. A home-based worker performing work on materials or goods furnished by the employer could be considered a statutory employee. Statutory employees receive W2 Form from the employer. Statutory employees are not liable for self-employment tax because their employers must treat them as employees for social security tax purposes.

Tort: a tort occurs when someone deliberately or through carelessness causes harm or loss to another person or their property.

References

1. 61 Am. Jur. 2d *Physicians and Surgeons* #205 (1981).

2. Garner BA (ed.). *Black's Law Dictionary*, 7th Edition. Eagan, MN: West Publishing Company, 1991.

3. Hall MA, Ellman IM. *Health Care Law and Ethics in a Nutshell.* Eagan, MN: West Publishing Company, 1990.

4. Southwick AF. *The Law of Hospital and Health Care Administration*, 2nd Edition. Chicago: Health Administration Press, 1988.

HIPAA

To provide effective treatment, healthcare providers must have comprehensive, accurate, and timely medical information. The automation of medical information permits the collection, analysis, storage, and retrieval of vast amounts of medical information that is not only used but also shared with other providers at remote locations. The increasing demand for access to medical information by providers and others, such as insurance companies, has led to increasing concern about patient privacy and confidentiality, resulting in the enactment of the privacy and security provisions of the Health Insurance Portability and Accountability Act of 1996 (HIPAA).

There are seven patient rights under HIPAA:

1. Right to a notice of privacy practices.

2. Right to access PHI.

3. Right to request amendment to PHI.

4. Right to request alternative means of communicating PHI.

5. Right to request restrictions on PHI.

6. Right to an accounting.

7. Right to complain about privacy practices.

The privacy rule regulates the use and disclosure of "protected health information" (PHI) by certain entities. Protected health information is information transmitted or maintained in any form—by electronic means, on paper, or through oral communications—that: (1) relates to the past, present, or future physical or mental health or condition of an individual, the provision of health care to an individual, or the past, present, or future payment for the provision of health care to an individual; and (2) identifies the individual or with respect to which there is a reasonable basis to believe the information can be used to identify the individual. Information that has been de-identified in accordance with the rule's stringent de-identification criteria is not considered protected health information and is not subject to the rule.

The Life of a Medical Report

It may help to understand how the privacy rule relates to medical transcription by examining the life of a transcribed report as it moves through the healthcare system. It begins with a patient encounter. Whether that encounter occurs in a hospital, a physician office, or an outpatient clinic, health information is collected to create the transcribed report; this information is **protected health information**, according to HIPAA. The healthcare provider collecting the information is a **covered entity**. Once the information has been collected by the provider, it is transmitted in some form for transcription. This is considered a permitted **disclosure** of the information, as long as only the minimum amount of information necessary for transcription is disclosed. If the information has been transmitted from a provider to an MT business for transcription for the covered entity, that MT business is considered a **business associate** of the **covered entity** (the healthcare provider).

Organizations *directly* subject to the HIPAA privacy rule are those that typically generate individually identifiable patient health information and therefore have primary responsibility for maintaining the privacy and confidentiality of such information. These **covered entities**, as defined by HIPAA, are: (1) most health plans; (2) healthcare clearinghouses; and (3) healthcare providers that transmit any health information in electronic form in connection with certain administrative transactions related to payment for health care. Employees of covered entities generally are not themselves covered entities but effectively must comply with the rule, because improper uses and disclosures of information by employees may be imputed to employers. Thus, medical transcriptionists who work as employees of hospitals, clinics, private physician offices, and other covered entities should follow the policies and procedures established by those organizations with respect to the handling of protected health information.

As a general matter, a covered entity may use or disclose protected health information only: (1) with an individual's written "consent" for treatment, payment, and healthcare operations; (2) with an individual's written "authorization" for purposes unrelated to treatment, payment, or healthcare operations; and (3) without consent or authorization for certain purposes enumerated by the rule, such as research and public health, if specified conditions are met. Except for disclosures made to healthcare providers for treatment purposes and certain other disclosures identified by the rule, a covered entity may use or disclose only the minimum protected health information necessary to accomplish the intended purpose. The rule generally requires covered entities to grant individuals access to records containing protected health information about them, as well as the opportunity to request amendments to such records. Covered entities also must comply with a host of administrative requirements intended to protect patient privacy. For instance, each covered entity must appoint a privacy officer who is responsible for ensuring that the entity develops and implements written policies and procedures designed to safeguard individuals' privacy.

The HIPAA privacy rule also applies *indirectly* to **business associates** of covered entities. Business associates are individuals and organizations who are not employees of covered entities but who provide services on behalf of covered entities, which involve the receipt or disclosure of protected health information. An MT business that provides transcription services for a covered entity is a business associate of that covered entity. The privacy rule requires covered entities to enter into a written agreement with each business associate—known as a "business associate agreement"—that limits the latter's ability to use and disclose the protected health information and that includes numerous other provisions. Significantly, the business associate may not use or disclose the protected health information other than as permitted or required by the business associate agreement or as required by law. Thus, an MT business generally may not use or disclose protected health information for a purpose unrelated to the provision of transcription services—unless the covered entity authorizes the MT business through the agreement to make uses or disclosures for that purpose. The specific requirements of business associate agreements are discussed further below.

Medical transcriptionists who are *employees* of healthcare providers or other HIPAA "covered entities" are affected by HIPAA, but they should go to their employers for guidance regarding HIPAA compliance. However, even these MTs should also be aware of the issues, in case they consider going into business for themselves, even on a part-time basis, at some point in the future. Consider the fact that "doing a little work on the side" makes one an independent contractor and thus a business owner.

MTs who are *subcontractors* to MT businesses will be required to agree contractually to essentially the same restrictions and conditions that apply to MT businesses with respect to handling patient information and, therefore, may also find this document useful.

REVIEW EXERCISES

REGULATORY REQUIREMENTS & JCAHO

1. Abbreviations and symbols can only be used when
   A. the dictator identifies them.
   B. abbreviations and symbols are never used.
   C. they are found in a medical dictionary.
   D. they have been approved for the medical staff policy and procedure manual.

2. Accreditation by JCAHO is voluntary for private and not-for-profit hospitals and is
   A. required in all states.
   B. unnecessary.
   C. conducted annually.
   D. required for reimbursement for certain patient groups.

3. Which of the following is required for confidentiality purposes?
   A. a keyboard locking system
   B. a special computer screen to block side viewing
   C. a paper shredder
   D. a special trash receptacle

4. JCAHO defines authentication as
   A. proof of authorship.
   B. a complete clinical record.
   C. a complete consultation report.
   D. recording a clinical event as soon as possible.

5. Identification of authors cannot be accomplished by
   A. a written signature.
   B. identifiable initials.
   C. a computer key.
   D. a check mark at the signature line.

6. JCAHO requires a history and physical report to be completed
   A. within 24 hours of hospital admission.
   B. within 24 hours of hospital discharge.
   C. only if the patient is admitted for surgery.
   D. immediately after surgery.

7. Which is most applicable? JCAHO states that when economically feasible and appropriate, medical entries should be typed to assist in
   A. legibility.
   B. timeliness.
   C. completeness.
   D. clinical pertinence.

8. JCAHO Accreditation is important because
   A. accreditation meets Medicare conditions of participation for reimbursement.
   B. the government requires all hospitals to undergo accreditation.
   C. the public demands it.
   D. physicians have requested it.

9. JCAHO means
   A. Joint Commission Association of Healthcare Organizations.
   B. Joint Commission on Accreditation of Healthcare Organizations.
   C. Joint Commissioners Association of Healthcare Organizations.
   D. Joint Commission on Acute Healthcare Organizations.

10. Joint Commission grants accreditation for a maximum of
    A. one year.
    B. three years.
    C. two years.
    D. eighteen months.

HIPAA

1. HIPAA stands for
   A. Health Insurance Portability and Accident Act.
   B. Health Information Portability and Accountability Act.
   C. Health Insurance Portability and Accountability Act.
   D. Health Information Portability and Insurance Act.

2. A breach in confidentiality of patient information can occur
   A. when a report is being transcribed on a digital system.
   B. when a doctor dictates a patient's health information into the transcriptionist's answering machine.
   C. when a transcriptionist uses a headset to play back information.
   D. when a doctor sees a patient.

3. Organizations that have the primary responsibility for protecting individually identifiable patient health information are called covered entities. Which below would constitute an example of a covered entity?
   A. business associate
   B. hospital administrator
   C. personal friend
   D. health plan

4. Medical transcriptionists who are employees of a covered entity must follow
   A. the HIPAA regulations.
   B. the people involved in billing for healthcare.
   C. business associate agreement with the healthcare provider.
   D. the policies and procedures established by the organization with respect to the handling of protected health information.

5. Failure of a covered entity to comply with HIPAA standards can result in
   A. civil monetary penalties of up to $200 for each accidental violation.
   B. civil monetary penalties of up to $100 for each accidental violation.
   C. imprisonment for 20 years for selling PHI.
   D. civil monetary penalties of up to $250,000 per year.

6. A medical transcriptionist working as an independent contractor should have
   A. a list of all social security numbers for patients.
   B. direct access to the U.S. Government HIPAA clearinghouse.
   C. a Business Associate agreement with accounts, policies, and procedures on maintaining confidential information and access to information necessary to do the job.
   D. a list of all business associates for healthcare providers.

7. In the case of disaster, which of the following is not part of a contingency plan?
   A. data backup
   B. disaster recovery
   C. emergency mode operation
   D. indemnification policy

8. MTs should retain protected health information only as long as it is necessary to do business; that is, no longer than necessary to
   A. verify records and authenticate by originator.
   B. verify information, distribute, and bill for services provided.
   C. provide information to patients.
   D. complete billing and transmission back to healthcare provider.

9. When physically transporting protected health information, an MT business would be violating confidentiality by
   A. using a bonded commercial courier for transport and having them sign a confidentiality agreement.

B. leaving PHI in an unprotected location for pick up, such as in a mailbox or front door.

C. delivering documents personally in a sealed, tamper-proof container.

D. covering patient identifiable information that is visible on the outside of the envelope.

10. Ways to protect identifiable patient information when faxing include all of the following except

A. having a cover sheet informing recipient of confidentiality of information being faxed and providing a warning to any recipient not authorized to have access to such information.

B. maintaining the fax machine in an easily visible and accessible location.

C. preprogramming frequently used fax numbers to avoid mistakes.

D. keeping the fax machine in a secure area of the business to prevent access by unauthorized individuals.

11. In the HIPAA privacy rule, PHI generally refers to

A. individually identifiable health information.

B. a patient's social history.

C. how many times a patient has been in the hospital.

D. a business associate.

12. Electronically transferred files containing PHI

A. should only be transferred using FTP protocol.

B. should be encrypted regardless of mode of transmission.

C. can be sent safely by email.

D. only need to be password protected.

13. For the home-based MT, the computer used for work needs to be secure. The computer is not secure if

A. the computer is password protected.

B. the computer is kept in a locked, secure room to prohibit access.

C. the computer is used by all family members.

D. the password is changed every 30 days.

14. According to HIPAA regulations, which one of the following is incorrect?

A. all inpatients must be listed in the patient directory

B. psychotherapy notes that document or analyze the contents of conversation during a counseling session are kept separate from the rest of the patient's medical record

C. information such as address, age, social security number, and phone number is protected health information

D. passwords should include both letters and numbers or other special characters

15. One of the patient's rights under HIPAA is

A. right to change their PHI.

B. right to access their PHI.

C. right to eliminate their PHI.

D. right to change physicians.

RISK MANAGEMENT

1. Which function is not included in a risk manager's main duties?

A. liability claims management

B. participating in safety and security programs

C. loss prevention and reduction

D. medical staff evaluation

2. If a policy and procedure manual does not reflect current practices, this can be referred to risk management because

A. time is wasted in correcting the manual.

B. new personnel will not be trained properly.

C. the manual represents the normal course of business.

D. changes must be cleared by the risk manager.

3. Dictated information that indicates potential risk to the patient or to the institution, including personnel, should be reported to

A. the director of health information management (medical records).

B. the physician.

C. the CFO.

D. the appropriate institutional personnel, as identified in the institution's program policies.

4. AAMT recommends that independent MTs and MT businesses retain any healthcare records for a period of

A. six months.

B. only as long as is necessary for verification, distribution, and billing purposes.

C. two weeks.

D. seven years (the legal standard).

5. Risk management is defined as

A. healthcare institution activities designed to prevent patients suing the hospital and reducing financial loss.

B. healthcare institution activities that identify, analyze, evaluate, reduce, or eliminate the risk of possible injury and loss to patients, visitors, staff, and the institution itself.

C. activities to monitor medical transcriptionists as to the quality of work submitted.

D. protecting the hospital's reputation.

6. The doctor dictating an operative report on the right knee changes to the left knee in the middle of the report. The transcriptionist would

A. type as the doctor dictated.

B. type as the doctor dictated and make a note of it.

C. type as dictated and send to quality assurance for review.

D. flag the report and bring to the attention of the supervisor or the report's originator for resolution.

7. Professional liability insurance is also called

A. malpractice insurance.

B. licensing insurance.

C. errors and omission insurance.

D. loss prevention insurance.

8. Which of the following is not one of the three basic objectives of a healthcare organization risk management program?

A. to create and maintain a safe, healthy environment and enhance the quality of care

B. to protect the physicians from malpractice suits

C. to minimize risk of medical or accidental injuries and losses

D. to provide cost-effective techniques to ensure against financial loss

9. Audit trails contribute to risk management and are also known as

A. paper trails.

B. documentation trails.

C. cookie trails.

D. sample trails.

10. A comprehensive risk management program contains three components. They are

A. risk identification, risk control, and risk financing.

B. risk identification, continuity of care, and risk financing.

C. providing safe environments, medical staff credentialing, and risk identification.

D. infection control reports, risk control, and risk financing.

ANSWER KEY

REVIEW EXERCISES

REGULATORY REQUIREMENTS & JCAHO

1. D
2. D
3. C
4. A
5. D
6. A
7. A
8. A
9. B
10. B

HIPAA

1. C
2. B
3. D
4. D
5. B
6. C
7. D
8. B
9. B
10. B
11. A
12. B
13. C
14. A
15. B

RISK MANAGEMENT

1. D
2. C
3. D
4. B
5. B
6. D
7. C
8. B
9. B
10. A

Appendices

Normal Lab Values

Background

The laboratory consists of two major sections: Clinical Pathology and Surgical Pathology. Within Clinical Pathology, there are three major departments: Microbiology, Hematology, and Chemistry, as well as specialty areas within each department. Surgical Pathology includes the histology department.

The entire laboratory is directed by a pathologist who is a medical doctor specializing in laboratory medicine. The lab is staffed by technologists and technicians, histologists, phlebotomists, and clerks.

A full-service laboratory will process many types of specimens, the most common being blood, urine, sputum, and stool, but also any other body fluid or tissue obtained through aspiration, biopsy, excision, or amputation.

Blood is drawn into specialized tubes which come in various sizes and shapes. Most blood collection tubes contain an anticoagulant which prevents the blood from clotting. The tops of the collection tubes are color-coded to indicate the type of anticoagulant. For example, green-top tubes contain sodium heparin, purple-top tubes contain EDTA, and blue-top tubes contain sodium citrate. Samples drawn with an anticoagulant will never clot (if properly collected). Tubes with red tops or red and black "tiger" tops do not contain an anticoagulant, and the blood will immediately begin to clot within the tube. It is important that the blood sample be collected in the tube specified for the test, because the wrong anticoagulant can interfere with the test results.

Tests are performed on either whole blood, serum, or plasma. In order to separate the cells from the liquid portion of the blood, the tubes are placed in a centrifuge for 5–10 minutes, forcing the cells and platelets to the bottom of the tube. The watery portion of the sample is called "plasma" if the sample has been anticoagulated and "serum" if the sample has been allowed to clot. Plasma appears slightly cloudy because it still contains clotting factors (proteins). Serum, on the other hand, is normally clear and straw-colored, since the clotting proteins form fibrin strands that entrap cells and platelets in the clot and therefore are no longer a component of the watery portion of the blood.

Common Laboratory Studies

The following tests are the most common laboratory tests performed. Most test results must be evaluated in the context of other laboratory studies and physical findings, as one test is rarely diagnostic for any one disease. For convenience and diagnostic purposes, tests are often grouped together as panels or profiles to assess a particular body system or disease, but these categories are not strict and there is much overlap.

The tables below include only the most common reasons for abnormal test results. Also, each laboratory sets their own reference (normal ranges) based on the methodology being used. These ranges will vary slightly from one laboratory to the next. Normal values for many tests also vary according to age and gender. If values vary, those listed here are for adult males.

Electrolytes and Acid/Base Balance

Sodium, potassium, chloride, and bicarbonate interact to help the body maintain normal fluid levels in the intracellular and extracellular spaces, maintain acid-base balance, and maintain muscle contractility. The kidneys, and to a certain extent the lungs, play the most critical roles in maintaining proper concentrations of these positively and negatively charged molecules, although many metabolic disorders and diseases can disrupt electrolyte balance.

TEST NAME	COMMENT	NORMAL RANGE	NORMAL RANGE (SI)
Na+ (sodium)	Elevated levels are indicative of dehydration. Hyponatremia may be caused by excessive fluid retention (dilutional effect) or by sodium loss through sweating, vomiting, or renal disease.	136 to 145 mEq/L	136 to 145 mmol/L
K+ (potassium)	Decreased levels associated with some diuretics, renal disease, or GI loss through diarrhea or vomiting. Increased levels are seen in renal disease or from rapid breakdown of muscle or red cell lysis.	3.5 to 5 mEq/L	3.5 to 5 mmol/L
Cl$^-$ (chloride)	Elevated levels seen in dehydration or renal disease. Decreased levels result from fluid retention (dilutional effect) or from increased excretion from renal disease, diuretic therapy, or vomiting.	100 to 106 mEq/L	100 to 106 mmol/L
HCO$_3$ (bicarbonate)	May also be referred to as CO_2 because bicarbonate is measured indirectly by measuring CO_2 levels. Bicarbonate buffers the blood to maintain pH. Abnormal levels must be evaluated in the context of other electrolyte levels and physical symptoms.	24 to 30 mEq/L	24 to 30 mmol/L
pH	Normal range must be maintained through buffering system of bicarbonate and electrolytes.	7.35 to 7.45	7.35 to 7.45
CO_2	High levels indicate ingestion/retention of bicarbonate or excessive loss of acids as in vomiting or hypoventilation. Decreased levels seen in diabetic acidosis, renal failure, or diarrhea.	22–26 mEq/L	22–26 mmol/L
Anion Gap	Used to assess metabolic acidosis and indirectly measures the total of anions from sulfates, phosphates, proteins, ketones, and lactic acid using the equation $Na - (Cl + HCO_3)$	12 to 20 mEq/L	12 to 20 mmol/L

Minerals

Minerals such as calcium, magnesium, and phosphorus (in the form of phosphates) are critical for maintaining bones and teeth. Phosphorus also plays an important role in energy utilization, red cell function, and overall metabolism. Calcium and magnesium play an important role in muscle contraction, and calcium is an integral component of the coagulation system. Calcium and phosphorous levels are inversely proportional and are primarily under the control of the parathyroid glands. Excretion and retention of these minerals is controlled by the kidneys. These minerals have some electrolytic activity but traditionally are not considered a part of an "electrolyte panel."

TEST NAME	COMMENT	NORMAL RANGE	NORMAL RANGE (SI)
Ca (calcium)	Elevated levels may indicate hyperparathyroidism, acute or chronic bone disease (e.g., metastasis), or renal disease. Hypocalcemia may result from parathyroid disease, malabsorption, or renal failure.	8.2 to 10.2 mg/dL	2 to 2.5 mmol/L
Mg (magnesium)	Elevated levels, if not caused by over-ingestion (e.g., milk of magnesia) are often due to renal failure. Decreased magnesium may indicate chronic alcoholism.	1.5 to 2.3 mg/dL	0.6 to 1.0 mmol/L
P (phosphorus)	Phosphates are abundant in foods, so typically decreased levels are due to over-excretion by the kidneys. Elevated levels may be due to release from injured bones.	2.5 to 4.5 mg/dL	0.8 to 1.5 mmol/L

Studies Related to Iron Metabolism

Iron is an integral part of hemoglobin and myoglobin molecules which the body uses to bind and transport oxygen. Iron is absorbed from the intestine and carried through the blood to the bone marrow bound to transferrin. Iron is stored bound to a protein called ferritin. The iron binding capacity represents the amount of iron that the body is capable of transporting through the blood by way of transferrin.

TEST NAME	COMMENT	NORMAL RANGE	NORMAL RANGE (SI)
Fe (iron)	Serum iron is decreased with malabsorption and/or malnutrition or with chronic blood loss. Elevated serum iron may be due to excessive dietary intake or hemochromatosis, pernicious anemia, or hemolytic anemia.	50 to 160 mEq/dL	9.0 to 28.8 mcmol/L
Ferritin	Ferritin levels are indicative of stored iron. Decreased levels are typically due to chronic iron deficiency. Levels may be elevated in liver disease, iron overload, infection, or inflammation.	20 to 200 ng/mL	20 to 200 mcg/L
TIBC (total iron binding capacity)	Increased in anemia caused by hemorrhage or iron deficiency. TIBC is decreased in hemochromatosis, nephrotic syndrome, or liver disease.	250 to 350 mcg/dL	45 to 63 mcmol/L
Transferrin	Decreased levels may be due to inadequate production because of liver damage. Elevated levels are common in severe iron deficiency as the body tries to capture more iron.	250 to 425 mg/dL	2.5 to 4.2 g/L

Studies Related to Kidney Function

The kidneys are responsible for filtering water-soluble waste products from the blood as well as maintaining the correct level of electrolytes, proteins, and glucose for fluid balance throughout the body. Water naturally passes through membranes toward higher concentrations of sodium and other dissolved molecules; therefore the proper osmolality (concentration) is needed to keep fluid levels balanced between the intracellular and extracellular spaces. Kidney disease is marked by an inability to properly regulate levels of minerals, proteins, glucose, and nitrogenous wastes.

Blood enters the kidney and is first filtered by the glomeruli, where all but cells, platelets, and large protein molecules are allowed to pass through the glomerular membrane. The filtrate passes through the renal tubules which reabsorb the necessary amounts of glucose and electrolytes, and excrete the excess molecules as well as the wastes into the urine.

BUN is used to assess glomerular filtration because BUN is not reabsorbed by the tubules. Whatever amount passes through the glomerulus is excreted in the urine. Creatinine is also used to assess glomerular function in the same way, only it is considered a more accurate assessment. The GFR (glomerular filtration rate) is dependent upon blood pressure, blood volume, and the resistance of the glomerular membrane.

TEST NAME	COMMENT	NORMAL RANGE	NORMAL RANGE (SI)
BUN (blood urea nitrogen)	Increased in renal disease or impaired blood flow to the kidneys due to decreased blood volume/pressure and also due to renal obstruction. BUN is decreased in severe protein deficiencies.	5 to 20 mg/dL	1.8 to 7.1 mcmol/L
Creatinine	Metabolic production of creatinine remains fairly constant, so increases in creatinine are almost always due to renal impairment or decreased blood pressure/volume passing through the kidneys.	0.6 to 1.2 mg/dL	50 to 100 mcmol/L
24-hour creatinine clearance-measure of glomerular filtration rate	Calculated by comparing creatinine excreted in the urine over 24 hours relative to blood levels of creatinine. GFR is decreased in shock, obstruction of blood flow to kidneys, or kidney disease.	90 to 135 ml/min/1.73m^2	0.86 to 1.3 ml/sec/m^2

Studies Related To Liver Function (LFTs)

The liver performs many metabolic tasks, including detoxification and protein production. The liver is responsible for manufacturing albumin, which is needed to maintain proper osmolality, and many of the carrier proteins (globulins) needed to transport non-water-soluble molecules through the blood. The liver also clears the blood of drugs, environmental chemicals, and metabolic wastes. Liver disease shows up in three ways: increased levels of liver enzymes found in the plasma due to spillage from damaged liver cells; decreased plasma proteins due to impaired ability manufacture needed molecules; and increased waste products (e.g. ammonia, bilirubin, drugs) in the blood due to inability to detoxify and metabolize.

TEST NAME	COMMENT	NORMAL RANGE	NORMAL RANGE (SI)
ALT (SGPT)	Enzyme spills into blood when cells are damaged. Increased levels are seen in liver disease or degenerative muscle diseases.	8 to 45 U/L	8 to 45 U/L
AST (SGOT)	Enzyme spills into blood when cells are damaged. Increased in active liver disease and pancreatitis. May also be increased with damage to myocardial or skeletal muscle damage.	<35 U/L	<35 U/L
Alkaline phosphatase ("alk phos")	Increased in biliary obstruction, hepatic and bone disease, including metastasis.	20 to 120 U/L	20 to 120 U/L

TEST NAME	COMMENT	NORMAL RANGE	NORMAL RANGE (SI)
Total protein	Includes all serum proteins but mostly albumin and globulins. Decreased in malnutrition, chronic disease, and with liver diseases which impair protein production.	6.4 to 8.3 g/dL	64 to 83
Albumin	Decreased in liver disease, malnutrition, and chronic infection.	3.5 to 5.0 g/dL	35 to 50 g/L
Globulin	Includes carrier proteins such as ceruloplasmin, haptoglobin, transferrin, lipoproteins, and the immunoglobin class of proteins (e.g. IgG, IgM, etc.)	1.5 to 3.0 g/dL	15 to 30 g/L
A/G ratio (albumin/ globulin ratio)	Ratio is reversed when albumin is decreased and globulin is increased.	1.5 to 3.0	1. to 3.0
Ammonia (NH$_3$)	Byproduct of protein metabolism which is normally converted to urea by the liver. Ammonia increases in hepatic failure.	15 to 45 mcg/dL	11 to 32 mcmol/L
Total bilirubin	Bilirubin is the breakdown product of hemoglobin. Increased levels are seen in hemolysis, newborns, and liver disease.	0.2 to 1.3 mg/dL	3.4 to 22.1 mcmol/L
Direct bilirubin	Measures bilirubin which has been processed by the liver to be excreted in the bile. Increased levels indicate obstruction in the biliary system.	0.1 to 0.4 mg/dL	1.7 to 6.8 mcmol/L
Indirect bilirubin	Measures bilirubin which has not been processed by the liver. Increased levels indicate liver impairment or hemolysis causing bilirubin levels to rise faster than the liver can process.	0.1 to 0.9 mg/dL	1.7 to 15.3 mcmol/L
GGT	Increased in biliary obstruction, liver disease, pancreatitis, and alcoholism.	<65 U/L	<65 U/L
Haptoglobin	Protein molecule which transports hemoglobin when not bound within the red cell. Levels are decreased in liver disease (impaired production) and increased in cases of chronic hemolysis.	40 to 180 mg/dL	0.4 to 1.8 g/L
LH (LDH, lactate dehydrogenase)	Enzyme found in liver cells and red cells. Increased levels in serum due to hepatitis or hemolytic anemia.	<110 U/L	<110 U/L

Tests Related to Glucose Metabolism

Glucose is the primary form of energy used by all cells. Insulin is required to move glucose from the blood into the cells. Elevated glucose levels stimulate the release of insulin. Abnormal glucose levels may result from too little insulin, too much insulin, or from resistance to the effects of insulin.

TEST NAME	COMMENT	NORMAL RANGE	NORMAL RANGE (SI)
Glucose	Elevated in diabetes, metabolic syndrome, or chronic states of stress. Decreased in acute inflammation, diabetic crisis, starvation/ fasting, or reactive hypoglycemia.	60 to 115 mg/dL (fasting)	3.3 to 6.4 mmol/L
Insulin	Increased levels seen in hyperglycemia and hyperinsulinism.	5 to 25 mcU/mL	24 to 172 pmol/L
Hemoglobin A$_{1c}$ (glycosylated hemoglobin)	Increased in states of sustained elevation of blood glucose over previous 4–6 weeks.	4 to 7%	4 to 7 %

Nonspecific Tests for Inflammation

Inflammation causes an increase in serum proteins, including albumin, globulins, and C-reactive protein. The sedimentation rate, i.e., the time it takes for red cells to fall out of solution, is affected by the increased levels of inflammatory proteins.

TEST NAME	COMMENT	NORMAL RANGE	NORMAL RANGE (SI)
ESR (erythrocyte sedimentation rate) Westergren and Wintrobe methods	Elevated values are associated with inflammation and autoimmune disorders.	Westergren method 0 to 20 mm/hr Wintrobe method 0 to 15 mm/hr	
CRP (C-reactive protein)	Elevated levels associated with states of inflammation.	<0.5 mg/dL	<5 mg/L

Arterial Blood Gas Studies

(Compare to studies above which evaluate venous blood.) These tests are evaluated together to assess the pulmonary gas exchange in patients with respiratory or circulatory disease. Because gases can be compressed, it is difficult to measure gases in terms of volumes, so they are measured according to the amount of pressure they exert (torr) and/or, the percent saturation. You may also hear the term "partial pressure" since each individual gas exerts a "part" of the overall gas pressure.

TEST NAME	COMMENT	NORMAL RANGE	NORMAL RANGE (SI)
pH (hydrogen ion concentration)	Respiration cannot occur outside this strict pH range.	7.35 to 7.45	7.35 to 7.45
HCO_3 (bicarbonate ion)	Controlled by the kidneys and acts as a buffer to maintain strict pH range.	22 to 26 mEq/L	22 to 26 mmol/L
sO_2 or O_2 sat (oxygen saturation)	Indicates percentage of hemoglobin molecules bound with oxygen.	94% to 100 %	0.94 to 1
pO_2 or PaO_2 (pressure of oxygen)	Measures the lungs' ability to oxygenate the blood.	80–100 mmHg	10.6 to 13.3 kPa
pCO_2 or $PaCO_2$ (pressure of carbon dioxide)	Measures the lungs' ability to exchange O_2 for CO_2.	35 to 45 mmHg	4.7 to 5.3 kPa

Cardiovascular/Cerebrovascular Risk or Disease

Cardiovascular tests can be separated into two major categories, those that assess risk of disease and those that diagnose disease and/or trauma. Cholesterol and lipid studies are used to assess a patient's risk of atherosclerotic disease of the heart (myocardial infarction, angina), brain (stroke), or peripheral arteries (peripheral vascular disease). Several other studies which evaluate inflammation and metabolic traits also add to risk assessment. Enzyme studies as well as other biologically active proteins which appear in the blood as a result of cardiac damage are used to assess a recent or acute infarction.

Cholesterol and lipids (fatty acids) are not water soluble, so they must be carried in the blood bound to protein molecules called lipoproteins. Elevated levels in the blood cause deposits to form within arterial walls called plaques, which narrow the lumen of the arteries, reducing or even obstructing flow.

Enzymes and other intracellular components are released into the blood when muscle cells are damaged. Rates of liberation of intracellular components vary, and the patterns of rising and falling levels are diagnostic. When cardiac muscle damage is suspected, serial blood evaluations are performed at defined time intervals.

TEST NAME	COMMENT	NORMAL RANGE	NORMAL RANGE (SI)
Total cholesterol	Total of all cholesterol fractions. Elevated levels are a risk factor for atherosclerosis.	<200 mg/dL	<520 mmol/L
LDL (low density lipoprotein)	Elevated levels are associated with higher risk of atherosclerosis.	40–130 mg/dL, less than 70 mg/dL	1–3 mmol/L
HDL (high density lipoprotein)	"Favorable" form of cholesterol. Higher levels reduce risk of atherosclerosis.	35–80 mg/dL	1–2 mmol/L
VLDL (very low density lipoprotein)	Elevated levels are associated with higher risk of atherosclerosis.		
Triglycerides	Elevated levels increase risk of atherosclerosis.	<160 mg/dL	<1.8 mmol/L
Homocysteine	Elevated levels are associated with increased risk of atherosclerosis.	<1.6 mg/dL	<12mcmol/L
hsCRP (high sensitivity C-reactive protein)	Elevated levels indicate vascular inflammation, increasing risk of atherosclerosis.	0.02 to 0.8 mg/dL	0.2 to 8.0 mg/L
BNP (brain natriuretic peptide)	Mildly elevated levels seen immediately following MI; grossly elevated levels indicative of damage to left ventricle as in congestive heart failure.	<50 pg/mL	<50 ng/L
troponin I	Elevated levels are seen early after myocardial infarction.	<1.5 ng/mL	<1.5 mcg/L
CK (CPK, creatine phosphokinase)	Levels increase with skeletal or cardiac muscle damage.	15 to 105 U/L 0 to 7 ng/mL	15 to 105 U/L 0 to 7 mcg/L
CK-MB	Isoenzyme specific for cardiac muscle damage. Levels increase in the first 24 hours following MI.		
Myoglobin	Levels elevated with muscle damage, not specific for cardiac muscle.	14–51 mcg/L	0.8–2.9 mil/L
LH (LDH, lactate dehydrogenase)	Serum levels rise after muscle damage, although not specific for cardiac muscle.	100 to 190 U/L	100 to 190 U/L

Thyroid-Related Studies

The thyroid gland secretes hormones which regulate metabolism. These hormones have far-reaching effects on many body systems. Thyroid hormones are regulated by feedback loops. A decrease in T_3 or T_4 causes thyroid stimulating hormone levels to rise, increasing T_3 and T_4. As levels rise, TSH goes back down. Of the two, T_3 is more metabolically active than T_4, but it binds loosely to thyroid binding globulin (TBG) so it is quickly removed from the blood. T_4 binds more tightly to TBG so it survives in the blood for a longer period, but very little is "free" to exert an effect on cells.

TEST NAME	COMMENT	NORMAL RANGE	NORMAL RANGE (SI)
T_4 (thyroxine)	Increased in Graves disease and acute thyroiditis.	4.5 to 12 mcg/dL	58 to 154 nmol/L
Free T_4	Decreased in iodine deficiency and chronic disease.	0.8–2.7 ng/dL	10.3–35 pmol/L
T_3	Elevated levels indicative of hyperthyroidism; decreased in hypothyroidism when TBG is normal.	70–190 ng/dL	1.1 to 2.9 nmol/L
Free T_3	Not bound to TBG, metabolically active form of T_3	260 to 480 pg/dL	4.0 to 7.4 pmol/L
TSH (thyroid stimulating hormone)	Increased in primary hypothyroidism. Decreased in primary hyperthyroidism.	0.4 to 4.2 mcU/mL	0.4 to 4.2 mU/L
T_3 uptake	Used to indirectly measure TBG (thyroid binding globulin).	25 to 38%	0.25 to 0.38
Antithyroid antibodies	Elevated in Hashimoto thyroiditis.	None	
TBG (thyroid binding globulin)	Abnormal levels affect metabolically active fraction of T_3 and T_4.	1.25 to 2.5 mg/dL	12 to 25 mg/L

Parathyroid Studies

The parathyroid glands maintain the balance of calcium, magnesium, and phosphorous between the blood and bones.

TEST NAME	COMMENT	NORMAL RANGE	NORMAL RANGE (SI)
PTH (parathyroid hormone)	Increased PTH results in hypercalcemia, and conversely decreased PTH causes hypocalcemia and increased serum phosphorus.	11 to 54 pg/mL	1.2 to 5.6 pmol/L

Immune System

Tests of the immune system include assays for cell markers, complement levels, and antibodies. For example, white blood cells have specific proteins on the outer surface. These proteins can be used to identify white cells. Antibodies are reported in ratios or titers, which are determined by testing serial dilutions (concentrations) and reporting the end point (the highest dilution that shows a reaction.) Also, since antibodies are very specific, they work well for tagging proteins so they can be measured. This concept is the basis of ELISA and fluorescent antibody tests.

TEST NAME	COMMENT	NORMAL RANGE	NORMAL RANGE (SI)
CD4	Used to monitor HIV infection. Decreased CD4 levels correlate with increased viral activity.	5 to 1500 cells/mm^3	0.5 to 1.5 $\times$ 10^9 cells/L

TEST NAME	COMMENT	NORMAL RANGE	NORMAL RANGE (SI)
ANA (antinuclear antibodies)	Increased levels of antibodies against nuclear elements are common in autoimmune diseases such as SLE.	Negative	
Anti-ds-DNA (antibodies against double-stranded DNA)	Increased levels of antibodies against DNA are seen in autoimmune diseases.	Negative	
RF (rheumatoid factor)	Seen in 80% of patients with rheumatoid arthritis	Negative	

Cancer Markers

Cancer markers include serum proteins and genetic markers which are expressed in some forms of cancer. The serum markers are used to screen for disease and then to monitor remission or progression of confirmed disease. Genetic markers are used to screen for risk of disease or to characterize known disease.

TEST NAME	COMMENT	NORMAL RANGE	NORMAL RANGE (SI)
PSA (prostate specific antigen)	Levels increase in prostatitis and prostate cancer.	<4 ng/mL	<4 mcg/L
CEA (carcinoembryonic antigen)	Elevated values may indicate carcinoma of the lung, digestive tract, or pancreas.	<5.0 ng/mL	<5.0 mcg/L
AFP (alpha-fetoprotein)	Elevated levels seen in hepatocellular cancer, hepatic disease, embryonal cancers, and in the maternal serum of a fetus with a neural tube defect (e.g., spinal bifida).	<15 ng/mL	<15 mcg/L
CA-125	Elevated levels associated with ovarian and digestive tract carcinomas	<35 U/mL	<35 kU/L
CA-19-9	Elevated values associated with digestive tract carcinomas.	<37 U/mL	<37 kU/L
BRCA-1, BRCA-2	Genetic markers associated with breast, prostate, and ovarian cancer		

Hematology

Samples used by the hematology lab are collected into purple-top tubes (also called lavender-top) and are not allowed to clot or separate from the serum as in most chemistry tests. Whole blood with intact cells is needed in order to obtain accurate cell counts and platelet counts. A small portion of the sample may be centrifuged in a microcentrifuge in order to determine the hematocrit, although this value is most often calculated indirectly using red cell counts and indices.

CBC (Complete Blood Count)

The CBC is one of the most common tests ordered, yet a diagnosis is rarely made based on the results of a CBC alone. A CBC must be interpreted along with other diagnostic and physical findings.

A CBC enumerates the formed elements of the blood, including white cells, red cells, and platelets. A CBC also includes specific information about the size and composition of red cells, called indices (MCV, MCH, MCHC, RDW). Platelets are actually small, extruded fragments of megakaryocytes and therefore are not actually cells. Platelets are integral to coagulation as they release factors which initiate clot formation as well as physically create barriers for sealing cuts and abrasions.

TEST NAME	COMMENT	NORMAL RANGE	NORMAL RANGE (SI)
WBC	Mild to moderate elevations seen in infection, pregnancy. Moderate to severe elevations can indicate leukemoid reaction, severe infection, or leukemia. Decreased levels seen in overwhelming infection, viral infection, bone marrow suppression, and immunodeficiency disease and status post chemotherapy and radiation therapy.	5000 to 10000/mm^3	5 to 10 $\times$ 10^9 cells/L
RBC	Increased in polycythemia vera, pulmonary disease and to compensate for high altitudes. Decreased levels seen in acute or chronic hemorrhage, decreased hemoglobin synthesis, aplastic anemia, bone marrow suppression, leukemia, and status post chemotherapy and radiation therapy.	4.8 to 5.6 $\times$ 10^6/mm^3	4.8 to 5.6 $\times$ 10^{12}/L
Hgb (hemoglobin)	Elevated levels are seen in polycythemia vera, dehydration, and compensation for reduced oxygen concentration in higher altitudes. Levels are reduced in malnutrition, iron deficiency, thalassemia, hemorrhage, leukemia, and anemia of chronic disease.	12 to 16 g/dL	7.5 to 10 mmol/L
Hct (hematocrit)	The percentage of whole blood composed of red blood cells. Reduced values coincide with reduced RBC. Normally, the hematocrit will be equal to roughly 3 times the hemoglobin value.	40% to 48%	40% to 48%
MCH (mean corpuscular hemoglobin)	Average weight of hemoglobin contained per red cell.	27 to 31 pg/cell (picogram)	27 to 31 pg/cell (picogram)
MCHC (mean corpuscular hemoglobin concentration)	Average concentration of hemoglobin per red cell. Decreased levels (hypochromia) associated with iron-deficiency anemia, hereditary anemias, chronic blood loss.	32 to 36 g/dL	320 to 360 g/L
MCV (mean corpuscular volume)	A measure of the size of red cells. Decreased values (microcytosis) are associated with iron deficiency and/or chronic blood loss (and many other conditions). Higher values (macrocytosis) may be due to B12 and/or folic acid deficiency or liver disease.	82 to 92 mcm^3	82 to 92 fL (femtoliter)

TEST NAME	COMMENT	NORMAL RANGE	NORMAL RANGE (SI)
RDW	A measure of the degree of variation in the size of red cells (anisocytosis). The higher the number, the less uniformity, indicating stress on the bone marrow. Seen in many conditions and diseases.	<15%	<15%
Platelets	Increased levels are seen in essential thrombocytosis, some forms of leukemia, and polycythemia vera. Reduced numbers (thrombocytopenia) seen in idiopathic thrombocytopenia (autoimmune disease), adverse drug reactions, aplastic anemia, disseminated intravascular coagulation (DIC), bone marrow suppression (e.g. chemotherapy and radiation).	150,000 to 400,000/mm^3	150 to 400 $\times$ 10^9/L

Differential

The differential separates the white cells into their various subtypes and reports each subtype as a percentage of the total. Traditionally, a differential is performed by staining a smear of peripheral blood and evaluating a total of 100 white cells under a microscope, reporting the percentage of each type of cell seen. The names of the white cell subtypes are based on their staining characteristics using a Wright stain. The granulocytes were so named because the granules contained within the cells stain various shades of pink, purple, and blue. Eosinophils have the typical small granules and also large granules which stain darkly with eosin, an intense red dye. Basophils likewise have large granules which stain heavily with the basic dye (dark bluish purple) contained in the Wright stain. Although many differential counts are still performed on stained blood smears, automated cell counters are also used to count white cell subtypes. An absolute count of each white cell is determined by multiplying the percentage in the differential by the total white count.

TEST NAME	COMMENT	NORMAL RANGE	ABSOLUTE COUNT
Granulocytes	Includes segmented neutrophils (mature), band neutrophils (less mature), basophils, and eosinophils.		
Segmented neutrophils ("segs"), also called polymorphonuclear leukocytes ("polys")	Increased in bacterial infection, pregnancy, some forms of leukemia. Decreased in some cases of poisoning, some viral infections, some leukemias, and status post chemotherapy and radiation.	40% to 70%	2000 to 6500/mm^3
Bands, also called stabs	Elevation in band neutrophils may also be referred to as a "left shift." Elevations seen in acute and severe infections.	4% to 8%	200 to 800/mm^3
Basophils	Increased in chronic myelogenous leukemia and polycythemia. Decreased in hyperthyroidism and bone marrow suppression.	0–1%	40 to 60/mm^3
Eosinophils	Increased in allergic reactions, parasitic infections, and chronic myelogenous leukemia.	0–5%	100 to 400/mm^3
Monocytes	Increased in some viral infections, monocytic leukemia, and some collagen diseases. Decreased in bone marrow suppression.	5% to 8%	200 to 600/mm^3

TEST NAME	COMMENT	NORMAL RANGE	ABSOLUTE COUNT
Lymphocytes	Usually increased in viral infections and some forms of leukemia. Greater than 10% atypical lymphocytes are characteristic of infectious mononucleosis. Decreased counts are seen in AIDS and autoimmune disorders.	25% to 40%	1250 to 4000/mm³
Blasts	Very immature white cells. Diagnostic for leukemia when seen in the peripheral blood.	None	

Abnormal Red Cells Seen On Peripheral Smear

Reticulocytes (immature red cells) can be noted on a Wright-stained peripheral smear but are more accurately counted and reported as a percent of total red cells using a methylene blue stain. Red cell morphology (shape) can be indicative and sometimes even diagnostic for certain diseases (e.g. sickle cells). The presence of these various red cell types are graded 1+ (10% of cells affected) through 4+ (greater than 75% of cells affected).

TEST NAME	COMMENT	NORMAL RANGE
Reticulocytes ("retics")	Elevated numbers are seen during recovery of severe anemia or in chronic anemia, as the stressed bone marrow pushes red cells into the peripheral blood prematurely.	None to 1+
Macrocytes	Large red cells, correlate with elevated MCV.	None to 1+
Microcytes	Small red cells, correlate with decreased MCV.	None to 1+
Nucleated RBC (nRBC) (normoblast)	Very immature red cells still containing remnants of a nucleus. Seen in some leukemias or severe anemias where the bone marrow is stressed to produce adequate RBCs.	None
Polychromasia	Seen as larger, more purplish red cells on Wright stain. Correlate with elevated reticulocyte count and elevated MCV.	None to 1+
Sickle cells	Sickle-shaped cells seen in sickle-cell disease, caused by abnormal hemoglobin molecules which distort the normal cell shape.	None
Poikilocytosis (subtypes tear drop, dacryocyte, elliptocyte, acanthocyte)	Variation in shape of red cells. Especially seen in thalassemia, liver and kidney disease, but this is a nonspecific finding seen in many conditions.	None to 1+
Anisocytosis	Variation in size of red cells. Correlates with RDW on CBC. Nonspecific finding seen in many conditions.	None to 1+
Schistocytes	Remnants of destroyed red cells, indicative of mechanical "shredding" of the red cell membrane (prosthetic heart valves), or from hemolytic anemia (uremia, disseminated intravascular coagulation).	None
Target cells	Named for their characteristic "target" appearance. Associated with hemoglobinopathies, especially thalassemia, and liver disease. May be a nonspecific finding.	None to 1+
Spherocytes	Spherical red cells which have lost their typical concave shape. Can be a nonspecific finding. Large numbers indicative of hereditary spherocytosis or spherocytic anemia.	None to 1+

Coagulation Studies

Coagulation studies are used to diagnose coagulopathies and monitor anticoagulation therapy. In contrast to many laboratory studies, PT and PTT tests do not measure actual concentrations of coagulation factors; rather, these tests measure their activity. Abnormalities in PT or PTT may lead to further studies to diagnose deficiencies of one of the many factors making up the coagulation system.

TEST NAME	COMMENT	NORMAL RANGE	NORMAL RANGE (SI)
PT (prothrombin time or "pro time")	Measures the time required for a clot to form. Prolongation may indicate hepatic disease, deficiency in vitamin K, Factor V, Factor VII, Factor IX, or fibrinogen. Also prolonged by coumarin therapy.	11 to 13 seconds	11 to 13 seconds
PTT (partial thromboplastin time)	Also measures the time required for a clot to form. Prolongation may indicate deficiency of fibrinogen or Factor IX, X, XI or XII.	21 to 35 seconds	21 to 35 seconds
INR (International Normalized Ratio)	The potency of thromboplastin used to perform the PT varies from one batch to another, so each batch of thromboplastin is assigned a sensitivity index value. The PT result is multiplied by the index value to arrive at a standarized number which can be interpreted the same regardless of the laboratory, methodology, or test reagents. The INR is important for monitoring coumarin therapy.	Normal ratio is 1. Target ranges for INR vary according to the underlying disease. DVT prophylaxis 1 to 1.5. Recurrent DVT 3 to 4. Atrial fibrillation 2 to 3.	
D-dimer	Product of clot lysis (breakdown). Values are elevated in DIC, MI, venous thrombosis.	<250 mcg/L	<1.37 nmol/L
FSP (fibrin split product or fibrin degradation product)	Breakdown product of fibrin clot. Elevated levels are indicative of DIC.		
Fibrinogen	Fibrinogen is converted to fibrin by clot initiation factors. Levels decrease with active clot formation. Fibrinogen is also an acute phase protein and is elevated in infection and inflammation.	200 to 400 mg/dL	2 to 4 g/L

Urinalysis

A urinalysis is much like a CBC in that it is used to screen for abnormalities, but rarely can a diagnosis be made on the results of a urinalysis alone. The urinalysis has three major components: the dipstick, macroscopic examination, and microscopic examination.

The macroscopic examination is simply observing the urine for color and clarity and any sediment large enough to be seen by the naked eye. Urine is normally straw colored to dark yellow and clear. Abnormal colors include brown, red, amber, or even very dark yellow. Drug metabolites may change the color of urine to bright orange or even green. Elevated proteins or large numbers of white or red cells or drug metabolites may cloud the urine.

Dipstick Test

The dipstick is a narrow plastic strip with as many as 10 different test pads. Each test pad reacts by changing colors, and the color and intensity are indicative of the results. After the stick is dipped into a urine sample, it is placed on a reader which detects the color changes.

TEST NAME	COMMENT	NORMAL RANGE
pH	Decreased (acidosis) in diabetic ketosis, UTI. Alkaline urine (increased pH) is seen with UTI, chronic renal failure, vomiting, and hyperventilation.	4.6 to 8.0
Protein	Protein appears in the urine in renal disease, diabetes mellitus, and infection.	None
Glucose	Glucose is normally reabsorbed by the renal tubules, but elevated blood glucose can overwhelm the kidneys, causing glucose to spill into the urine. Glucose may also appear in the urine in liver disease, impaired tubular reabsorption, and uncontrolled diabetes mellitus.	None
Ketones	Ketones are an end-product of fat metabolism. Ketones appear in the urine in diabetic ketoacidosis, low-carbohydrate diets, and starvation.	None
Blood	Blood may be detected in the urine as intact cells or as hemoglobin. Hematuria (intact cells in the urine) may result from infection, malignant hypertension, or trauma. Hemoglobinuria is present in burn victims, transfusion reactions, intravascular hemolysis, and DIC.	None
Bilirubin	Bilirubin appears in the urine under any circumstance that causes increased RBC destruction, with liver impairment, or biliary obstruction.	None
Urobilinogen	Bilirubin is acted on in the gut by bacteria to produce urobilinogen, which is reabsorbed and metabolized by the liver. It appears in the urine when bilirubin is increased.	None
Nitrite	Nitrates, normally excreted in the urine, are converted to nitrites by bacteria. Positive nitrite is indicative of bacterial UTI.	None
Leukocyte esterase	Leukocyte esterase is detectable in the urine when the urine contains white cells. Typically, a positive esterase test indicates a UTI.	None.
Specific gravity	This is a measure of the kidneys' ability to concentrate urine. The value is decreased (dilute urine) in diabetes insipidus, glomerulonephritis, and renal damage. Elevated values (concentrated urine) may be seen in dehydration, diabetes mellitus, and congestive heart failure.	1.005 to 1.030

Microscopic Examination

The microscopic part of the examination involves centrifuging the urine sample and placing a drop of the concentrated sediment under a microscope to examine the specimen for formed elements. Results are reported as the average number of elements seen in either the low-power or high-power field of the microscope (written *hpf* for high-power field and *lpf* for low-power field).

TEST NAME	COMMENT	NORMAL RANGE
WBC	Intact white cells may be seen in the urine sediment, indicating an infection within the urinary tract.	0 to 4 cells/hpf (should correlate with dipstick results)
RBC	Intact red cells may originate from anywhere within the urinary tract. See above for possible implications.	0 to 3 cells/hpf (should correlate with dipstick results)
Epithelial cells	Epithelial cells throughout the urinary tract slough off and appear in the urine under normal circumstances. Very large numbers may indicate trauma within the urinary tract.	Renal tubule epithelial cells: 0 to 3 cells/hpf Bladder and squamous epithelial cells are normal.
Bacteria	Very small numbers of bacteria may be seen in urine when the sample is contaminated during collection. Large numbers indicate infection.	

TEST NAME	COMMENT	NORMAL RANGE
Casts (red cell, white cell, hyaline, granular, waxy, broad, or fatty)	Clumps or masses of cells (red, white, or epithelial cells) or proteins that form in the renal tubules are called casts. They are seen in cases of renal tubular disease or glomerular disease.	None
Crystals	Crystals may form in the urine as metabolites crystalize under acidic or alkaline conditions. Many have little to no clinical significance, but some form as a result of increased levels of metabolites in the urine. Calcium oxalate and triple phosphate are the most common abnormal crystals seen.	Amorphous urates, sodium urate, calcium carbonate, ammonium biurate, calcium phosphate, amorphous phosphates are reported when present. Any number is considered abnormal.

Medical Soundalikes

FREQUENTLY CONFUSED TERMS

ABDUCT to move away from	**ADDUCT** to move toward
AIDE an assistant	**AID** to provide assistance
	ADE a drink (lemonade)	
ANATOMIC relating to the human anatomy or body location	**ATOMIC** nuclear particles
ANTERIOR before	**INTERIOR** within
APPRAISED to determine the value (property appraisal)	**APPRISED** to inform (the patient was apprised of her diagnosis)
ASCITIC a collection of fluid in the abdomen	**ACIDIC** an acid-like substance
ATOPIC relating to atopy (allergy)	**ECTOPIC** out of place (ectopic pregnancy)
AURA subjective symptoms often occurring prior to a seizure or migraine	**ORA** plural of os (mouth)
AWL instrument for making holes	**ALL** the whole, everybody, everything
AXIS a line through the center of an organ	**ACCESS** to obtain entrance into
CAROTID the artery in your neck	**PAROTID** the gland in your jaw
CARRIES plural form of the noun carry (e.g., the receiver had 5 carries in this game)	**CARIES** decayed teeth (carious)

CIRCUMSCRIBED
bound by line, limited or
confined (well-circumscribed
border)

CIRCUMCISED
excision of penile foreskin
(diagnosis: phimosis)

CIRRHOSIS
interstitial inflammation
of an organ,
especially the liver

XEROSIS
abnormal dryness, especially
of the hands or feet

COLLABORATE
to work jointly with others

CORROBORATE
to support with evidence

COMPLEMENT
lab test or something that fills up
or completes

COMPLIMENT
kind remark

CONSTIPATION
difficulty passing stools

OBSTIPATION
extreme constipation

CONTRACTIONS
rhythmic muscle movements
(contractions during labor)

CONTRACTURES
retraction of muscles
(from disuse/deconditioning)

CORD
long rope-like structure
(vocal cord, etc.)

CHORD
musical note which
combines more than one
individual note

CORNEAL
pertaining to the
cornea of the eye

CORNUAL
pertaining to an area of the
fallopian tube

COURSE
moving in a path from point to point

COARSE
loose or rough texture or harsh,
raucous tone

CREATINE
occurs in muscle tissue
as phosphocreatine
(high in urine suggests MD)

CREATININE
a component of urine
(final product of creatine
catabolism)

DISCREET
showing good judgment
(ability to be silent)

DISCRETE
distinct separation
(as in a discrete lesion)

DIVERTICULUM
singular

DIVERTICULA
plural

DYSPHAGIA
difficulty swallowing

DYSPHASIA
difficulty speaking

EFFECT
to cause to happen (verb)
or
an outward sign (noun)

AFFECT
to produce an effect upon;
influence (verb)
the subjective aspect of an
emotion, as in a flat affect
(noun)

EFFUSION
collection of fluid in tissue

INFUSION
introduction of fluid into a vein

ELUDE
evade or escape notice

ALLUDE
to refer indirectly

ELUTE
to remove absorbed material (e.g., drug)
by means of a solvent (drug-eluting stent)

EMIGRATE
to leave one country to settle
  in another

IMMIGRATE
to come into a country to take up
  residence

ETIOLOGY
cause of disease

IDEOLOGY
a belief system

FACIAL
pertaining to the face or
  facial region

FASCIAL
a sheet of fibrous tissue

FISSURE
a cleft or groove

FISHER
usually a surname or
  "one who fishes"

FORNICATION
illicit coitus

FORMICATION
sensation of insects crawling on
  the skin

FOSSA
general term for a hollow or
  depressed area
  (plural = fossae)

FOCI
plural of focus (more than one point
  of convergence)

GATE
an opening in a fence

GAIT
walking stride

HABITUS
physical characteristics

HABITAT
environment in which a species lives

HEAL
to make well

HEEL
posterior portion of the foot

HEROIN
an illicit drug

HEROINE
a woman having the qualities of a hero

ILIUM
hip bone

ILEUM
intestine

ILLICIT
illegal

ELICIT
to bring out

INCISE
to cut into

EXCISE
to cut out

INCISION
to cut into or through

EXCISION
to cut out or remove

INSTALLATION
the act of placing something into
  position for service

INSTILLATION
to impart gradually, as in a fluid
  drop by drop

INSURE
to provide insurance for
  or to underwrite

ENSURE
to make certain (ensure compliance)

JOULES
a unit of work or energy
  (300 joules delivered)

JEWELS
diamonds, rubies, etc.

LAY
to put or place
  (lay the book on the table)

LIE
to recline or to speak an untruth
  (lie down on the table)

LOOP
a circle of suture

LOUPE
a magnifying instrument

LUHR mandibular plating system needles,	**LUER** brand name of curet, forceps, retractors, rongeurs, etc.
MARSHAL an officer having charge of prisoners	**MARTIAL** relating to an army or military life

MELENIC
dark stools due to
    presence of blood
	MELANOTIC
	characterized by black
	    pigmentation

MUCOUS
secreting or containing
    mucus (adj)
	MUCUS
	material produced by the
	    mucous membrane (noun)

OPPOSED to place opposite or against	**APPOSED** fitted together (as in edges of wounds)
ORAL pertaining to the mouth	**AURAL** pertaining to the ear
OVERT obvious behavior	**EVERT** to turn out (evert a suture line)

PEELING
to strip off (as in peeling skin or
    peeling back a catheter)
	PEALING
	loud ringing of bells
	    (think of Big Ben)

PERFUSE
to cause blood to flow
    (through an artery or
    lumen of a tube)
	PROFUSE
	pouring forth abundantly
	    (diaphoresis)

PERINEAL
relating to the perineum—
    the area between the vulva and anus
    (female) and scrotum and anus (male)
	PERONEAL
	relating to the lateral
	    fibula and the muscles
	    attached thereto

PLAIN ordinary (an x-ray without contrast)	**PLANE** two-dimensional flat surface (sagittal, coronal, etc.)
PLURAL more than one	**PLEURAL** pertaining to the lungs

PROSTHETIC
referring to artificial (prosthetic
    heart valves, penile implants)
	PROSTATIC
	referring to the male prostate
	    gland

PROSTRATE
to lie prone in adoration

REFLEX
an involuntary response
    to external stimuli
    (patellar reflex)
	DEFLEX
	repositioning of an infant's
	    head to aid vaginal delivery

REGIMENT squadrons of military personnel	**REGIMEN** a program of medical treatment

REGIME
a form of government

RHONCHI
a transmitted chest sound
   heard on auscultation

BRONCHI
plural of bronchus

ROOT
the lower part or base
   (portion of a tooth
   inside the gum line)

ROUTE
a planned method of travel
   (method of drug delivery)

SACK
a bag to carry things

SAC
a pouch, often containing fluid

SEAMEN
U.S. Navy personnel
   (men on the sea)

SEMEN
male ejaculate

SEEDING
radioactive seed placement
   (treatment for prostate CA)

SEATING
designated seating
   (as in a theater)

SERIAL
in a series (e.g., serial EKGs)

CEREAL
Frosted Flakes, oatmeal, etc.

SHOTTY
feels like buckshot
   (shotty lymph nodes)

SHODDY
hastily or poorly done

SITE
a place or location
   (operative site)

SIGHT
the ability to see
   (her sight was adequate)

SPICULATION
small spike-like projection

SPECULATION
to think or wonder about

TETANIC
marked muscular contractions
   (heard in OB/GYN reports)

TITANIC
a big boat on the bottom of
   the North Atlantic ocean

THECAL
pertaining to the thecal sac

FECAL
pertaining to feces

TICK
a blood-sucking animal

TIC
an involuntary movement
   (as in Tourette's syndrome)

TINEA
fungal infection of the skin

TENIA
tapeworm

TRACT
a pathway (urinary tract)

TRACK
mark or series of marks
   (needle tracks in IVDA)

TRIAL
as in a trial of medication

TRAIL
a path to follow

TYMPANIC
relating to the tympanic
   membrane

TYMPANITIC
a sound quality (as in striking a
   tympany drum) (a tympanitic
   abdomen)

UNKEMPT
lacking neatness
   (unpolished)

UNKEPT
no such word, according
   to Webster

VARICOSE
veins that are dilated
   or thrombosed

VERY CLOSE
something in close proximity
   to another

VENOUS
pertaining to veins
   rather than arteries

VENUS
the planet named for the
   Roman goddess of love

VERSUS
in contrast to or as the alternative of

VERSES
lines in a poem

VESICAL
pertaining to the bladder

VESICLE
a cyst or blister

VILLUS
a projection, especially from
   a mucous membrane (noun)

VILLOUS
shaggy, covered with villi (adj)

WANT
to desire

WONT
accustomed to, inclined, or apt

WAVE
to motion with hands or a
   swell on the surface of
   the water

WAIVE
to give up claim to

WAVER
to fluctuate one's opinion

WAIVER
a document giving up
   claim

WHEAL
a raised area of skin
   from an intradermal
   injection

WHEEL
round tool invented by
   cavemen

Pharmacology

GENERIC DRUG IDENTIFIERS

Did you know that many generic drugs contain prefixes and suffixes that identify them by type or action? Knowing these suffixes can assist you in readily identifying a drug with which you may not be familiar. A number of brand names also retain the identifiable suffix, enabling you to determine their use as well. *Examples:* Accupril, Xylocaine, Streptase, Compazine, Norpramin, Wycillin, Cefotan, Retrovir.

GENERIC SUFFIX	DRUG TYPE	EXAMPLES
-ane	inhalational anesthetic	halothane isoflurane sevoflurane
-ase	enzyme	amylase, lipase streptokinase urokinase
-azepam	benzodiazepine	diazepam halazepam lorazepam
-azine	phenothiazine antipsychotic	fluphenazine prochlorperazine thioridazine
-azole	antifungal	econazole ketoconazole oxiconazole
-azosin	alpha$_1$ blockers	doxazosin prazosin terazosin
-barbital	barbiturate	butabarbital pentobarbital phenobarbital
-caine	local/regional anesthetic	benzocaine lidocaine bupivacaine procaine

GENERIC SUFFIX	DRUG TYPE	EXAMPLES
-cillin	penicillin	amoxicillin ampicillin cloxacillin methicillin penicillin
-curium, - curonium	neuromuscular blocking agent	doxacurium mivacurium pancuronium vecuronium
-cycline	tetracycline antibiotic	doxycycline methacycline tetracycline
-floxacin	fluoroquinolone antibiotic	ciprofloxacin levofloxacin norfloxacin
-iazide	thiazide diuretic	chlorothiazide hydrochlorothiazide polythiazide
-ipine	calcium channel blocker	amlodipine nicardipine nifedipine
-micin, -mycin	aminoglycoside or macrolide antibiotic	gentamicin streptomycin tobramycin azithromycin erythromycin
-olol	beta blocker	atenolol metoprolol propranolol
-olone	corticosteroid	clocortolone fluocinolone prednisolone triamcinolone
-onide	corticosteroid	amcinonide desonide halcinonide
-phylline	bronchodilator	aminophylline dyphylline oxtriphylline theophylline
-pramine	tricyclic antidepressant	desipramine imipramine trimipramine
-pril	ACE inhibitors for CHF	captopril enalapril lisinopril
-profen	NSAID	fenoprofen ibuprofen ketoprofen
-sone	corticosteroid	betamethasone dexamethasone hydrocortisone

GENERIC SUFFIX	DRUG TYPE	EXAMPLES
-terol, -terenol	bronchodilator	albuterol isoproterenol metaproterenol pirbuterol salmeterol
-tidine	H2 blocker for PUD	cimetidine famotidine ranitidine
-triptyline	tricyclic antidepressant	amitriptyline nortriptyline protriptyline
-tropin	gland-stimulating hormone	follitropin gonadotropin menotropin urofollitropin
-vir	antiviral	acyclovir indinavir ganciclovir

Resource: *Understanding Pharmacology for Health Professionals, 3rd Edition, Susan M. Turley, Prentice Hall, 2002.*

JCAHO Dangerous Abbreviations

EFFECTIVE JANUARY 1, 2004

ABBREVIATION	POTENTIAL PROBLEM	PREFERRED
U (for unit)	Mistaken as zero, four, or cc	Write "unit"
IU (for international units)	Mistaken as IV or 10	Write "international unit"
O.D. or Q.O.D.	Mistaken for each other. The period after the Q can be mistaken for an "I" and the "O" can be mistaken for "I"	Write "daily" and "every other day"
Trailing zero (x.0 mg) (Note: Prohibited only for medication-related notations); Lack of leading zero (.X mg)	Decimal point is missed	Never write a zero by itself after a decimal point (X mg), and always use a zero before a decimal point (0.X mg)
MS MSO$_4$ MgSO$_4$	Confused for one another. Can mean morphine sulfate or magnesium sulfate	Write "morphine sulfate" or "magnesium sulfate"
μg	Mistaken for mg (milligrams) resulting in one thousand-fold dosing overdose	Write "mcg"
H.S. (for half-strength or Latin abbreviation for bedtime)	Mistaken for either half-strength or hour of sleep (at bedtime), q.H.S. mistaken for every hour. All can result in dosing errors.	Write out "half-strength" or "at bedtime"
T.I.W. (for three times a week)	Mistaken for three times a day or twice weekly resulting in an overdose	Write "3 times weekly" or "three times weekly"
S.C. or S.Q. (for subcutaneous)	Mistaken as SL for sublingual, or "5 every"	Write "Sub-Q," "subQ," or "subcutaneously"
D/C (for discharge)	Interpreted as discontinue whatever medications follow (typically discharge meds)	Write "discharge"
c.c. (for cubic centimeter)	Mistaken for U (units) when poorly written	Write "mL" for milliliters
A.S., A.D., A.U. (Latin abbreviation for left, right, or both ears)	Mistaken for OS, OD, and OU, etc.	Write "left ear," "right ear," or "both ears"

NOTE: The trailing zero is omitted for all medication orders and other medication-related documentation. However, in reporting laboratory values and in certain other numeric notations, the precision of the numeric value is indicated by the digits after the decimal point, even when that trailing digit is a zero. For example, a serum potassium level might be reported as 4.0 mEq/Liter, not 4 mEq/Liter. Similarly, sizes for endotracheal tubes and other clinical equipment are often specified numerically with one place after the decimal point. This is acceptable, even when the number after the decimal point is a zero.

JCAHO also recommends using the above-noted abbreviations whether the abbreviations are typed in capital letters, lower case letters, with or without periods between the letters.

The safety of the patient comes first. As a long-term objective, ambiguous and otherwise dangerous forms of notation should be eliminated from all health care documentation.

FINALLY: Please refer to the Institute for Safe Medication Practices (ISMP) website at http://www.ismp.org/ for a complete list of dangerous abbreviations relating to medication use that it recommends be explicitly prohibited.

Also, refer to *The AAMT Book of Style for Medical Transcription*, 2nd Edition, pp. 461 to 464. This listing contains the ISMP recommendations as of 2001.

Sources: http://www.ismp/org/ and http://www.jcaho.org/accredited+organizations/patient+safety/04+npsg/04_faqs.htm#abbreviations

How to Take a Test/ Test-Taking Tips

During the learning process, the brain still controls all bodily functions including reason, thinking, movement, sensory perception, and our emotions. The cerebral cortex controls the brain's highest-level functions such as sight, hearing, memory, and thought. In preparing to study for a test, it is important to understand these processes as well as the process of critical thinking and how it is used to process information.

Diet

The mind-body connection is of critical importance. Maintaining good health allows you to learn more efficiently. Maintaining a well-balanced diet and an appropriate amount of fluids and electrolytes is critical. Preparing for the CMT exam is no time to go on a restrictive diet. Your brain needs amino acids to repair and replace tissues, neurons, and chemicals in the brain. It needs glucose for energy, and it needs vitamins and minerals to keep neurotransmitter activity healthy. Here are a few guidelines regarding "brain food."

Vitamin B₁ (thiamine) is important because a deficiency can cause confusion, depression, fatigue, or memory loss. Severe deficiency can cause irreversible brain damage.

Vitamin B₂ (riboflavin) is important because a deficiency can cause depression and lethargy.

Vitamin B₆ (pyridoxine) is vital because low levels can worsen premenstrual tension, cause depression, irritability, fatigue, and poor serotonin (a neurotransmitter that promotes relaxation) production.

Vitamin B₁₂ (cobalamin) is critical because a deficiency can contribute to bipolar disorder, chronic fatigue, confusion, insomnia, irritability, memory loss, paranoia, phobias, and restlessness.

Vitamin C deficiency can cause anxiety, depression, excitability, fatigue, and hysteria.

A lack of **folate** (folic acid) can result in depression and lethargy. A **niacin** deficiency can cause anxiety, depression, fatigue, or memory loss. A short-term lack of **calcium** can cause tremors and/or confusion. Difficulties in learning or comprehending can result from an **iron** deficiency. Low levels of **magnesium** in the brain can result in agitation, confusion, irritability, or tremors, and low levels of **zinc** in the brain can impair memory.

In the weeks prior to sitting for the CMT exam, it is recommended that you eat a variety of foods every day, including vegetables, fruits, grains, and low-fat proteins. Choose low-fat foods, especially those low in saturated fat, trans-fats, and cholesterol. Use sugars, salts, and vegetable oils in moderation, and drink plenty of water to maintain proper hydration and flushing out of impurities.

Research has found that no single food can boost your brainpower, but high-carbohydrates, such as pasta, can help improve your mood, thus putting you in the best state of mind for learning. Carbohydrates are easily converted into glucose, which is a simple sugar that provides energy to the brain. Glucose in turn triggers the production of serotonin, which strongly affects mood and emotions. Serotonin helps you stay calm and relaxed and improves your ability to concentrate. Conclusion: Eating pasta can help improve your studying skills.

Learning Styles
There are various styles of learning, including visual, auditory, and kinesthetic. If you are an individual who learns best by watching how something is done or by reading about it, you are a visual learner. To make the most of this learning style, read everything you can find in preparation for the exam (see *Appendix 6: References for Further Study*). You can also make yourself flash-cards and get your family involved in your learning process or leave notes to yourself regarding difficult concepts on your bathroom mirror, refrigerator, etc. You can also watch medical documentaries on TV or browse Internet medical sites for additional information.

If you learn best by hearing things, then you are an auditory learner. To make the most of this learning style, use as much auditory information as possible. Dictate sample questions into your own tape recorder and play them back in your car or join a study group that meets regularly to share ideas. You can also attend medical lectures in your community and play dictation tapes in your car or on your tape recorder. (*Note: Dictation tapes from previous CMT exams can be purchased directly from AAMT.*)

If you prefer to jump right in and learn by doing, you are a kinesthetic learner. To make the most of this style of learning, you should attend workshops, go on field trips, participate in group projects, tutor, mentor, or teach others. You can definitely learn by teaching others. If you have difficulty speaking in front of a group of people, try mentoring on a one-to-one basis. Share your knowledge with another MT less experienced than yourself, and you, in turn, will improve your knowledge as well.

Attitude and Motivation
Other important factors in learning are attitude and motivation. The approach you take to a particular task is your attitude, and your interest in a particular task or how meaningful it is to you is reflected in your attitude. If you have set a goal for yourself to sit for and pass the CMT exam, then your attitude is positive toward the task at hand. Now you need to develop the strategies necessary to see this goal become a reality. One teacher relates that there are invariably a few people in each new MT class whose attitude starts out as defeatist. One particular, otherwise intelligent, professional woman left the first class in tears saying, "I am not smart enough to learn this!" Of course, I convinced her she was indeed smart enough. She just needed to take it one step at a time. She needed to break down the tasks at hand into manageable forms and learn them (not memorize). When all of the individual tasks are put together as a whole and critical thinking is added, the "big picture" emerges and a new medical language specialist is created.

Motivation can be looked at as the proverbial "light at the end of the tunnel" that inspires you to keep going, no matter how difficult the process seems, until you reach your goal of becoming a certified medical transcriptionist. There are two types of motivation: intrinsic and extrinsic. Intrinsic includes a general desire to learn, a sense of curiosity, a willingness to take risks, an interest in the subject to be studied, and the desire to excel at something. Extrinsic motivation includes the desire for improved self-esteem, a sense of fulfillment, increased competence, reaching one's goal, valuable credentials on your resume, and hopefully a better job with a higher salary.

Concentration and Memory

Let's talk about concentration and memory. In order to adequately concentrate on the task at hand (studying for the CMT exam), you must keep distractions to a minimum. Try to clear your mind of external influencing factors, which prevent you from concentrating as you study. Turn off that television and put the children to bed (and your significant other too, if necessary). Use earplugs if needed to create a silent study cocoon for yourself, if this is what you need to optimize your concentration and learning. Make sure you are not hungry, angry, tired, or sad. Use a comfortable chair, but not too comfortable—you don't want to fall asleep—and be sure you have task lighting if needed.

It is important that you study when the time is right for you. Everybody is different. Some people are morning people and some are late night people. Find a study time that fits your work and life schedule. Study in a familiar place, utilizing incandescent light rather than fluorescent light, which can cause eyestrain. Of course, you can study outside in natural sunlight if this fits your lifestyle and climate. Set realistic goals for your study session, make a "to-do list" if it helps you stay centered, and focus on one topic at a time. Drink water throughout your study session to maintain hydration, take short breaks every 45 minutes to 1 hour, and vary your study activities by reading some, taking a few notes, or quiet thinking about what you have just read to keep your study process active rather than passive. Some individuals like "white noise" in the background when studying. This "noise" is a low-level background sound that masks outside distractions. This could include soft music, which obliterates the sound of a clock ticking or a noisy air conditioner. Earplugs will work here, too.

Many people report the benefits of "power napping" wherein one takes a short nap of 5 to 15 minutes (but no longer), saying this rejuvenates the body and mind. Other people prefer cardiovascular exercise like brisk walking, StairMaster, treadmill, etc., prior to a study session to get their juices flowing. Still others prefer yoga or a Pilates-type exercise (low impact) to "center" the body prior to a period of prolonged concentration. Each person is different, and you need to know yourself and what works for you.

Once you have improved your concentration abilities, now you need to commit what you are learning to memory. How your brain processes information determines what you remember and what you forget. There are three basic stages involved in information processing. These are registration, short-term memory, and long-term memory.

In registration, information is received and may eventually be understood and selected to be remembered. This process involves reception, perception, and selection. In reception, you sense something but you do not recognize what it means. For instance, you might auscultate someone's heartbeat but not be able to describe it accurately. In perception, you recognize what you have heard and attach a meaning to it. Now, when hearing that same heartbeat, you are able to determine if the beats are those of sinus rhythm and perhaps even hear a murmur. The final phase is registration, and this involves choosing to remember information so that the next time you hear the same heartbeat you will recognize what it is and what it means.

When new information is selected to be remembered, it automatically goes into short-term memory, which can last a little as 15 seconds. Research has determined that short-term memory can hold five to nine bits of information, depending on how well that information is grouped. For example, we've all heard dictated, "Recall was 5 out of 5 after 1 minute, and 3 out of 5 after 5 minutes." This means the patient's short-term memory is working just fine but his/her long-term memory is deficient. A good memory is a skill that can be developed through practice.

Long-term memory is stored in an organized manner in the brain, but its duration there depends on how completely the information has been processed and how long you use it. An example here might be an individual who learns conversational Spanish. If he uses it on a daily basis he will not only retain that knowledge but will advance it as well. However, should that same individual stop using this skill on a regular basis, over a period of time the skill can be lost completely.

Therefore, learning medical language and utilizing medical language on a daily basis is critical to being able to retrieve that knowledge when needed, as in a testing situation. Make medicine a part of your whole life, not just during your work time each day. Watch medically based television shows, converse with other MTs, attend AAMT functions locally and nationally, and immerse yourself in your profession.

Summary

The skill set required to be a successful, certified medical transcriptionist encompasses much more than just typing, as we all know, and certification tells the world that you are indeed a professional. Your CMT credential means you are a goal-directed individual who takes pride in your profession and expects to be paid as such.

Therefore, the evening before your scheduled exam, get a good night's sleep, eat a healthy breakfast (containing carbohydrates and protein), take your vitamins, drink plenty of water, drive yourself to the testing center, and complete your CMT exam comfortable in the knowledge that you have done everything you can to make your dream of being a certified medical transcriptionist a reality.

We take the liberty of adding our CONGRATULATIONS to all those who understand what it takes to reach this goal and how important it is, not only to you, but to our profession as a whole.

Source: Some material from *Studying & Test Taking Made Incredibly Easy*. Philadelphia: Lippincott Williams & Wilkins, 1999.

References for Further Study

Berkow R. *The Merck Manual of Diagnosis and Therapy*, 16th ed. Whitehouse Station, NJ: Merck & Co., 1992.

Blauvelt CT, Nelson FRT. *A Manual of Orthopaedic Terminology*. Philadelphia: C.V. Mosby, 1998.

Boegli EH. *Prentice Hall Health's Complete Review of Surgery Technology*, 2nd ed. Upper Saddle River, NJ: Prentice Hall Health, 2005.

Chabner D-E. *The Language of Medicine*, 7th ed. Philadelphia: Saunders, 2004.

Crowley LV. *An Introduction to Human Disease: Pathology and Pathophysiology Correlations*. Boston: Jones and Bartlett, 2001.

Dirckx JH. *H & P: A Nonphysician's Guide to the Medical and History Examination*. Modesto, CA: Health Professions Institute, 2001.

Dirckx JH. *Human Diseases*. Modesto, CA: Health Professions Institute, 2003.

Dirckx JH. *Laboratory Tests & Diagnostic Procedures in Medicine*. Modesto, CA: Health Professions Institute, 2004.

Dorland's Illustrated Medical Dictionary, 30th ed. Philadelphia: W.B. Saunders Company, 2004.

Drake R, Drake E. *Saunders Pharmaceutical Word Book*. Philadelphia: Saunders, 2005.

Fetrow CW, Avila JR. *Professional's Handbook of Complementary & Alternative Medicines*, 3rd ed. Philadelphia: Lippincott Williams & Wilkins, 2003.

Goldberg B. *Alternative Medicine: The Definitive Guide*. Fife, Washington: Future Medicine Publishing, Inc., 1995.

Hamann B. *Disease: Identification, Prevention and Control*, 2nd ed. New York: McGraw Hill, 2001.

HIPPA for MTs. American Association for Medical Transcription (www.aamt.org), 2002.

Hughes P (ed). *The AAMT Book of Style for Medical Transcription*, 2nd ed. Modesto: AAMT, 2002.

Judson K, Hicks SB. *Glencoe Law & Ethics for Medical Careers*, 3rd ed. New York: McGraw-Hill, 2002.

Lance LL. *Quick Look Electronic Drug Reference*. Baltimore: Lippincott Williams & Wilkins, 2005.

Levien DH. *Introduction to Surgery*, 3rd ed. Philadelphia: W.B. Saunders, Co., 1999.

Lunsford AA. *The St. Martin's Handbook*, 5th ed. New York: Bedford/St. Martin's, 2003.

Marieb, EN. *Essentials of Human Anatomy & Physiology*. San Francisco: Benjamin-Cummings, 2002.

McWay DC. *Legal Aspects of Health Information Management*, 2nd ed. Clifton Park, NY: Thomson Delmar Learning, 2002.

Merriam Webster's Collegiate Dictionary, 10th ed. Springfield, MA: Merriam-Webster, 1997.

Murray M, Pizzorno J. *Encyclopedia of Natural Medicine*. New York: Prima Publishing, 1998.

Novelline RA. *Squire's Fundamentals of Radiology*, 6th ed. Cambridge, MA: Harvard, 2004.

Phillips N. *Berry & Kohn's Operating Room Technique*, 10th ed. Philadelphia: C.V. Mosby, 2003.

Sabin WA. *The Gregg Reference Manual*, 10th ed. Burr Ridge, IL: McGraw-Hill/Irwin, 2004.

Shaw DL. *Anatomy and Physiology Glossary*. Thorofare, NJ: Slack, 1990.

Sheldon H. *Boyd's Introduction to the Study of Disease*. Philadelphia: Lippincott Williams & Wilkins, 1992.

Stedman's Abbreviations, Acronyms & Symbols, 3rd ed. Baltimore: Lippincott Williams & Wilkins, 2003.

Stedman's Alternative & Complementary Medicine Words, 2nd ed. Baltimore: Lippincott Williams & Wilkins, 2005.

Stedman's Anatomy & Physiology Words, 2nd ed. Baltimore: Lippincott Williams & Wilkins, 2002.

Stedman's Cardiovascular & Pulmonary Words, 4th ed. Baltimore: Lippincott Williams & Wilkins, 2004.

Stedman's Dermatology & Immunology Words, 3rd ed. Baltimore: Lippincott Williams & Wilkins, 2005.

Stedman's Emergency Medicine Words. Baltimore: Lippincott Williams & Wilkins, 2003.

Stedman's Endocrinology Words. Baltimore: Lippincott Williams & Wilkins, 2001.

Stedman's GI & GU Words, 4th ed. Baltimore: Lippincott Williams & Wilkins, 2005.

Stedman's Guide to Idioms. Baltimore: Lippincott Williams & Wilkins, 2005.

Stedman's Illustrated Dictionary of Dermatology Eponyms. Baltimore: Lippincott Williams & Wilkins, 2005.

Stedman's Internal Medicine & Geriatric Words. Baltimore: Lippincott Williams & Wilkins, 2002.

Stedman's Medical & Surgical Equipment Words, 4th ed. Baltimore: Lippincott Williams & Wilkins, 2004.

Stedman's Medical Dictionary, 27th ed. Baltimore: Lippincott Williams & Wilkins, 2000.

Stedman's Medical Eponyms, 2nd ed. Baltimore: Lippincott Williams & Wilkins, 2005.

Stedman's Medical Terminology Flashcards. Baltimore: Lippincott Williams & Wilkins, 2005.

Stedman's Medical Terms and Phrases. Baltimore: Lippincott Williams & Wilkins, 2004.

Stedman's Neurology & Neurosurgery Words, 3rd ed. Baltimore: Lippincott Williams & Wilkins, 2003.

Stedman's OB/GYN & Pediatric Words, 4th ed. Baltimore: Lippincott Williams & Wilkins, 2005.

Stedman's Oncology Words, 4th ed. Baltimore: Lippincott Williams & Wilkins, 2003.

Stedman's Ophthalmology Words, 3rd ed. Baltimore: Lippincott Williams & Wilkins, 2004.

Stedman's Organisms & Infectious Disease Words. Baltimore: Lippincott Williams & Wilkins, 2001.

Stedman's Orthopaedic & Rehab Words, 4th ed. Baltimore: Lippincott Williams & Wilkins, 2002.

Stedman's Pathology & Lab Medicine Words, 3rd ed. Baltimore: Lippincott Williams & Wilkins, 2002.

Stedman's Plastic Surgery/ENT/Dentistry Words, 3rd ed. Baltimore: Lippincott Williams & Wilkins, 2003.

Stedman's Plus Spellchecker 2004. Baltimore: Lippincott Williams & Wilkins, 2004.

Stedman's Psychiatry Words, 3rd ed. Baltimore: Lippincott Williams & Wilkins, 2002.

Stedman's Radiology Words, 4th ed. Baltimore: Lippincott Williams & Wilkins, 2003.

Stedman's Surgery Words, 2nd ed. Baltimore: Lippincott Williams & Wilkins, 2002.

Stedman's Medical Word of the Day Calendar. Baltimore: Lippincott Williams & Wilkins, 2005.

Tamparo CD, Lewis MA. *Diseases of the Human Body*. Philadelphia: F.A. Davis, 2000.

Tessier C. *The Surgical Word Book*, 3rd ed. Philadelphia: Saunders, 2004.

Turabian KL. *A Manual for Writers of Term Papers, Theses, and Dissertations*. Chicago: University of Chicago Press, 1996.

Turley SM. *Understanding Pharmacology for Health Professionals*. Upper Saddle River, NJ: Prentice Hall Health, 2002.